Stereotactic Biopsy and Brachytherapy of Brain Tumors

Stereotactic Biopsy and Brachytherapy of Brain Tumors

Peter Dyck, M.D., F.A.C.S.

Clinical Professor of Neurosurgery
University of Southern California
Los Angeles, California

Introduction by
Professor Dr. Fritz Mundinger

University of Freiburg
Freiburg, West Germany

University Park Press • Baltimore

University Park Press
International Publishers in Medicine and Human Services
300 North Charles Street
Baltimore, Maryland 21201

Sponsoring Editor: Larry W. Carter
Production Manager: Berta Steiner
Design: Caliber Design Planning, Inc.
Cover illustration by Ted Bloodhart

Typeset by Kingsport Press
Manufactured in the United States of America by Halliday Lithograph

Library of Congress Cataloging in Publication Data
Main entry under title:

Stereotactic biopsy and brachytherapy of brain tumors.

Includes index.
1. Brain—Tumors—Radiotherapy. 2. Radioisotope brachytherapy. 3. Brain—Biopsy, Needle. 4. Stereo-encephalotomy. I. Dyck, Peter James. [DNLM: 1. Brain neoplasms—Radiotherapy. 2. Brachytherapy—Methods. 3. Stereotaxic—Methods. 4. Brain—Radiography. 5. Biopsy —Methods. WL 358 S838]
RC280.B7S8 1983 616.99′2059 83–14500
ISBN 0–8391–1926–7

This book is dedicated to the patients whose hope against overwhelming odds brought about this endeavor.

Contents

Introduction

In spite of the many great strides in medicine in recent decades, neurosurgeons have continued to express trepidation when approaching deep-seated intracranial lesions, even when they are cystic. Similar pessimism prevails towards recurrent cerebral neoplasms, particularly those that have failed teletherapy. Olivecrona, among many others, was of the opinion that nothing more could be done at this point.

Palliative shunting of obstructed ventricular systems caused by midline tumors is widely available, and modern anesthesia, microsurgical technics, and corticosteroid therapy have improved overall the prospects of brain tumor patients. However, the prognostic outlook for patients with deep-seated, recurrent tumors remains unfortunately poor. It was not too long ago that Paul Bucy said that cerebral gliomas in general are incurable. Nevertheless, a handful of neurosurgeons have not been dissuaded by the prevailing pessimism, and they continued to explore various avenues that might improve the dismal lot of these unfortunate patients with midline or recurrent neoplastic lesions.

Shortly after Roentgen's discovery of X-rays, the salutary effects of irradiation of brain tumors became apparent. In 1922 Tönnis implanted radium needles or paraffin capsules containing radium into residual gliomas after subtotal resection. By 1935, Harvey Cushing drew attention to this technic in North America, while Kroll, Jäger and Kessel rigorously pursued this eventually disappointing endeavor in Germany.

Resurgence of interest in interstitial radiation grew in the early 1950s. Artificially produced radioisotopes with favorable clinical and physical characteristics and the ability to deliver high radiation doses to a tumor without injury to surrounding brain became widely available.

Georg von Hevesy, from the University of Freiburg im Breisgau, was among the pioneers in this field. A radioactive source was administered orally or intravenously in an attempt to concentrate the radionuclide within a tumor by taking advantage of the disrupted blood-brain barrier produced by the pathologic process. Iodine-121 and its therapeutic role in thyroid neoplasia served as the therapeutic leit motif of this endeavor.

In 1949, Selverstone and Ericson, and two years later Sweet, advocated the use of radiophosphorus (P-32) as a therapeutic adjunct. Sodium-24 and potassium-42 were proposed by Locksley in 1949; Tipser and Freedberg advocated rubidium-86; I proposed wismut-106 in 1958; and finally in 1961 Browell suggested the use of dysprosium-165 EDTA. A number of other isotopes were also tried. Although an increased concentration of the isotope within the neoplasm could be proven, it could not be verified that the regional interstitial radiation was not detrimental to surrounding healthy structures. Hence, these early endeavors were abandoned.

It appeared logical that direct interstitial radiation with an implanted radionuclide might prevent injury to surrounding normal brain, yet deliver therapeutic range of radiation to the offending lesion. Now arose the question of whether interstitial radiotherapy (curietherapy) should be protracted or short lived (brachycurietherapy). The answer in part lay in the cell kinetics of the neoplasm.

How best to adapt the principles of radiobiology and hence arrive at an acceptable teletherpeutic dosimetry for a brain tumor has been a long-standing topic of discussion in neurosurgical circles. Cystic gliomas and craniopharyngiomata were treated with intracavity instillation of phosphorus-32 by Klar (1953) and by Obrador, Spiegel and Wycis (1956). Colloids of gold-198 and yttrium-90 were also recommended for this purpose.

In 1951, Phillip and I utilized phosphorus-32-molybdenum compound, encased in a plexiglass capsule, as intracavity radiotherapy following radical excision of the lesion. In 1955, a graphite macrosuspension of gold-198 was employed subsequent to reoperation on a tumor; it was deposited into the cavity.

In 1957, we began using tantalum-182. I also introduced iridium-192 as an interstitial radioimplant. Fragmented cobalt-60 wire was also employed by me as well as by Klar and Scheer in 1952. Brachytherapeutic principles only were applied in this instance, for obvious reasons.

When cesium-157 and especially iridium-192 came on the market, interstitial radiation concentrated over a short period of time gained a foothold in the treatment of brain tumors. The Gamma-Med® developed by Sauerwein and myself in 1963 remains an available brachycurietherapeutic tool at our institution to the present day. With it, high-intensity regional radiation is delivered to a highly anaplastic lesion within minutes.

In spite of the fact that interstitial radiation of brain tumors has been hesitantly accepted, our results and the data of others support a basis for optimism. Yet it must be underscored that not all institutions offer a favorable environment for the development of modern stereotaxis and present day interstitial radiotherapy.

It was soon learned that radionuclides inserted intraoperatively at craniotomy did not necessarily remain where they were placed, and it was difficult to arrive at dosimetric computations. Also, when cobalt-60 or cesium-157 were employed, the radiation precautions to the hospital crews proved extremely costly. Such undertakings were soon abandoned.

Radiotherapists who handle radioisotopes are constantly aware of the environmental dangers. In order to minimize this danger, Henschke, after extensive personal experience, developed a sophisticated radionuclide application technic for iridium-192. Hilaris then developed an iodine-125 application technic in 1975.

The utilization of stereotaxis for interstitial radiotherapy greatly enhanced targeting accuracy. Although stereotaxy, as introduced by Spiegel and Wycis in 1947, occupied itself then primarily with functional neurological disorders, today it emphasizes localization of nonfunctional intracranial mass lesions. Traugott Riechert and I performed the first stereotactically guided radioimplant of a cerebral cyst in 1953.

In the early 1950s, it was not the deep-seated intracerebral lesions, but rather pituitary neoplasms that received most of the curietherapeutic attention. We were involved in such an endeavor for more than two decades. At first we used phosphorus-32. Then in 1959, Molinatti advocated the use of yttrium-90 seeds. Two years later Joplin proposed the use of gold-182; that same year, 1961, I suggested the use of iridium-192 wires. In February, 1979, I employed iodine-125 to irradiate the tumor of an acromegalic patient. Excellent short- and long-term results have been reported all over the world with this form of interstitial radiotherapy of pituitary tumors.

Rediscovery of the transphenoidal surgical approach to the pituitary fossa, advocated by Jules Hardy and presently in vogue, has modified indications for interstitial radiotherapy of pituitary tumors as well. Yet, interstitial radiotherapy of other cerebral neoplasms has recently received greater attention, albeit in only a few institutions in the world.

The advent of microsurgery, laser technic, modern teletherapy, and high voltage, neutron and proton therapy, combined with corticosteroids and chemotherapy, at first appeared to offer a ray of hope for patients suffering from malignant intracranial lesions. Yet in the past few years, regional and international studies suggest that this is not necessarily the case. In fact, when compared with data from the period 1941–1978, present survival is only slightly improved and useful survival may actually be decreased.

With the introduction of CT-aided stereotaxy and modern radiodosimetric computations, more encouraging prognostic results are in the offing. As of May 19, 1983, we have interstitially radiated 1502 intracranial lesions. Most of our experience is with iridium-192, but iodine-125, made available to us by Hilaris in 1979, also has been widely utilized. Favorable physical properties, including a steep drop in the radiation radius of iodine-125, make it a desirable isotope in the therapeutic armamentarium. And both iridium-192 and iodine-125 comply with national guidelines for radiation safety. Present clinical experience and dosimetric standardization based on CT data, volume reformat and neuropathologic data will inevitably lead to further refinements. Basic research in this field, assimilating available data and further expanding investigation, is needed.

Clinically it is stereotaxy coupled to the CT scanner that has brought about the resurgence of interest in interstitial radiotherapy of nonresectable intracranial lesions. This optimism has been supported by a low complication rate and a high degree of accuracy in diagnosis.

The contemporary spectrum for therapy of brain tumors includes total resection, excision biopsy, curietherapy, teletherapy, and a combination of the latter two. The aggressiveness of the lesion and its histologic type determine the mode of treatment.

After a long period of professional dormancy, interstitial radiation of brain tumors is again receiving its due attention. And with meticulous attention to modern stereotaxis and radiotherapeutic principles, interstitial radiotherapy will find its rightful niche, to the benefit of some patients.

This book is a forum for national and international expression by experts in stereotaxy. Its purpose is to gather pertinent data that impact on modern interstitial radiotherapy of brain tumors. Peter Dyck has taken on not only the arduous task of editing, but also of contributing from his own experience in this field. Thanks to his far-sightedness, neurosurgeons, neurologists, radiotherapists, oncologists and students now have a competent guide to CT-aided stereotaxic biopsy and brachytherapy of brain tumors.

Prof. Dr. Fritz Mundinger
Freiburg im Breisgau
West Germany
May, 1983

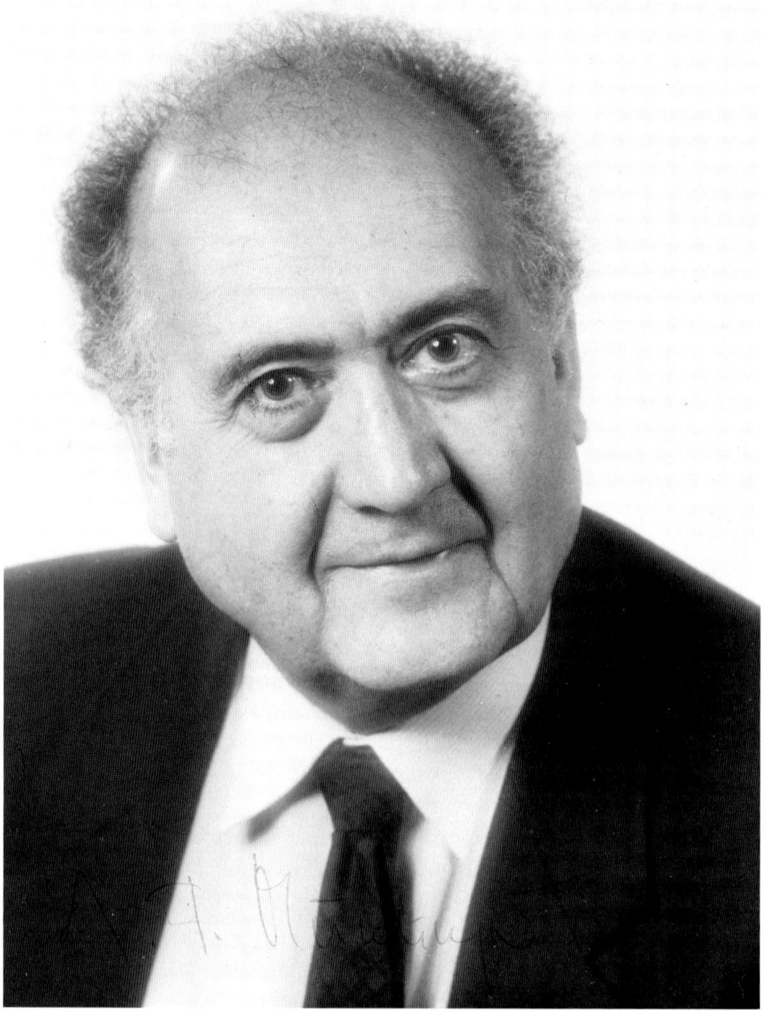

Preface

The current renaissance of interest in human stereotaxy is due to new developments primarily in three areas of medicine: computerized tomography of the brain, computer processing of stereotactic data, and increasing awareness of inadequacies of chemotherapy and teletherapy.

Of foremost importance is the modification of CT targeting systems to allow artifact-free, CT-guided stereotaxis. But even with the current precision and expediency of computerized tomography, our contemporary stereotaxic systems approach an accuracy that challenges the resolution capabilities of the CT scanner itself. Professor Dr. Fritz Mundinger of the University of Freiburg, West Germany, has remained one of the forerunners of this frontier. Much of his experience, as well as that of Leksell and others, is covered in these pages. A completely new development is stereotaxis performed with the patient in the CT-scanner.

Computer processing of stereotaxic data is now readily available. Armed with a hand-held calculator and an appropriately programmed magnetic card, the stereotactician is able not only to plan a precise trajectory to the lesion, but also to compute the iodine-125 or iridium-192 dosimetry before the patient leaves the operating theatre. Armand Bouzaglou explains the details of making these calculations in his chapter on radiotherapy.

These technical developments would have dubious value to the surgery of brain tumors were it not for a clinical need. We live in a period of *Sturm und Drang* of brain tumor therapy. Doubt has been expressed recently about the role of chemotherapy in useful survival. Even more alarming is the fact that chemotherapy may potentiate teletherapeutic injury to surrounding normal brain.

It is well known that radiation is not selectively injurious to neoplasms only, but affects also healthy brain tissues. In this therapeutic circumstance, is teletherapy without tissue diagnosis ever justified? It would seem that the answer is no since modern stereotaxis allows biopsy of almost any lesion of the brain with an acceptable risk to the patient.

A substantial body of knowledge suggests that in certain circumstances, interstitial radiation is equal to if not superior to teletherapy. However, a great deal of prospective data-gathering is needed, preferably on a national or global basis. The immediate future of modern stereotaxy is very exciting because it fills an urgent clinical need. At the same time, it offers the stereotactician a chance to take a step forward in the twentieth century with Aesculapius at his side.

In compiling this book, I endeavored to make this step forward less troublesome for the reader than it was for me. In bringing together existing knowledge from so many sources, it has become clear that several areas of our knowledge of this procedure are decidely inadequate. I anticipate that the reader will encounter some controversial issues in these pages; these are due not to bias or imperiousness, but possibly to incomplete fact.

My ultimate hope is that this book will not only inform the reader, but will stimulate the acquisition and publication of new information that will bring about improved results in our treatment of brain tumors. Time will tell.

Peter Dyck, M.D., F.A.C.S.
La Cañada-Flintridge, California
17 May 1983

Acknowledgments

According to John Donne, "No man is an island entire of itself." This becomes apparent early when one endeavors to edit a book.

First I express my gratitude to my colleagues, Armand Bouzaglou, M.D., Livia Solti-Bohman, M.D., and Philip Gruskin, M.D. They comprise the primary team.

I express my gratitude to Robert J. McKenna, M.D., President-Elect of the Society of Surgical Oncology and Barry Sakulsky, M.D., Cancer Research Director, St. Vincent Medical Center, for sharing my dream.

I thank John Gardner, President of Queen of Angels Medical Center and that institution's research foundation and the Cosler Cancer Fund. The same gratitude is extended to Vincent F. Guinan, President, St. Vincent Medical Center, and its public relations staff.

The CT-scanner and operating room crews' industry and loyalty will not be forgotten.

It was the graciousness of Robert Sloane, President, Los Angeles Orthopaedic Hospital, that allowed photographic and audiovisual recording of this project under the directorship of Alfred Benjamin, the SLR camera of Eloise Smith and the video mastery of Abe Thomas.

I would like to thank Franz Isak for his friendship and uncanny capacity to make tangible precision built objects from casual sketches.

My deepest gratitude goes out to Larry Carter, Senior Editor of University Park Press for his indefatigable patience and faith in me.

Yet I suspect this entire project would have come to naught were it not for Martha Aparicio who rolled with the punches and kept the whole project together, with a smile.

My family will see more of me!

Collaborators and Contributors

Collaborators

Armand Bouzaglou, M.D., A.C.R. Assistant Clinical Professor of Radiology, University of Southern California; Chief Radiation Oncologist, Wilshire Oncology Medical Group, Los Angeles, California

Peter Dyck, M.D., F.A.C.S. Clinical Professor of Neurosurgery, University of Southern California, Los Angeles, California

Philip Gruskin, M.D., F.A.C.P. Associate Clinical Professor of Pathology, University of Southern California; Associate Director of Pathology, St. Vincent Medical Center, Los Angeles, California

Livia G. Solti-Bohman, M.D., M.A.B.R. Assistant Clinical Professor of Radiology, University of California at Los Angeles; Staff Radiologist, St. Vincent Medical Center, Los Angeles, California

Contributors

Jörgen Boëthius, M.D. Professor of Neurosurgery, Karolinska Sjukhuset, Stockholm Sweden

Joseph N. Carberry, M.D., F.A.C.P. Clinical Professor of Pathology, University of Southern California; Director of Pathology, St. Vincent Medical Center, Los Angeles, California

William V. Glenn, Jr., M.D. Multi-Planar Diagnostic Imaging, Inc., Torrence, California

Patrick J. Kelly, M.D. Associate Professor of Neurosurgery, State University of New York at Buffalo, New York

Peter S. Kennedy, M.S., M.D. Assistant Clinical Professor of Medicine, University of Southern California; Medical Oncologist, Wilshire Oncology Group, Los Angeles, California

William W. Lo, M.D., F.A.B.R. Staff Radiologist, St. Vincent Medical Center, Los Angeles, California

Professor Dr. med Fritz Mundinger Chief of Stereotaxy and Nuclear Medicine, Department of Neurosurgery, University of Freiburg im Breisgau, West Germany

Michael L. Rhodes, Ph.D. Multi-Planar Diagnostic Imaging, Inc., Torrence, California

Kenneth L. Saeger, M.D., F.A.C.P. Assistant Clinical Professor of Pathology, University of Southern California; Associate Director of Pathology, St. Vincent Medical Center, Los Angeles, California

Roger A. Slater, M.D. Assistant Clinical Professor of Neurosurgery, University of California at Irvine, California

Stereotactic Biopsy and Brachytherapy of Brain Tumors

1 Historical Review

Peter Dyck

It is generally believed that Albert Einstein's genius lay not only in his capacity for original thought but also in his uncanny ability to assimilate diversified knowledge into a meaningful whole. Contemporary computerized CT-guided stereotaxis and interstitial radiotherapy are also culminations of diversified fields in modern science coming together for the benefit of man. Mundinger and his colleagues at the University of Freiburg in Germany have been the catalytic hub for this activity (4,29,33,40). Mundinger's three decades of interest and contemporary preeminence in this field should earn him the title of the "father of stereotactic biopsy and interstitial radiotherapy" (29–31,33,34).

Stereotaxy

This is not to imply, however, that functional stereotaxis or its application to the treatment of brain tumors began and ended in Freiburg im Breisgau. In fact, it appears that Dittmer was the pioneer stereotactician (10), and Horsley and Clarke were the first to devise a stereotactic apparatus for use on monkeys and cats (19). Their device received widespread use and acclaim, and hence they are said to have founded the field of experimental stereotaxis. Human application of stereotaxy came 39 years later in 1947 when Spiegel et al. (48) introduced stereoencephalotomic thalamotomy for treatment of extrapyramidal disease.

Interest in stereotaxy grew and rapidly became worldwide. Hécaen et al. (17) and Guiot et al. (15) in France, Schaltenbrand and Bailey (43) and Riechert and Wolff in Germany (40), Leksell in Sweden (27), Gillingham in Great Britain (13), Krayenbühl and Yasargil in Zürich (25), Kandel and Cheboratyova (24) and Bechtereva et al. (1) in Russia, Laitinen and Toivakka in Finland (26), Bertrand and Jasper in Canada (3), Velasco-Suárez and Escobedo in Mexico (54), and last but not least Narabayashi in Japan (35) are among the pioneers of stereotaxy.

Clinical interest flourished and surgical indications multiplied in an almost explosive fashion, so that by 1965 25,000 stereotactic procedures had been performed (47). This number increased to 37,000 by 1969 (46).

Then the sword of Damocles fell on stereotaxy. First, L-dopa was introduced in the treatment of parkinsonism; and second, a public outcry over the use of stereotactic psychosurgery in man further dampened enthusiasm for its use. Experimental and clinical dormancy set in.

CT of the Brain

CT scanning of body structures is based on a simple principle. A collimated x-ray beam is passed through tissue and reflected by a scintillation crystal or other radiation detector. Its attenuation, or better, absorption at various distances can be calculated (37). It is at this point that computer science comes into play because the calculations required are staggering (51). The gantry field is divided into picture points, or "pixels," with an assigned anatomically accurate x-ray attenuation coefficient (37). This information can be recorded on a cathode ray tube or, more commonly now, on a television screen. By simultaneously rotating the x-ray source and its radiation detector, a two-dimensional plane is established; if the human head is then interposed, an axial "slice" of the brain is obtained (6,52).

Modern CT scanning equipment embodies multiples of this principle and thus speeds up the process. Hounsfield of EMI Ltd. developed the first CT scanner, which was installed at Atkinson Morley's Hospital in Wimbleton, England (21,22).

An endeavor to adapt these early axial slices for localization of intracranial structures then followed (11,18,23,38,42). When coronal reconstruction became feasible (41) and the softwear capabilities improved so that it was possible to roam around, if you will, on a computerized display of a slice of the brain in reference to a superimposed X-Y coordinate grid, axial localization during CT scanning was born (4,51). In order to allow a depth, or Z plane, determination, a measurement of the distance between the slice and 0-point of the gantry was built into the softwear. CT replaced conventional x-ray in stereotaxy almost overnight. A flurry of activity followed, mainly in an endeavor to adapt and modify existing stereotactic systems to CT scanning (4,5,7,28,36) or to devise new ones (8,14,44).

To complete the triple alliance—comprised of CT, stereotaxis, and finally brachytherapy—a brief historical comment about radioactive isotopes is in order. In contrast to teletherapy, interstitial radiotherapy is comprised of localized radiation produced by implanted isotopes (31). In 1901 Pierre Curie sealed radium in a small glass tube and gave it to a physician colleague, Danlos, to insert into a tumor (9). This was the birth of interstitial radiotherapy. Two years later Alexander Graham Bell gave similar advice to physicians in North America (2).

In 1914 Frazier was the first to implant a radioactive isotope into the brain (12). Using 50–100 mg of radium, such interstitial implantation was free-hand and temporary, usually lasting not more than 20 hrs. It was employed as an adjunct to teletherapy. By 1922 Frazier had treated 32 patients by this means (12).

Tönnis and Wilke revived interest in brachytherapy in 1960 when cobalt-60 became available (53). However, radiation hazards and a lack of safer isotopes held this activity at abeyance.

From 1952 to 1981, Mundinger stereotactically interstitially irradiated 1,263 patients harboring various intracranial tumors using differing isotopes (29–34). Szikla and co-workers have the next largest series (49,50). Poblete and Zamboni reported a small group as well (39). In the United States Gutin's group (16,20) and Slater (45) have reported small series. Our experience matches that of the latter two series; yet even when these data are combined there is no statistical significance because the numbers are too small and the treatment protocols too divergent. A few isolated reports, mostly unpublished, complete the sum of American experience in this area.

This then is modern CT guided-stereotactic radiotherapy of tumors. It is a fusion of stereotaxy, CT, and modern use of currently available isotopes. The combined application of all three modalities is an endeavor to alter the portent of doom that looms over patients harboring malignant disease of the brain.

References

1. Bechtereva NP, Bondartchuk AN, Smirnow VM, et al: Method of electrostimulation of deep brain structures in treatment of some chronic brain diseases. Confin Neurol 37:136–140, 1975
2. Bell AG: Letter to the editor. Arch Roentgen Ray 8:64, 1903
3. Bertrand G, Jasper H: Microelectrode recording of unit activity in the human thalamus. Confin Neurol 26:205–208, 1965
4. Birg W, Mundinger F: Direct target point determination for stereotactic brain operations from CT data and the setting parameters for polar-coordinate stereotactic devices. Appl Neurophysiol 45:387–395, 1982
5. Boëthius J, Bergström M, Greitz T: Stereotaxic computerized tomography with a GE 8800 scanner. J Neurosurg 52:794–800, 1980
6. Brooks RA, DiChiro G: Slice geometry in computer assisted tomography. J Comput Assist Tomogr 1:191–199, 1977
7. Brown RA: A computerized tomography-computer graphics approach to stereotaxic localization. J Neurosurg 50:715–720, 1979
8. Brown RA, Roberts SR, Osborn AG: Stereotaxic frame and computer software for CT directed neurosurgical localization. Invest Radiol 15:308–312, 1980
9. Danlos H: Considerationes cur le traitment des (dermatologique) par l'radium. J Physiother (Paris) 3:98–106, 1909
10. Dittmer C: Über die Lage des sogenannten Gefässzentrums in der Medullaoblongata: Berichte d. Sächsischen Gesellschaft der Wissenschaften. Leipz Math Phys Klasse 25:449–469, 1873
11. Feild JR, Lawrence JA, White TJ, et al: Scalp localization of supratentorial lesions demonstrated by computed tomography. Neurosurgery 6:164–175, 1980
12. Frazier CH: The effects of radium emanations upon brain tumors. Surg Gynecol Obstet 31:236–239, 1920
13. Gillingham FJ: Small localized lesions of the internal capsule in the treatment of dyskinesias. Confin Neurol 22:385–392, 1962

14. Glenn W: Personal communication, September 1982
15. Guiot G, Harty J, Albe-Fessard D: De'limitation precise des structures souscorticales et identification de noyaux thalamiques chez l'homme par l'electrophysiologie stéréotaxique. Neurochirurgia 5:1–18, 1962
16. Gutin PH, Phillips TL, Hosobushi Y, et al: Permanent and removable implants for brachytherapy of brain tumors. Int J Radiat Oncol Biol Phys 7:1371–1381, 1981
17. Hécaen H, Talairach J, David M, et al: Coagulations limitées du thalamus dans les algies du syndrome thalamique. Rev Neurol (Paris) 81:917–931, 1949
18. Hink VC, Clifton GL: A precise technique for craniotomy localization using computerized tomography. J Neurosurg 54:416–418, 1981
19. Horsley V, Clarke RH: The structure and function of the cerebellum examined by a new method. Brain 31:45–124, 1908
20. Hosobushi Y, Phillips TL, Stupar TA, et al: Interstitial brachytherapy of primary brain tumors: preliminary report. J Neurosurg 53:613–617, 1980
21. Hounsfield GN: Computerized transverse axial scanning (tomography) I. Description of system. Br J Radiol 46:1016–1022, 1973
22. Hounsfield GN: Picture quality of computed tomography. Am J Roentgenol 127:3–9, 1976
23. James HJ, Wells M, Alksne JF, et al: Needle biopsy under computerized tomographic control: a method for tissue diagnosis in intracranial lesions. Neurosurgery 5:671–674, 1979
24. Kandel E, Cheboratyova WM: Conray ventriculography in stereotaxic surgery. Confin Neurol 34:34–40, 1972
25. Krayenbühl H, Yasargil MG: Relief of intention tremor due to multiple sclerosis by stereotaxic thalamotomy. Confin Neurol 22:368–374, 1962
26. Laitinen L, Toivakka E: Locating brain tumor through deep EEG probes. Confin Neurol 34:101–105, 1972
27. Leksell L: The stereotaxic method and radiosurgery of the brain. Acta Chir Scand 102:316–319, 1951
28. Lundsford LD, Rosenbaum AE, Perry J: Stereotactic surgery using the therapeutic CT scanner. Surg Neurol 18:116–122, 1982
29. Mundinger F: CT-stereotactic biopsy of brain tumors. In: Tumours of the Central Nervous System in Infancy and Childhood, edited by D Voth, P Gutjahr, C Langmaid. Springer-Verlag, New York, 1982, pp 234–246
30. Mundinger F: Die stereotaktische interstitielle Therapie nicht resezierbarer intrakranieller Tumoren mit Ir-192 und Jod-125. In: Kombinierte chirurgische und radiologische Behandlung maligner Tumoren, edited by M Wannemacher, HW Schreiber, F Gauwerky. Urban & Schwarzenberg, Munich, 1981, pp 90–112
31. Mundinger F: Implantation of radioisotopes (curie-therapy). In: Stereotaxy of the Human Brain, edited by G Schaltenbrand, AE Walker. George Thieme Verlag, New York, 1982, pp 411–435
32. Mundinger F, Hoefer T: Protracted longterm irradiation of inoperable midbrain tumors by stereotactic curietherapy, using Ir-192. Acta Neurochir (Wien) [Suppl 21], 93–100, 1974
33. Mundinger F, Metzel E: Erfahrungen mit der lokalen Strahlenbehandlung inoperabler Zwischenhirn- und Basalganglien-tumoren mit der stereotaktischen Permanent-Implantation von $Iridium^{192}$. Arch Psychiatr Nervenkr 212:70–90, 1968
34. Mundinger F, Ostertag CB, Weigel K: Stereotactic treatment of brain lesions: biopsy, interstitial radiotherapy (Ir^{192}-I^{125}) and drainage procedures. Appl Neurophysiol 43:192–204, 1980
35. Narabayashi H: Beginning and development of stereotaxic surgery in Tokyo. Confin Neurol 37:363–373, 1975
36. Perry JH, Rosenbaum AE, Lundsford LD, et al: Computed tomography-guided stereotactic surgery: conception and development of a new stereotactic methodology. Neurosurgery 7:376–381, 1980

37. Phelps ME, Hoffmann EJ, Ter-Gossian MM: Attenuation coefficients of various body tissues, fluids and lesions at photon energies of 18–136 KEV. Radiology 117:573–583, 1975
38. Piskun WS, Stevens EA, LaMorgese JR, et al: A simplified method of CT assisted localization and biopsy of intracranial lesions. Surg Neurol 11:413–417, 1979
39. Poblete M, Zamboni R: Stereotactic implant of iridium-192 in brain tumors. In: Stereotactic Cerebral Irradiation: INSERM Symposium 12, edited by G. Szikla. Elsevier/North Holland Biomedical Press, Amsterdam, 1979, pp 321–328
40. Riechert T, Wolff M: Die Entwicklung u. klinische Bedeutung der gezielten Hirnoperationen. Med Klin 46:609–611, 1951
41. Rosenbaum HE: Three-dimensional computerized tomographic scans of brain: a new approach to intracranial diagnosis. Arch Neurol 34:386–387, 1977
42. Rushworth RG: Stereotactic guided biopsy in the computerized tomographic scanner. Surg Neurol 14:451–454, 1980
43. Schaltenbrand G, Bailey P: Introduction to Stereotaxis with an Atlas of the Human Brain. Thieme, Stuttgart, 1959
44. Sheldon CH, McCann G, Jacques S, et al: Development of a computerized microstereotaxic method for localization and removal of minute CNS lesions under direct 3-D vision. J Neurosurg 52:21–27, 1980
45. Slater R: Paper presented at the Western Neurological Society, Jackson Hole, Wyoming, October 1982
46. Spiegel EA: Indications for stereoencephalotomy. Confin Neurol 31:5–10, 1969
47. Spiegel EA: Methodological problems in stereoencephalotomy. Confin Neurol 26:125–132, 1965
48. Spiegel EA, Wycis HT, Marks M, et al: Stereotactic apparatus for operations on the human brain. Science 106:349–350, 1947
49. Szikla G, Betti O, Szenthe L, et al: L'experience actuelle des irradiations stereotaxiques dans le traitment des gliomes hémispheriques. Neurochirurgie 27:295–298, 1981
50. Szikla G, Paragut JC: Irradiation interstitielle des gliomes. Neurochirurgie [Suppl 2], 187–228, 1975
51. Ter-Pogossian MM: Computerized cranial tomography: equipment and physics. Semin Roentgenol 12:13–25, 1977
52. Thompson JL: Computerized axial tomography and the diagnosis of glioma: a study of 100 consecutive historically proven cases. Clin Radiol 27:431–441, 1976
53. Tönnis W, Wilke O: Die Behandlung von Hirntumoren mit radioaktirvem Kobalt (Co^{60}). Acta Neurochir (Wien) 8:456–467, 1960
54. Velasco-Suárez MM, Escobedo FR: Stereotaxic intracerebral instillation of dopa. Confin Neurol 32:149–157, 1970

2

Riechert-Mundinger Stereotactic Apparatus

Peter Dyck

Spiegel and Wycis are credited with introducing stereotactic surgery in man (13). The apparatus was modified a number of times before their fifth model became acceptable to them (12). Two years later, in 1949, Leksell devised a stereotactic apparatus comprised of an inner frame that attached to the skull and carried an outer bow (5). This bow anchored the instrument block and could be moved through two planes. Riechert designed his first apparatus in collaboration with Wolff in 1950 (11). The design was modified in 1955.

This 1955 model was adapted to computed tomography (CT) scanning with only minor modifications (10). These design changes were preoccupied with various modifications in skull fixation, employing different plastics, so as to allow CT scanning without hindrance from scatter artifacts produced by metals. These modifications are currently in use at the University of Freiburg im Breisgau but are not available commercially (3). Hence the equipment is described within the framework of these limitations.

As shown in Figure 2–1, with the trajectory set at zero the instrument arc, when swept through its entire X and Y planes, describes a hemisphere with a constant radius. By taking into consideration four angular variables in this polar coordinate system, any two points may be mathematically aligned so that a single linear trajectory may pass through both of them. Hence, practically speaking, a computer program can be written which allows one to choose any desired target within the brain and reach it through a predetermined trephination point (2).

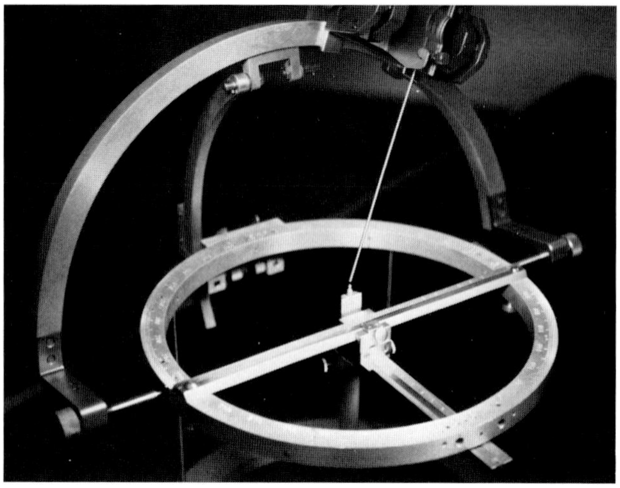

Figure 2–1 The Riechert-Mundinger stereotactic apparatus is based on mathematical principles, known as analytical geometry, described by René Descartes (1596–1650). In such a system any specific point may be represented by a designation in the X-Y plane. By adding a third dimension, or Z function, a three-dimensional representation becomes possible. This is illustrated here. Such coordinates can be represented by their cosines and numbers; hence mathematically any two such coordinates may be connected by a straight line (desired trajectory).

Birg has programmed a TI-59 hand-held calculator (Texas Instruments, Dallas, Texas) to accomplish this task (1). Its practical application is described in Chapter 4.

Base Ring

Figure 2–2 illustrates the aluminum alloy base ring anchored by pins to the skull. Because metal creates artifacts during CT scanning, the base ring is placed so that it is excluded from the CT gantry but still allows tomographic data gathering. This is accomplished in part by placing the base ring as close as possible to the orbitomeatal line, thus leaving maximal calvarial surface artifact-free and at the same time retaining

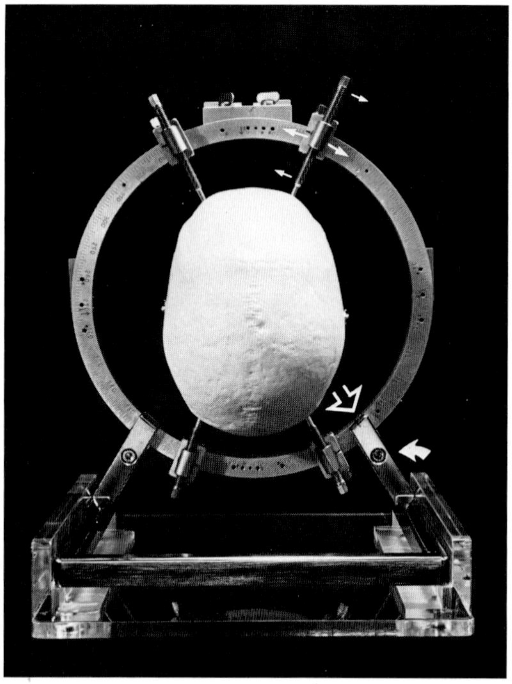

Figure 2–2 Skeletal fixation is obtained by metallic screws in the commercially available equipment. The base ring is aligned by calibration markers on the ringholder (*open arrow*) The ring is held in place by a cotter-key screw (*curved arrow*). The pin mount angle is adjustable on the base ring (*dark arrow*) and the desired pin swivel may be individually set (*small arrow*). For the best skeletal fixation the vectors of force in front should be identical to those applied to the back of the skull, as shown here.

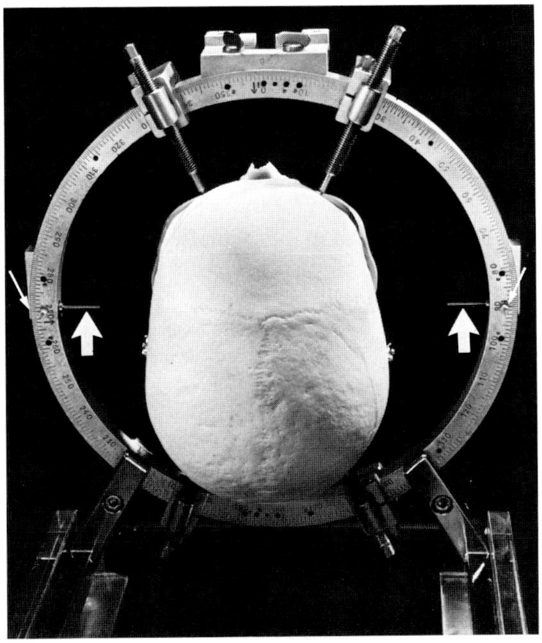

Figure 2–3 In order to horizontally align the stereotactic equipment within the CT scanner, reference pins are screwed into the base ring. Small pins, which become visible on the lateral CT scout films, are shown (*small arrows*). More accurate calibration is possible when the large pins, which were placed in the x plane (*large arrows*), become visible on axial sections through the base ring at the inception of tomography.

firm calvarial pin fixation. The commercially available stereotactic apparatus comes supplied with metallic mounts and fixation screws. An endeavor is under way to replace these with materials that are compatible with the CT scanner and yet still retain enough strength to provide rigid support. The base ring accommodates various attachments, including the arc device that carries the instrument block. The attachments are so designed as to almost abolish the possibility of error that might violate the geometric principles on which the stereotactic system is based. Two pins are screwed into the x plane to serve as calibration markers at the time of CT scanning. Similar marker pins are placed in the z plane, as shown in Figure 2–3. These markers aid calibration and are visible on the axial sections and lateral scout films during CT scanning (Figure 2–4). Three arcs of variable length attach to the base ring and are cali-

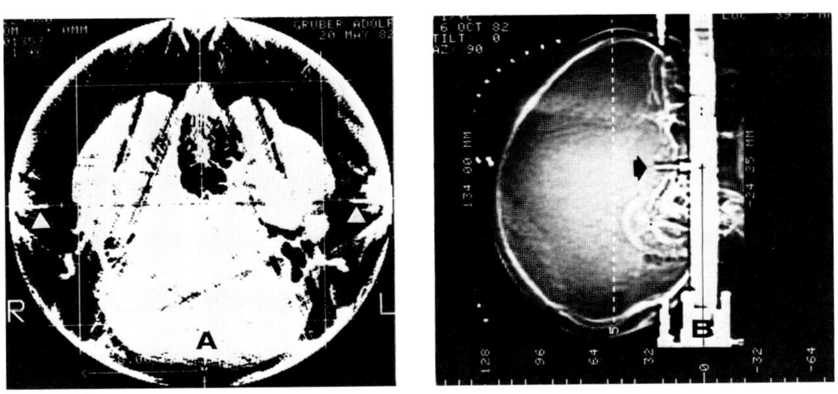

Figure 2–4 The axial section **(A)** illustrates that at the 0 level the base ring is visible and the horizontal pins on this ring are in alignment with the X-axis of the CT gantry (*solid white arrowheads*). This is further confirmed on the lateral scout views, which show superimposition of the right and left pins (*dark arrow*) projecting into the z plane of the base ring **(B)**.

brated in a manner so as to designate the horizontal angle of the arc device. The assembly of three arc components is possible in only one way, thus making them failproof.

Two etched marks on the base ring help align the ring in a horizontal plane of the X axis during CT scanning. Similar markings are present on the mount of the GE-T 8800 scanner. The operating table mount is similarly calibrated.

To help align the patient's head within the base ring, an occipital support, adjustable rubber-shod ear plugs, and a nasal bridge support are provided (Figure 2–5). However, because the exact position of the head within the base ring is not important, the head may be manually held while the calvarial pins are applied, thus avoiding a time-consuming step in the surgical procedure.

Base Ring Mount

The base ring mount fits into a plastic seat that is securely attached to the foot end of a conventional operating table, as shown in Figure 2–6. When stereotactically approaching the anterior two-thirds of the hemi-

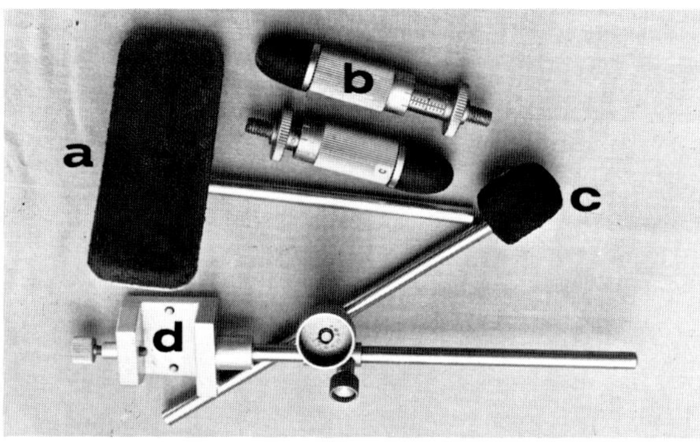

Figure 2–5 Components are available to assist in skeletal fixation of the head, which may be cradled in an occipital support (*a*). The ear plugs (*b*) serve as lateral stabilizers, and a nasal bridge support (*c*) helps stabilize the nose. A ring mount (*d*) is also shown. All these attachments may be replaced by a steady hand.

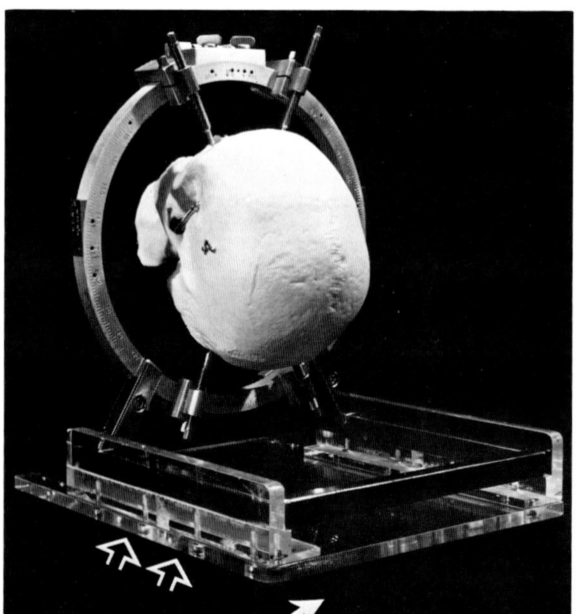

Figure 2–6 The plastic seat is securely bolted to the tail end of a standard operating table (*open arrows*). Because this design does not accommodate American grid cassettes, the x-ray film is placed below it (*curved arrow*).

sphere, conventional placement (Figure 2–7) is advised; but when posterior parietal or occipital lesions are approached, the ring mount placement is reversed (Figure 2–8) so as not to physically impede approach to this area. To facilitate surgical ease in the occipital area, the operating table may be raised and the surgeon seated.

Instrument Block and Arc Device

Commensurate with cartesian geometric principles of a sphere, the instrument arc is designed to allow any desired trajectory to pass through two predetermined points within the hemisphere with the base ring serving as a reference. To ensure this, the arc device attaches to the base ring in a noninterchangeable manner. Its horizontal angulation is measured in degrees, as indicated on the support bow. The length of the bow one chooses depends on the angulation desired. Hence the longest bow is employed for those lesions located in back.

The instrument block provides the remaining angular adjustments necessary to reach an intracranial target. The instrument block slides on an arc that allows a 150° approach to the hemisphere in a side-to-

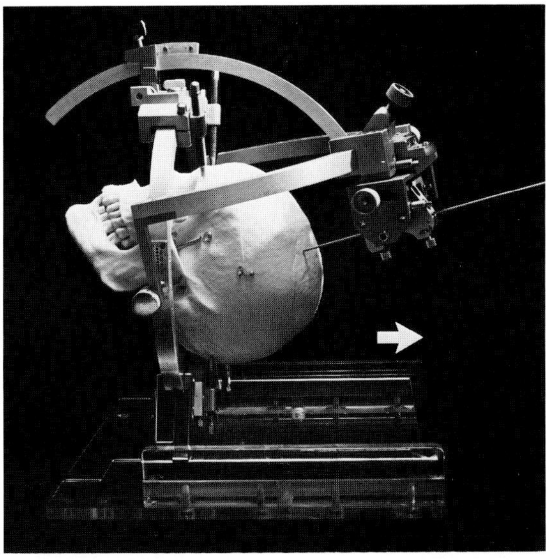

Figure 2–7 Traditional placement of the base ring mount, allowing ample access to the anterior two-thirds of the calvarium.

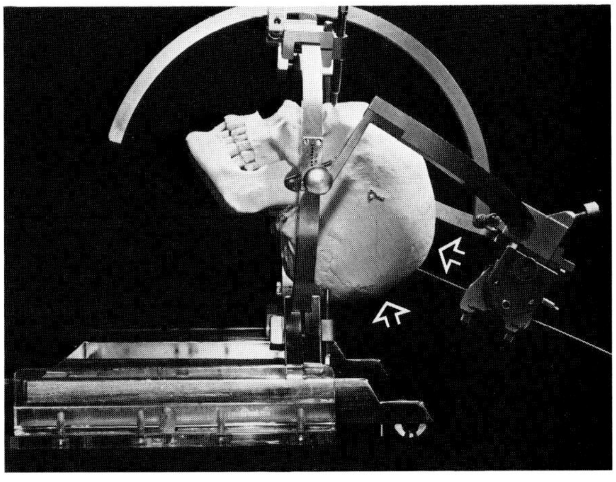

Figure 2–8 In order to facilitate a greater angle of access to the occipitoparietal brain, the base ring mount may be reversed and mounted as shown. Note that the plastic table mount remains unchanged but the metal base ring mount has been reversed. *Open arrows* point to the improved access provided by this maneuver.

side plane, or X plane. This arc is divided into two 90° sectors. The right sector is designated positive, the left negative.

Any trajectory that does not pass through the center of this geometric sphere is determined by vertical and horizontal vernier adjustments on the instrument block (Figure 2–9). A magnification lens attachment is provided to accommodate this fine calibration.

The biopsy guide and microdrive attach directly to the instrument block. Advance toward a target is determined by this means, as is the distance from target to arc. The instrument block also serves to hold the spline for an electrically driven *motorized perforator.* The commercially available *burr* is small but adequate for permanent implantation of isotopes but is considered unnecessarily risky by the authors; hence it has been replaced by a customized larger-diameter burr (Figure 2–10). The instrument guide provides three parallel horizontally aligned trajectory capabilities. Each is separated from the other by 4 mm (Figure 2–9).

The instrument arc and block assembly is durable and well designed. The microdrive could be improved and simplified, but it is functional and not particularly cumbersome.

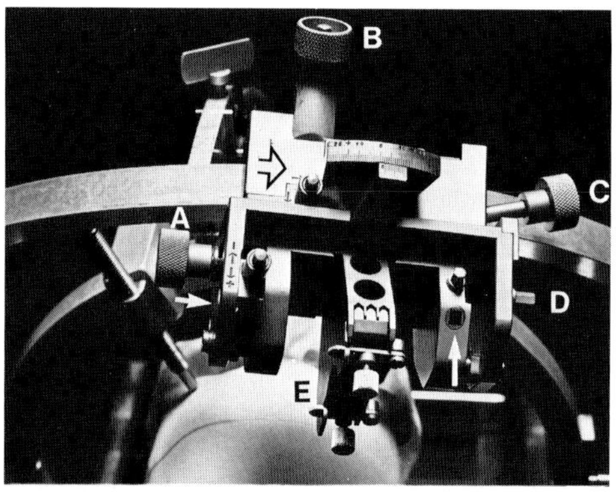

Figure 2–9 The instrument block is well designed, embodying means for instrumentation *guidance* (*e*). The *long arrow* points to a microdrive seating. Vernier adjustments in a vertical plane are indicated by a *short solid arrow,* and the same adjustments horizontally by the *open arrow.* To retain alignment, *A* anchors the vertical vernier setting and *C* the horizontal. When *B* is tightened, the lateral angle setting is ensured; when *D* is loosened it releases the spline that carries the instrumentation or anchors the electric power drill.

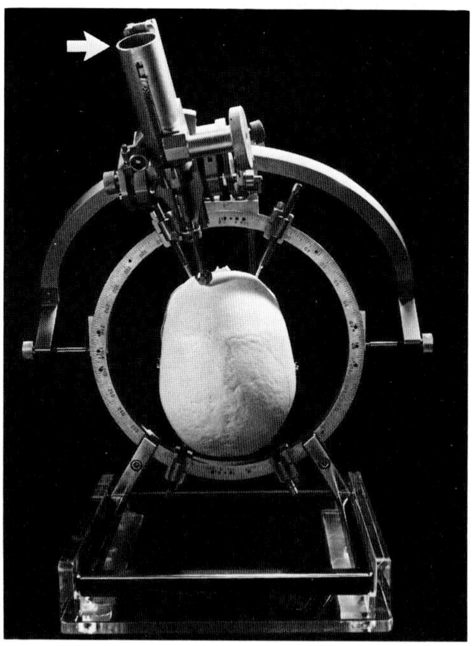

Figure 2–10 The commercially available *perforator* has been replaced by this 12 mm diameter burr (*arrow*), which allows better hemostasis of surface vessels.

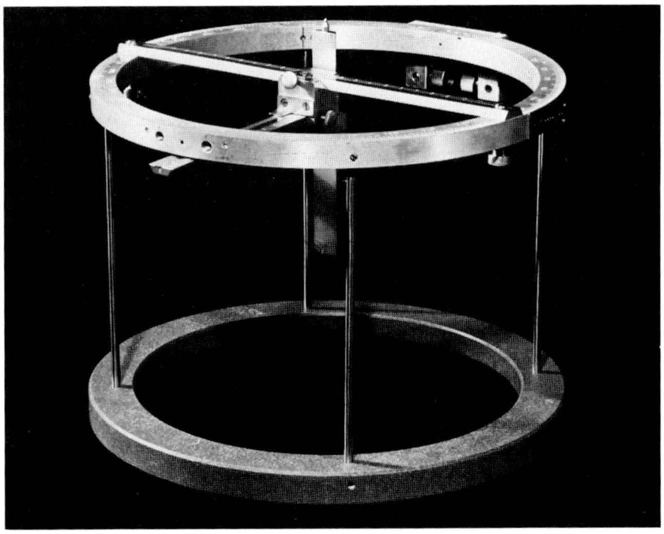

Figure 2–11 Phantom apparatus. See Figure 2–1 for details.

Phantom Device

The phantom apparatus is simply a base ring mounted on a ring stand (Figure 2–11). Attached to the base ring is an adjustable array which allows presetting of any target within the geometric hemisphere in question. This is made possible by a sliding block, which moves in both the X and Y planes and allows for calibration of the depth, or the Z function.

By convention, the horizontal plane is designated by X: positive to right, negative to left. The vertical plane is represented by Y, positive from center upward (toward the nose), negative downward. The Z plane indicates the depth of intrusion into the geometric hemisphere, or colloquially speaking, the tumor depth. Keeping this in mind, it becomes understandable why the position of a human head within the base ring has no geometric importance. It is important, however, that the stereotactic apparatus is so calibrated that the center of the base ring coincides with the center of the CT gantry. Hence frequent calibration is essential.

It must be remembered that this phantom device was originally designed to approach deep cerebral structures through the anterior half of the cerebral hemispheres, and so it is admirably suited for our purpose. It creates a problem, however, when stereotaxy involves the parietal and occipital brain, i.e., the posterior two quadrants. To represent them the phantom must be turned around, so that front becomes back and vice versa. The front of the phantom ring is designated 0° and the back 180°. When representing posterior quadrant lesions, the converse becomes true. The arc-fixing mount must be switched and attached at the 180° marking and then reversed again when the instrument arc is placed on the patient's base ring. This inconvenience could have been avoided had the X-Y subserving functions been mounted below the phantom reference ring.

Modifications in the design of the instruments are inevitable. For example, the ring stand comes painted, and it should not have been because when the equipment is autoclaved the paint comes off or blisters.

CT Scanner Mount

The CT scanner mount is sturdy and made of metal (Figure 2–12). Yet its sturdiness outweighs its usefulness. It serves well for head fixation during CT scanning of most supratentorial lesions but creates an impasse when the patient's base ring is attached high on the calvarium for scanning of brainstem structures or posterior fossa lesions. This will also inevitably be changed from metal to plastic so as to be compatible with CT while retaining sturdy geometrically reliable reference points for stereotaxy.

Biopsy Forceps

The biopsy forceps is well designed. It is, in essence, a mesoscopic "pituitary punch." Specimens obtained are adequate for smear and paraffin-mounting techniques. Being a punch, it can lacerate vessels—and therein lies the danger. Yet in the author's experience the best specimens are obtained when the forceps is advanced open-jawed for 2–3 mm before it is closed (Figure 2–13). Axial rotation of the forceps at the target site does not yield better specimens. Insulated cannulas should be made available so that in case of vessel laceration unipolar electrocoagulation may be attempted by introducing a metal stylet through them. Such cannulas are not yet commercially available.

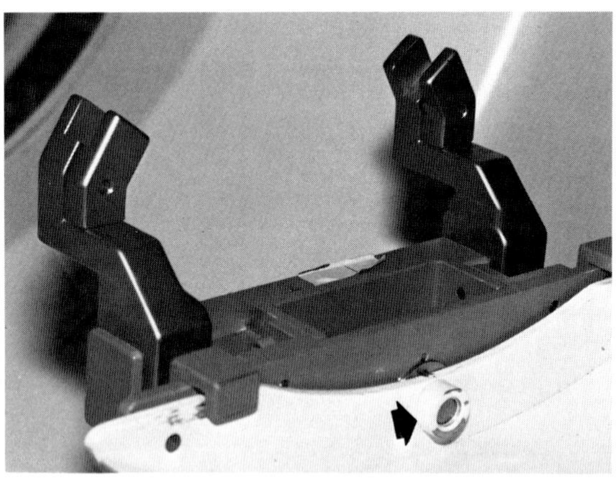

Figure 2–12 The CT table mount fits only the GE-T 8800 scanner. It has a vertical microdrive adjustment screw. The *arrow* points to a fixation screw that anchors it to the scanner table. It does not allow scanning of the posterior fossa because it is made of metal.

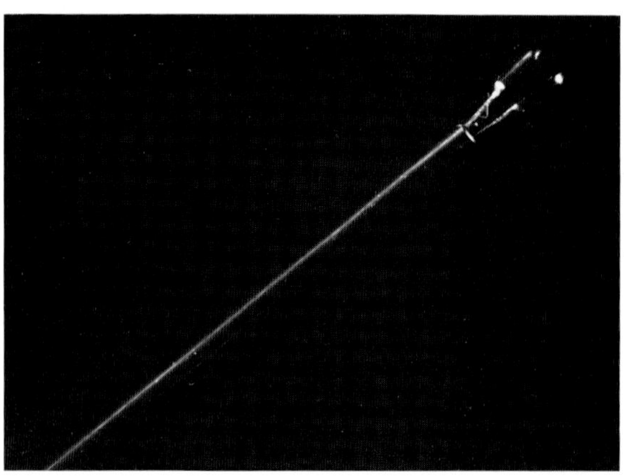

Figure 2–13 Biopsy forceps. The best tissue specimens are obtained if the forceps are advanced open-jawed for 2 mm prior to retrieval of tissue.

Special Stereotactic Approaches

Occipital Lesions

An occipital lesion presents formidable problems because the inferior 50° of a 180° vertical arc is stereotactically excluded from surgical approach, even with the base ring holder reversed. However, the patient may be placed face down on the operating table, thus exchanging the occipital for the frontal lobes, stereotactically speaking. It must be emphasized that the patient need not undergo CT scanning in this position even if surgical intervention is planned this way. This can be mathematically corrected by converting the Y function from minus to plus during computer calculations of the trajectory.

Diencephalic Lesions

Because the base ring cannot always be placed low enough on the skull to escape interference during CT scanning, the base ring may be reverse-mounted high on the calvarium, as shown in Figure 2–14. CT scanning is now possible if the CT scanner mount is made of plastic or carbon, once again a commodity that is not commercially available.

Posterior Fossa Lesions

As with diencephalic or temporal pole lesions which are beyond CT scanner reach with conventional skull fixation and available equipment, so it is with posterior fossa lesions. Commercially, this capability

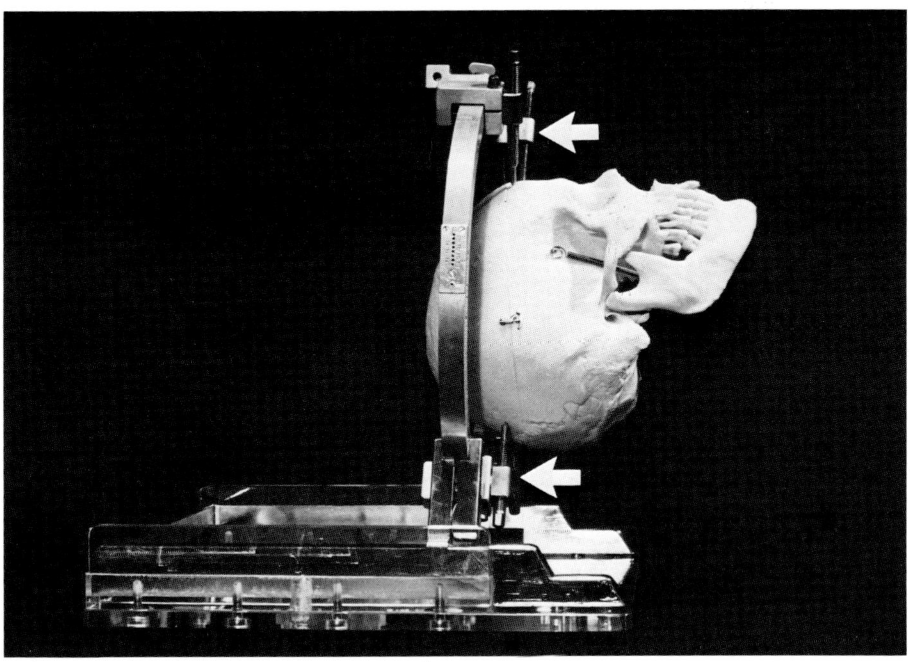

Figure 2–14 Reverse mounting of a base ring is shown. This maneuver should be avoided if possible because it introduces computerization problems and CT scanning difficulties unless customized equipment is available.

is not available at present but can be made so by simple redesign of the equipment to allow surgical access to the occiput or subocciput in a sitting position.

Although stereotactic practice is burdened by a preoccupation with horizontal fixation of the patient, this should be looked on as vestigial "collimated" vision from the x-ray era of stereotaxy. There is no reason why a patient must lie on an operating table in a perfectly horizontal and vertical plane anymore.

Hence patients with occipital or posterior fossa lesions could undergo stereotactic biopsy in a sitting position with the base ring stabilized by a customized adapter attached to a Mayfield head rest. This, rather than a face-down position, would be preferable to both patient and surgeon. Such a device is being designed.

Afterloading Catheters

Interstitial irradiation may be accomplished by permanent implantation of a radioactive source, which is known as curietherapy (7). Alternatively, it may be temporary isotopic irradiation by a retrievable source (6,9). Mundinger labeled this short-term irradiation "brachytherapy" (6,8). The author's experience is exclusively with the temporary form, employing iridium-192 as the radiation source. This isotope has a well-established track record in North America as an interstitial implant, and hence it was chosen in preference to others.

The afterloading catheter described by Gutin et al. has physical drawbacks (4). Slater's afterloading catheter (American Heyer-Schulte Corporation, Goleta, California) is not rigid enough nor is it readily available or cost-effective. Hence it was decided to employ a standard Pudenz-Schulte ventricular shunt catheter (Edward Wock & Company, Inc., Research Triangle Park, North Carolina) as a means by which to deliver the isotope ribbon to the tumor site. Such catheters are perforated and so allow egress of blood should hemorrhage or drainage of cyst fluid occur. Yet the surrounding irradiation is apparently intense enough to hamper bacterial replication. Hence serious infection is unlikely even if the catheters are exteriorized. Our limited experiences support this hypothesis to date.

Conclusion

The Riechert-Mundinger stereotactic apparatus is by no means unique or perfectly adapted to modern stereotaxy. Urgent modifications are needed. In spite of these drawbacks it offers a means by which intracranial lesions may be approached with minimal risk and acceptable degrees of accuracy. Also, in contrast to more contemporarily proposed CT stereotactic systems, the Riechert-Mundinger equipment is more versatile and better facilitates sterile technique.

Modification of the equipment to make it more compatible with CT scanning or nuclear magnetic resonance (NMR)-guided stereotaxy in the not too distant future provides ample room for improvement. Some of this was highlighted in this chapter. The phantom, for instance, needs to be redesigned to make it more versatile; yet the instrument arc and block are functional as they exist, generally speaking.

References

1. Birg W, Klar M, Mundinger F: Programmierbare Taschentechner bei stereotaktischen Hirnoperationen. Med Klin 72:135–136, 1977
2. Birg W, Mundinger F: Computer calculations of target parameters for a stereotactic apparatus. Acta Neurochir (Wien) 29:123–129, 1973
3. Birg W, Mundinger F: Direct target point determination for stereotactic brain operations from CT data and calculation of setting parameters for polar-coordinate stereotactic devices. Appl Neurophysiol 45:387–395, 1982
4. Gutin PH, Phillips TL, Hosobushi Y, et al: Permanent and removable implants for the brachytherapy of brain tumors. Int J Radiat Oncol Biol Phys 7:1371–1381, 1981
5. Leksell L: A stereotactic apparatus for intracerebral surgery. Acta Chir Scand 99:229–299, 1949
6. Mundinger F: Die stereotaktische interstitielle Therapie nicht resezierbaner intrakranieller Tumoren mit Iridium-192 und Jod-125. In: Kombinierte chirurgische und radiologische Therapie maligner Tumoren, edited by M Wannenmacher. Urban & Schwarzenberg, Baltimore, 1981, pp 90–112
7. Mundinger F: Implantation of radioisotopes (curietherapy). In: Textbook of Stereotaxy of the Human Brain, edited by G Schaltenbrand, AE Walker. Thieme Verlag, Stuttgart, 1982, pp 410–445
8. Mundinger F, Birg W: Stereotactic brain surgery with the aid of computed tomography (CT stereotaxy). Adv Neurosurg 10:17–24, 1982
9. Mundinger F, Osterlag CB, Birg W, et al: Stereotactic treatment of brain lesions, biopsy, interstitial radiotherapy (Ir-192 and I-125) and drainage procedures. Appl Neurophysiol 43:198–204, 1980
10. Riechert, Munginger F: Beschreibung und Anwendung eines Zielgerätes für stereotaktische Hirnoperationen (II Model). Acta Neurochir (Wien) [Suppl III], 308–337, 1955
11. Riechert T, Wolff M: Die Entwicklung und klinische Bedeutung der gezielten Hirnoperationen. Med Klin 46:609–611, 1951
12. Spiegel EA, Wycis HT: Stereoencephalotomy. II. Clinical and Physiologic Applications. Grune & Stratton, New York, 1962, p 2
13. Spiegel EA, Wycis HT, Marks M, et al: Stereotaxic apparatus for operations on the human brain. Science 106:349–350, 1947

3

CT-Guided Stereotaxy: Riechert-Mundinger Method

L. G. Solti-Bohman
W. W. M. Lo

Computerized axial tomography (CAT), better known as computerized tomography (CT), revolutionized neurodiagnosis when Hounsfield (14) of EMI, Ltd. developed the first CT scanner and Ambrose (1) demonstrated its diagnostic capabilities at Atkinson Morley's Hospital in Wimbledon, England. Endeavors to improve on its diagnostic capabilities were almost instantaneous. Among these was an attempt to better depict the relationship of an intracranial lesion to the calvarium (4). To accomplish this task, Hayman et al. anchored two crossed bobbypins to the patient's hair at the time of CT scanning (12). Levinthal et al. affixed a wire in the coronal plane to serve as a reference marker (17). Piskun et al. (20) in 1979 and Hinck and Clifton (13) in 1981 advised the incorporation of progressively longer radiographic markers between scalp and CT gantry. These markers were placed lateral to the head and were arranged with the base lying along the canthal-meatal line (radiopaque catheters taped to the x-ray film fulfilled this goal). These markers were spaced 1 cm apart and were increased in length by the same amount (20). Instead of dispersing them uniformly, Hinck and Clifton clustered the 12 catheters in groups of three (13). It stands to reason that the number of markers seen beside the intracranial lesion also aid its localization in reference to the side of the head. This was useful in planning a craniotomy, but these data supplied only a lateral reference point. By taping a circumferential radiomarker-impregnated band to the head, the CT scan would provide not only a lateral but also an anteroposterior reference for the target coordinate (7).

This logic has been extrapolated by Gildenberg et al. (8). They related the coordinates of a point of interest (e.g., a tumor) to the CT scan scout films and stereotactically approached 18 lesions in seven patients. In one case, four of six cerebral abscesses were aspirated by such means. Five glial tumors were also biopsied by this technique. It must be emphasized, however, that such an undertaking is possible only if the patient is cooperative, because any change in head position between scanning and procurement of scout films invalidates any comparison. Even if such an undertaking is more accurate than a free-hand technique, it is therefore by no means precise.

As CT scanners became more widely available, endeavors to modify and adapt traditional stereotactic equipment to it were inevitable. Mundinger and Ostertag were probably the first stereotacticians to accomplish this (18). Adaptation of the Leksell stereotactic apparatus was pioneered by Leksell in Sweden (2,3) and elsewhere (11). In some instances significant theoretical and design modifications resulted (19). The Riechert-Mundinger stereotactic apparatus was probably most drastically modified by Jacques et al. in order to accommodate the authors' investigative and clinical needs (15,16). In spite of these innovations, room for improvement remains.

Stereotactic surgical intervention while the patient remains in the CT scanner was pioneered by Glenn and associates (9,10,21). For such an undertaking the patient's head and the stereotactic apparatus are imaged simultaneously. Hence the coordinates of a firmly anchored structure may be related to the stereotactic frame and its attachments. The planar geometric (X and Y) values are derived from the scanner software. The Z value of structure is computed in reference to a diagonal (feducial) rod mounted between three pairs of vertical plastic rods. Such an arrangement provides three feducial points with specific cartesian coordinates which allow computation of the Z value of the intracranial structure with reference to these outside markers.

The Brown-Roberts-Wells stereotactic apparatus, although not employing an "in-scanner" technique, uses the same mathematical logic to arrive at the Z value for an intracranial X,Y coordinate (5,6). Perry's modification of the Leksell stereotactic apparatus similarly arrives at the Z value of an intracranial structure by the same feducial concepts (19).

Hence stereotactic equipment can be roughly divided into two types: that which utilizes externally mounted reference points to determine the depth (Z value) of the target, and that which arrives at these data by relying on the CT scanner itself. In the latter system, no markers need be placed between intracranial structures and the CT gantry, but the patient's head fixation in reference to the scanner gantry is essential. The Riechert-Mundinger apparatus follows this premise.

Principle

The Riechert-Mundinger head frame is adapted to the GE 8800 CT scanner so that the stereotactic fields of the two systems coincide. Any structure visualized on CT may then have its coordinates read on the scanner; the coordinates so obtained may be directly transferable to the stereotactic arc and the structure accordingly localized by the stereotactic probe. An essential requisite of this principle is that the patient's head remains firmly fixed to the stereotactic ring frame during scanning and the subsequent surgical procedure so that the spatial relationship of the head to the stereotactic base remains the same (Figure 3–1).

Requirements

Three stepwise requirements must be met to ensure that the stereotactic fields of the two systems coincide. First, assuming that the travel of the scanner table is horizontal, the scanning plane and the plane of the stereotactic ring to the scanner table must both be vertical. Second, the centers of the scan circle and of the stereotactic ring must coincide; and third, the X and Y axes of the two systems must superimpose.

Equipment

The Scanner

The GE 8800 CT scanner gantry and table are each supported by a pair of metallic plates. The surface of the four plates lie within 0.06 inch of a plane verified by carpenter's level and surveyor's transit to be horizontal at installation.

The gantry bearing on which the table and detector array are mounted can be tilted by motor up to 15° in a cranial and caudal direction on its horizontal base. The true vertical position of the bearing is confirmed with a level at installation. Subsequently that position may be reestablished by superimposing either one of two sets of steel rings, one member of each pair being attached to the tilting bearing and the other to the fixed base. These small rings are found where the bearing and

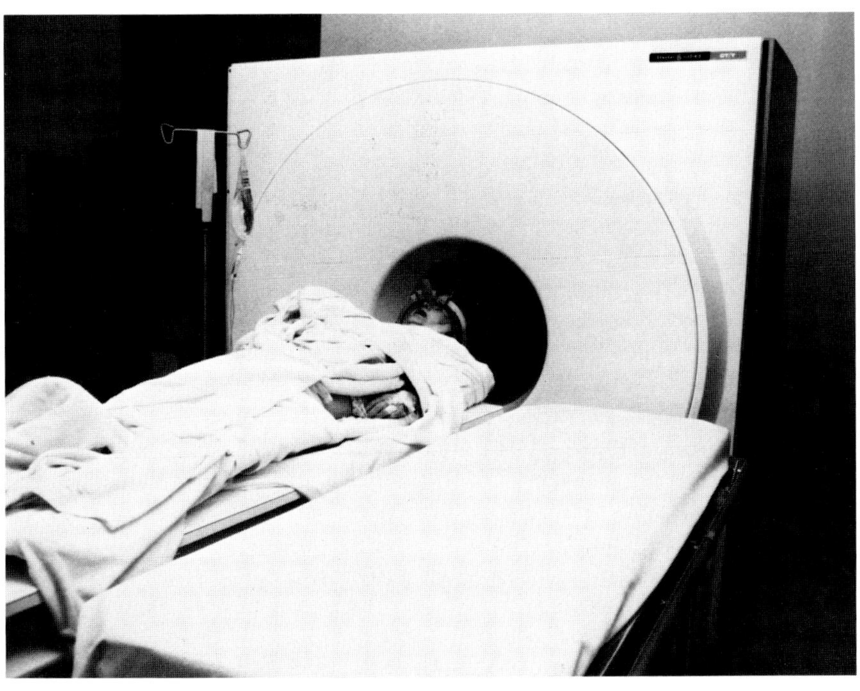

Figure 3–1 Patient has been transferred onto the scanner table with the stereotactic ring attached to the calvarium.

base meet after removing a side panel from the gantry enclosure. The table side readout is not sufficiently reliable to ensure that the gantry is truly vertical.

The scanner table is installed in a manner which allows the cradle to remain horizontal during travel. The table is motorized for cradle height adjustment and horizontal travel into the gantry. Driven by motor and belt, only the cradle height is imprecise. Fine adjustment for the height of the head frame therefore depends on the stereotactic table adaptor. Additionally regulated by an electronic encoder, the horizontal table travel is accurate to 0.5 mm. The table offers no side-to-side travel and no tilt.

In the electronic spatial coordinate system of the scanner, the horizontal (X) and vertical (Y) axes lie in the plane of the scanner circle through its center, and the Z axis lies perpendicular to the scan circle through its center.

Scanner Software

Two readily available capabilities of the GE 8800 CT scanner computer system are provided by the "grid" and "measure distance" software functions. Adaptation of the Riechert-Mundinger stereotactic frame to the CT scanner permits the use of these capabilities to obtain the X and Y coordinates of any point within the stereotactic field which lies within its reconstruction circle. The Z coordinate is obtained by noting the slice location readout. Depressing the grid button on the display console automatically places an intersecting vertical and horizontal line on the image on the screen. The horizontal and vertical lines are marked at 1-cm intervals. The intersection of these lines corresponds to the precise center of the reconstruction circle. Therefore at any axial level the actual center of the stereotactic system can be displayed. The "measure distance" capability allows deposition of cursors and gives, in addition to the measured distance to 0.01 cm precision, the value of the X and Y coordinates of both points. These coordinates are given in centimeters, with 0.04 cm precision. The first cursor is deposited on the center of the grid and the second cursor on the point in question. When the distance between these cursors is obtained, the X and Y coordinates of both points also appear on the screen. The slice location notation appearing on the upper left-hand side of the console gives the Z coordinate (Figure 3–2). According to scanning convention, the right side of the body is displayed on the left side of the screen and vice versa. Therefore points to the left of the Y axis have negative numerical values. Because the conventional neurosurgical approach path is the mirror image of this system, the stereotactic system gives positive values to structures seen to the left of the Y axis and negative values to those seen to the right. Structures anterior to the X axis are positive, whereas those posterior are negative. The value of the Z coordinate is positive. This convention remains valid for the most common neurosurgical approach when the stereotactic frame is placed at an axial level below the lesion. On those rare instances when the patient is actually scanned prone and the stereotactic head frame is attached cephalad to the posterior fossa lesion, thus providing for the stereotactic neurosurgical approach to the lesion from a position below the frame, the positive and negative notations of the numerical values of the stereotactic coordinates must be accordingly adjusted.

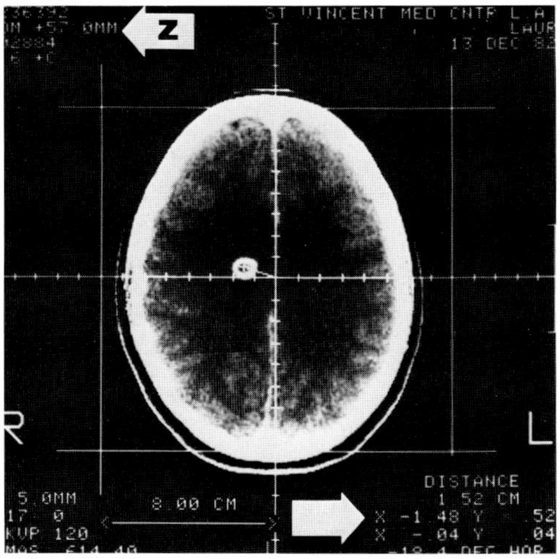

Figure 3–2 The Z value is displayed in the left upper corner. In the right lower quadrant the *arrow* points to the X-Y coordinate values (X = 1.48 and Y = 0.52).

Note that positioning the head within the stereotactic frame does not require precise centering of the calvarium to the stereotactic frame. For this reason, once the skull is fastened into the stereotactic base ring, references to the right or left quadrants do not necessarily correspond to right or left hemispheres because the position of the falx had not been precisely aligned with the Y axis (Figure 3–3).

Head Frame

The stereotactic head frame is a steel ring which is attached with steel pins to the patient's calvarium. The ring bears outer surface markings for 0°, 90°, 180°, and 270° points as well as markings for alignment

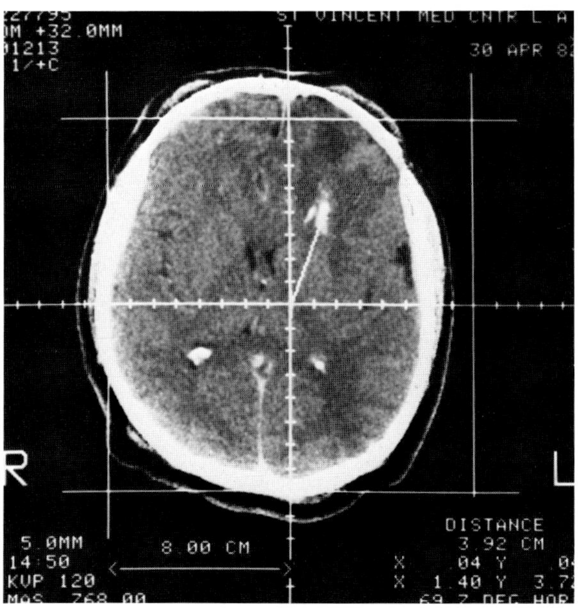

Figure 3–3 Note that the head has been anchored about 15 mm to the left of the midline.

with the GE 8800 CT table adaptor apparatus. The 0° and 180° markers on the surface of the ring are placed exactly at the zero equatorial plane. Thus when the lateral alignment laser light crosshair falls on the 180° marker point of the vertically positioned stereotactic frame ring, the horizontal and vertical planes of the stereotactic ring and that of the CT scanner gantry are superimposed.

Adaptor Mechanism

An adaptor was made by Fischer to be temporarily attachable to the head end of the scanner table after removal of the standard head holder (Figure 3–4). The adaptor is manufactured to hold the stereotactic ring vertically, and it is centered to the vertical plane, which passes through the center of the scan circle. The adaptor is equipped with fine vertical adjustment screws to facilitate movement along the Y axis of the system and to aid in superimposing the centers of the stereotactic and scanner systems. The stereotactic ring may be rotated in the adaptor until its X and Y axes superimpose on that of the scan circle.

Laser Positioning Device

The GE 8800 CT system includes two ruby laser beams as aids for patient positioning: a horizontal crosshair from one side wall of the room to the other (lateral laser), and a vertical crosshair from the ceiling to the floor. The crosshairs lie in a plane parallel and 470 mm caudal to the gantry circle (external landmark). They are intended to lie along the X and Y axes of the scanner stereotactic system. We use only the lateral laser crosshair for ascertaining the position of the stereotactic ring. After the proper stereotactic ring height has been found, the lateral laser beam crosshair may be used as a future positioning aid. We mark the location of the laser crosshair on the opposite wall for ready reference.

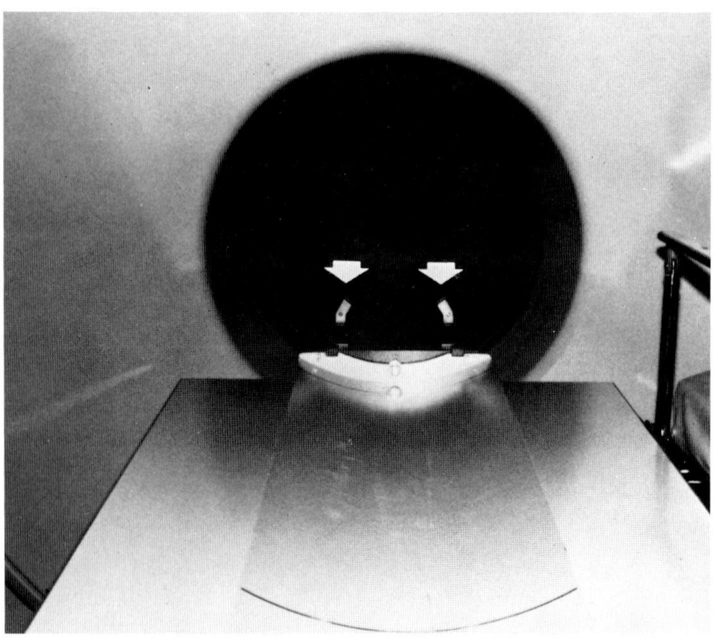

Figure 3–4 An empty CT scanner is shown. The *arrows* point to the table adaptor designed for the GE 8800 CT.

The vertical laser light is not used because there is no side-to-side table adjustment.

The horizontal and vertical beams (crosshair) of the lateral laser positioning light have been adjusted to lie in the horizontal and vertical planes of the vertical CT scanner gantry. The vertical light defines the vertical plane exactly 470 mm away from the center point of the gantry, and the horizontal beam defines the horizontal plane passing through the center of the gantry.

Verification

To ensure that the stereotactic ring can be reliably and quickly centered to the gantry when the patient arrives from the operating room, the lateral scanner alignment laser light is calibrated to the zero point of the gantry before the actual stereotactic procedure. The phantom attachments (phantom coordinate ring and substructure) are used for fine calibration, necessitating that the calibration be performed before sterilization of these tools.

To fulfill the requirements which follow from the principle of this system, the centering of the stereotactic phantom ring to the CT scanner gantry circle must be accomplished with high precision. The requirements are: 1) the center of the phantom ring must be placed at the exact center of the scanner circle (reconstruction circle); 2) the ring must be positioned so that its X and Y axes coincide with those of the reconstruction circle; and 3) the equatorial plane of the ring must be parallel to the scan plane (Figure 3–5). These parameters are achieved by superimposition of the horizontal and vertical beams of the lateral (external landmark) laser with markings placed on the surface of the phantom coordinate ring at the point defining the intersection of the zero point of the horizontal and vertical axes (Figure 3–6). In addition, true vertical position of the gantry can be confirmed by removing the side panel and observing the steel rings attached to the gantry at its base. Clockwise or counterclockwise rotation of the stereotactic ring determines the X and Y planes of the stereotactic system. The X plane must lie along a horizontal plane, and so ring rotation must be eliminated.

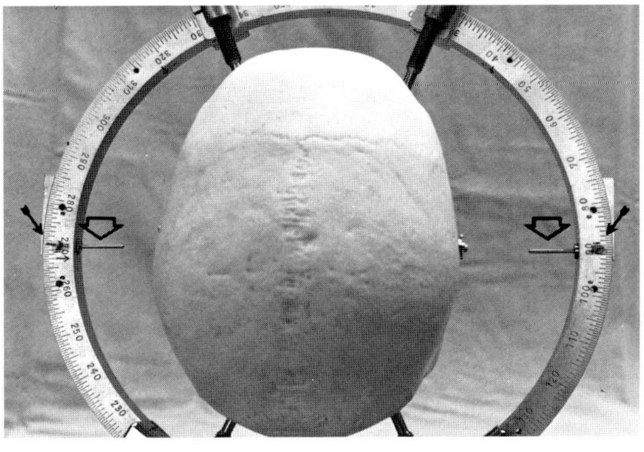

Figure 3–5 This skull mounting illustrates the X plane (*open arrows*) and the Z plane (*solid arrows*) pin placement. These serve to confirm the horizontal alignment with the CT scanner gantry.

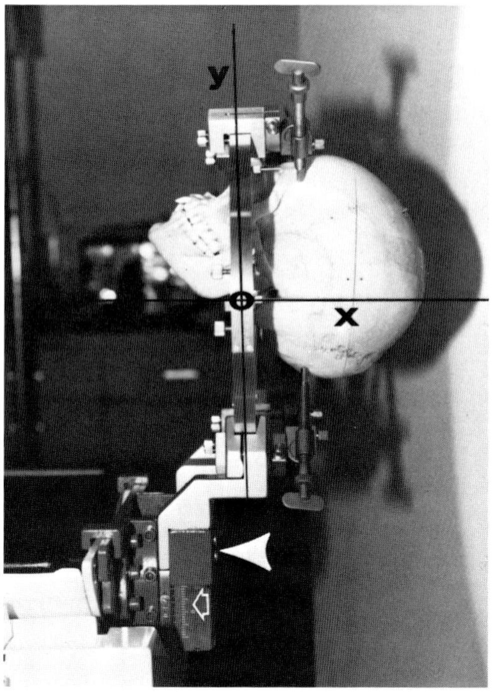

Figure 3–6 Note how the lateral laser beam crosshair serves to align the horizontal and vertical axes of the stereotactic ring with those of the CT gantry. The *arrowhead* points to the table adaptor and the *open arrow* to a microdrive that can be adjusted manually.

The actual calibration is achieved as follows. The conventional head-holder apparatus of the GE 8800 CT scanner table is removed, and the stereotactic table adaptor is placed in its location. The stereotactic phantom coordinate ring (which is identical to the stereotactic ring to be placed over the patient's skull but also contains the phantom superstructure) is fastened into the table adaptor. The gantry must be vertical and

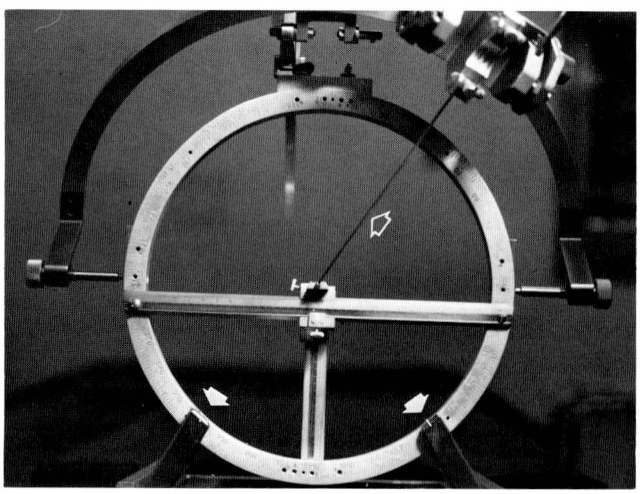

Figure 3–7 The phantom coordinate ring has been placed in the CT scanner adaptor. The cannula (*open arrow*) points to the center of the ring, where both X and Y = 0. To avoid artifact from the phantom ring during CT scanner, the Z value is set at 50 mm. Etched markings (*closed arrows*) on both ring and table holder expedite alignment. (The surgical probe carrying the arc device is removed when scanning begins.)

parallel to the plane of the stereotactic ring, which is positioned perpendicular to the table top. After the phantom ring has been properly placed in the table adaptor by alignment of markers, the lateral laser light crosshair points to the center mark of the ring. The external landmark is set (by pressing the EL = 470 mm button) for the table position, and the table is then moved to scan (achieved by pressing the "move to scan" button). The phantom substructure is set to carry arbitrary (known) spatial coordinates (Figure 3–7). Scanning the phantom tip with the thinnest available slice thickness (1.5 mm) yields a point image on the console screen. Confirmation of the point location is achieved by placing a grid on the image and measuring the distance of the center of the grid from the point. The numerical value of the X,Y,Z coordinates thus obtained should coincide with the known and arbitrarily set coordinates of the phantom point. For example, if the phantom carries coordinates of X = 0, Y = 0, and Z = 50 mm, scanning the phantom tip at 49.5 mm table location should yield a point image which superimposes on the center of the zero point of the X and Y coordinates. The X and Y axes are visually demonstrable on the screen by depressing the grid button on the display console. A scan at the 50.5 mm location should yield a blank screen (no image). These simple tests ensure that the laser crosshair is parallel to the X and Y planes of the reconstruction circle, the table movement is horizontal, and the slice location determination is precise.

If a discrepancy is noted in the position of the point image in relation to the center of the image display grid, fine adjustment in the position of the laser light is done and the calibration is repeated until satisfactory results are achieved. The vertical position of the stereotactic ring and the zero rotation of its X and Y planes are confirmed during calibration as well as immediately prior to the actual stereotactic localization.

We have not yet encountered table-movement slice location discrepancies. Table movement is periodically checked and the necessary adjustments made by scanner service personnel.

Procedure

Placement of the Stereotactic Ring

An intravenous contrast infusion is started prior to placement of the stereotactic ring. The start of the infusion precedes the ring placement in order to avoid emesis when the stereotactic head frame is attached. The contrast infusion consists of 42 g of iodine.

At our institution the stereotactic ring is placed on the patient's head in the operating room. Ring placement is performed with the tumor location in mind. The axial plane of the base ring is ideally 32 mm below the lowest point of the lesion. This requirement should be met so that the scans of the lesion are free from metal artifacts caused by the ring and cranial attachment pins. This apparatus extends 31 mm above the zero axial plane of the ring. Supratentorial lesions, which comprise most of our cases, are easily accommodated by this requirement. Low occipital or cerebellar lesions are approached with the patient prone and the stereotactic ring attached to the calvarium above the level of the lesion. This approach, with the current metallic table to ring adaptor system, throws metallic artifacts on the scans. We are in the process of developing a radiolucent table adaptor. In addition in these cases, care must be exer-

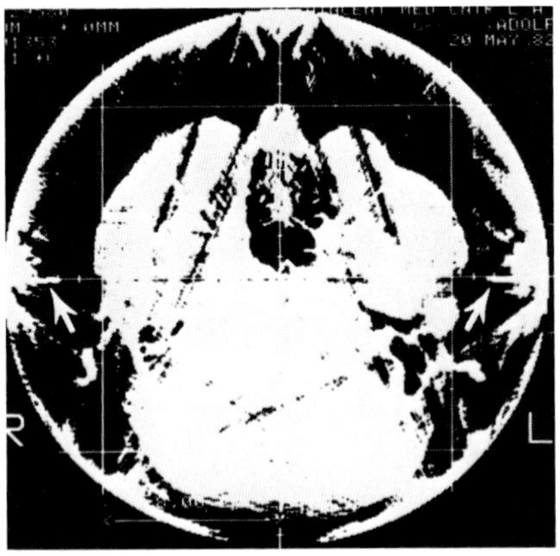

Figure 3–8 A tomographic section through the stereotactic ring shows perfect alignment of the reference pins (*arrows*) and the horizontal axis.

cised when assigning positive or negative values to the numerical values of the chosen points.

Prescanning Tests

Upon arrival of the patient from the operating room with the base ring firmly attached to the head, we perform two quick tests to confirm the proper positioning of the stereotactic ring. One documents the exact perpendicular position of the ring with respect to the table top (lining up the axial scan plane with the equatorial plane of the base ring); the other aligns the coronal (X) axis of the ring along the horizontal plane in order to rule out clockwise or counterclockwise rotation of the ring. The first test is performed with the aid of a lateral scout view of the base ring apparatus and the "measure distance" capability. The lateral scout view of the apparatus is displayed on the satellite display console (SDC). One cursor is deposited at the center point of the ring and a second cursor is deposited at the zero point of the table position scale, appearing at the bottom of the screen. A measurement of the distance between these two points yields the angulation as well. The angle should

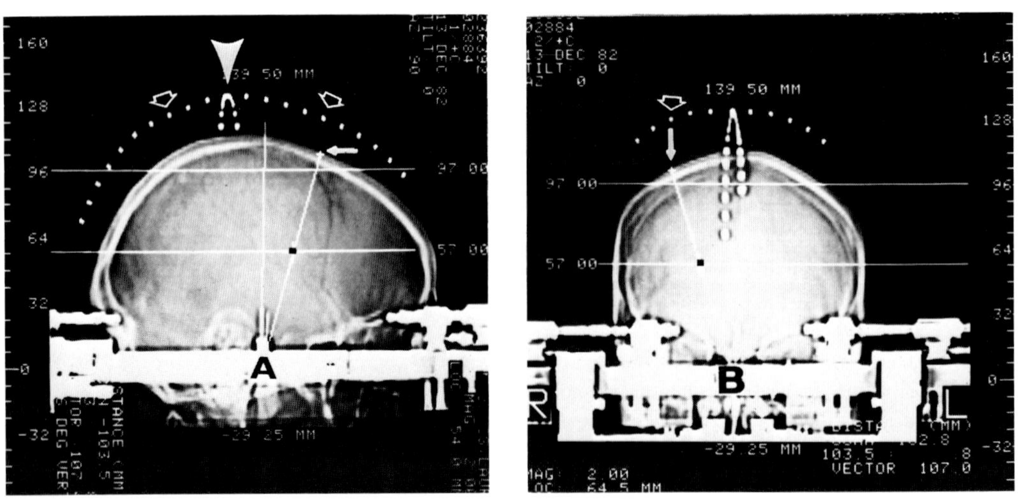

A B

Figure 3–9 Lateral (**A**) and frontal (**B**) scout films are shown. The *arrowhead* points to the center of the scalp reference. The *small solid arrow* indicates the Y value of the trephination point. The X value for the same function is displayed in **B**.

be zero. The second of these tests—confirmation of superimposition of the X and Y axes of the stereotactic and scanner fields—is performed by scanning the stereotactic ring at zero table location. A 25-cm calibration file is used with a round reconstruction circle, allowing visualization of the entire stereotactic ring. Two pins are present along the X axis on the inner surface of the stereotactic ring at the 0° and 180° positions. Although many artifacts are seen because of the metallic frame, the pins are displayed within the ring circle (Figure 3–8). The grid is placed on the image. The two horizontal pins at 0° and 180° should superimpose on the X axis of the grid. If not, appropriate height adjustment and/or rotation of the ring should be made. Ring markers at 0° and 180° are also an equal distance from the center if the adaptor has been correctly installed. If not, readjustment is necessary.

Scanning

Scanning may now begin. To aid in determining the approximate location of the subsequent burrhole, surface localization markers are attached to the patient's calvarium. These are two perpendicular plastic strips which contain small metallic markers at 1-cm intervals. No significant artifacts are encountered from these during scanning. The scout scans are performed in the lateral and frontal projections to show the surface localization strips.

Because the currently used ring contains metallic elements which extend above its equator, scanning begins at a level 1 mm above the attachment point of the metallic pins to the calvarium, 32 mm above the center of the stereotactic ring. Because of the relatively large size of the tumors, we elect to scan most of our cases with 5 mm thick contiguous sections. In cases where smaller lesions are scanned and 5 mm thick slices are used, the scans can be performed at 3-mm intervals, yielding overlapping cuts, providing a higher choice of axial levels along the Z axis for selection of target points. Alternatively, 1.5-mm slices may be used at 1.5-mm intervals, thus increasing further the number of slices that contain the lesion. Overlapping cuts or thinner slices are usually necessary only in small lesions. Scanning is performed from the top of the ring attachment apparatus to the vertex. The images are not magnified and not targeted. The scanning is performed at slow speed: 576 views in 9.6 sec per slice.

At the conclusion of scanning the intended target and trephination levels are marked on the scout views. Visualization of the localization beads and the position of the intended trephination level on the scout views assists in determining the approximate position of the burrhole on the skull, so the head may subsequently be shaved only in the intended surgical area (Figure 3–9). This completes the scanning portion of the stereotactic localization study.

Selection of Points

Based on the size and geometry of the tumor, one or several target and trephination point(s) are selected. One trephination point may serve as the entrance point to one or more target points (Figure 3–10). The target point is the intended location of the tip of the radiation loading catheter and usually the most distant biopsy site. The trephination point is the site where the burrhole is placed and the biopsy probe and subsequently the interstitial radiation catheter enter the skull (Figure 3–11). A line connecting the trephination and target points forms the approach path.

In patients who have solid spherical tumors the target point is usually selected at the far side of the tumor, away from the trephination point. Cystic tumors and those with necrotic centers we believe are best approached with the likely alteration of the structure in mind, because drainage of the liquid contents upon catheter entry to the tumor causes the tumor to collapse around the catheter. Thus in these cases it is advisable to place the target point slightly closer to the center of the lesion. It is also advisable to perform a scan on the patients after implant catheter placement to confirm the changes in geometry prior to loading the intended radiation dose into the catheters.

During selection of the target point the trephination point should be considered as well, so that the approach path would approximate a line passing through the central axis of the tumor along its longest diameter. This ensures a symmetrical radiation dose distribution to the tumor. Large tumors often require multiple radiation catheters. Usually these catheters lie in nearly parallel paths and do not intersect. Some tumor locations are not conducive to "optimal" target point selection. Nearby large vascular branches, whether normal or tumor vessels, must be avoided.

A line connecting the trephination and target points form the approach line, which should not traverse ventricles, large vessels, or the falx. Serial biopsies are taken along this line as the neurosurgeon advances his instruments, noting the sites of the biopsy points according to their distance from the inner table of the skull. The location of the tissues can then be correlated with their CT appearance. The serial biopsy technique can further inform the treating physicians regarding tumor characteristics.

Selection of the trephination point is also subject to a few guidelines. In addition to the obvious need to avoid areas such as the frontal sinuses, orbits, sagittal sinus, etc., we are restricted in our approach to the mass

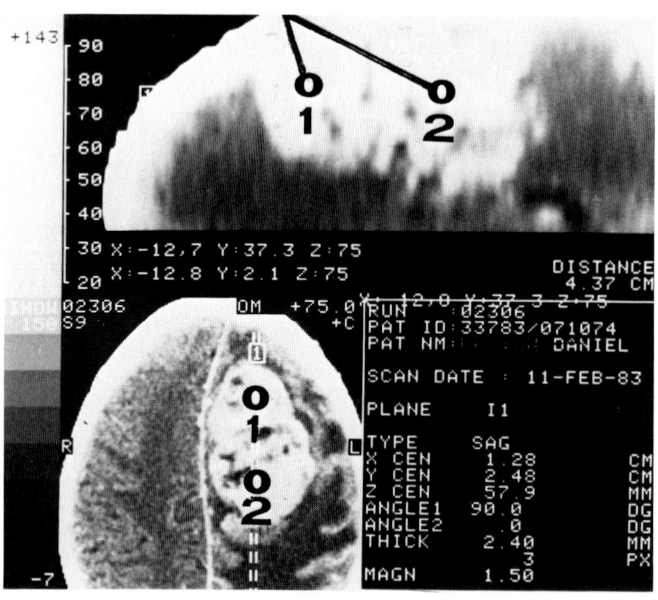

Figure 3–10 A single trephination point has been plotted to approach two target lesions. The ○ indicates the respective target locations, and the coordinate values are shown below. Both targets were reached through a single burrhole, as shown. Courtesy of Dr. Merten, Waldsee, Germany.

by the base ring itself. Likewise, important functioning regions (e.g., motor strip, visual cortex) must be avoided during selection of the trephination points. Wherever feasible, we use the preexisting burrholes and craniotomy defects. The presence of superficial vessels is slightly less important because these are visible on the surface. This topic is further detailed in later chapters in this volume.

Once target and trephination points have been selected and the approximate approach path is confirmed, the spatial coordinates are determined. The axial slice which corresponds to the selected target point is called up on the display console screen, and a grid is placed on this image. The cursor is then deposited at the intended target point, and the cursor is moved to the zero point of the grid. Using the "measure distance" software capability of the scanner computer, the distance between these two points is displayed on the screen along with the numerical value of the X and Y coordinates of both points. The value of the Z coordinate of the target point is read off the slice location notation of the same slice. The cursor is then placed again on the target point, and the axial slice of the intended trephination level is called up. With the cursor kept on the position of the actual target point, the trephination point selection is aided and an approximate idea of the approach path can be obtained. Placing the grid on this slice and depositing the cursor at the center of the grid and the intended trephination point again gives the numerical values of the X and Y coordinates when the "measure distance" button is depressed on the console. Once scanning is completed and all the slices are satisfactory, the coronal and sagittal reformatting program is called up. Most of our cases were performed with the "Exam" mode software. The same aim can be achieved with the new, faster "Arrange" reformatting software package. Once reformatting in the coronal (X,Z) and sagittal (Y,Z) planes is performed at the Y and X coordinates of the target point, respectively, the Z levels for the target and trephination points can be confirmed on these images. The approach path may also be visualized by oblique reformatting.

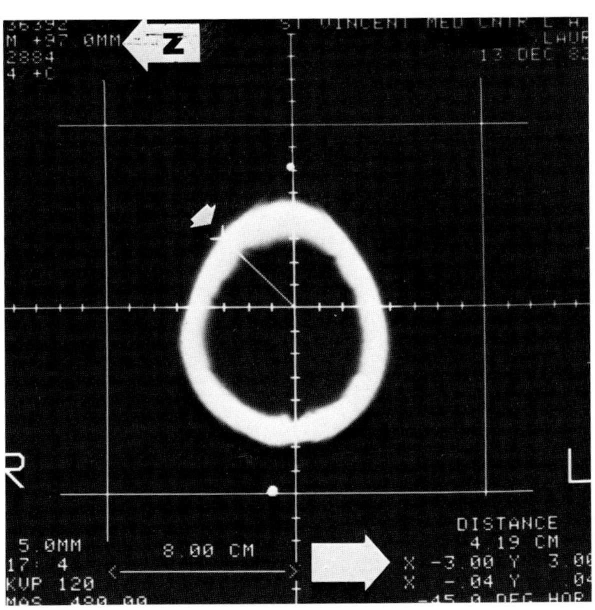

Figure 3–11 The trephination coordinates are displayed: X = +30 mm; Y = +30 mm; Z = 97 mm. The *arrow* indicates the trephination point in reference to the skull.

Once the numerical values (X, Y, Z) of the target and trephination coordinates are obtained, the appropriate positive or negative value is assigned to them as dictated by the neurosurgical stereotactic approach convention.

Once the X, Y, and Z coordinates for the selected target and trephination points are obtained, their values are fed into a Texas Instrument 59 calculator equipped with the Birk program. This computes the needle placement depth, height, and side angles, as well as the needle side and vertical adjustment angles. Equipped with these five values, the neurosurgical portion of the procedure can begin.

Conclusion

The CT scanner is quickly replacing the traditional anteroposterior and lateral roentgenograms of former stereotaxy. It is more accurate and often less cumbersome. This chapter describes the marriage between the Riechert-Mundinger stereotactic apparatus and the GE 8800 CT scanner. The reformatting capabilities of recent-generation scanners allow the quick visualization of various potential approach routes, thus aiding the optimal selection of the actual surgical and treatment paths.

References

1. Ambrose J: Computerized transverse axial scanning (tomography). 2. Clinical application. Br J Radiol 46:1023–1047, 1973
2. Bergström M, Boëthius J, Collins VP, et al: A combined study of computed tomography and stereotactic biopsy in gliomas. In: Neurological Surgery with Emphasis on Non-Invasive Methods of Diagnosis and Treatment. Excerpta Medica, Amsterdam, 1978, pp 45–50
3. Boëthius J, Bergström M, Greitz T, et al: CT localization in stereotactic surgery. Appl Neurophysiol 43:164–169, 1980
4. Bosch DA: Indications for stereotactic biopsy of brain tumors. Acta Neurochir (Wien) 54:167–179, 1980
5. Brown RA: A computerized tomography-computer graphics approach to stereotaxic localization. J Neurosurg 50:715–720, 1979
6. Brown RA, Roberts TS, Osborn AG: Stereotaxic frame and computer software for CT-directed neurosurgical localization. Invest Radiol 15:308–312, 1980
7. Field JR, Lawrence JA, White TJ, et al: Scalp localization of supratentorial lesions demonstrated by computerized tomography. Neurosurgery 6:164–175, 1980
8. Gildenberg PL, Kaufman HH, Krishna-Murphy KS: Calculation of stereotactic coordinates from the computed tomography scan. Neurosurgery 10:580–586, 1982
9. Glenn WV, Johnston RJ, Morton PE, et al: Further investigation and initial clinical use of an advanced CT display capability. Invest Radiol 10:479–489, 1975
10. Glenn WV, Johnston RJ, Morton PE, et al: Image generation and display techniques for CT scan data: thin transverse and reconstructed coronal and sagittal planes. Invest Radiol 10:403–416, 1975
11. Gutin PH, Phillips TL, Hosobushi Y, et al: Permanent and removable implants for the brachytherapy of brain tumors. Int J Radiat Oncol Biol Phys 7:1371–1381, 1981
12. Hayman LA, Evans RA, Hinck VC: Scalp markers for precise craniotomy siting, using computed tomography. J Comput Assist Tomogr 3:701–702, 1979

13. Hinck VC, Clifton GL: A precise technique for craniotomy localization using computerized tomography. J Neurosurg 54:416–418, 1981
14. Hounsfield GN: Computerized transverse axial scanning (tomography). I. Description of system. Br J Radiol 46:1016–1022, 1973
15. Jacques S, Sheldon CH, McCann GD: A computerized microstereotactic method for approach, 3-dimensionally reconstruct, remove and adjuvantly treat small CNS lesions. Appl Neurophysiol 43:176–182, 1980
16. Jacques S, Sheldon CH, McCann GD, et al: Computerized 3-dimensional stereotaxic removal of small CNS lesions in patients. J Neurosurg 53:816–820, 1980
17. Levinthal WS, Stevens EA, La Morgese JR, et al: A simplified method of CT assisted localization and biopsy of intracranial lesions. Surg Neurol 11:413–417, 1979
18. Mundinger F, Ostertag C: Computerized tomography in stereotactic interstitial curietherapy of cerebral midline tumors. In: Cranial Computerized Tomography, edited by W Lanksch, E Kazner. Springer-Verlag, New York, 1976, pp 110–113
19. Perry JH, Rosenbaum AE, Lundsfort LD, et al: Computed tomography-guided stereotactic surgery conception and development of a new stereotactic methodology. Neurosurgery 7:376–381, 1980
20. Piskun WS, Stevens EA, La Morgese JR, et al: A simplified method of CT assisted localization and biopsy of intracranial lesions. Surg Neurol 11:413–417, 1979
21. Rhodes ML, Glenn WV, Azzusi YM, et al: Stereotactic neurosurgery using 3-D image data from computed tomography. J Med Sci 6:105–119, 1982

4

Computerized Stereotactic Surgical Planning

Peter Dyck

In spite of the advanced scientific sophistication in computerized tomography (CT)-guided stereotaxis in recent years, medicine will always remain both an art and a science. Although this chapter focuses on only a small segment of contemporary neurosurgery, it serves to illustrates how inextricably art and science are interrelated.

Modern technology allows one to stereotactically pinpoint any intracranial structure with high precision. Still required is an understanding of the intervening neuroanatomy that separates the target from its approach route. Therein lies the art! For example, an insular lesion is closer to the temporal squama than any other bony confines of the skull on a CT scan; yet this lesion can be reached by this route only at the expense of possible injury to major middle cerebral vessels if one takes the shortest route. Hence such intervention is not wise. A thalamic, or third ventricular, mass might be most expeditiously reached, mathematically speaking, by a parasagittal approach, but violation of a partially obstructed ventricular system may not be advisable. This again requires surgical judgment.

An endeavour is made in this chapter to outline clinical modus operandi to various intracranial structures, hopefully in a manner that is of assistance to the reader.

Zipro-T Computerized Program

The in-house computer programs at the University of Freiburg im Breisgau that deal with stereotaxis are known as "Zipro." Birg (see Chapter 5) has made available similar data capabilities by providing solid-state software for the TI-59 programmable calculator (Texas Instruments, Inc., Dallas, Texas). Its mathematical principles are described elsewhere (1). The Riechert-Mundinger stereotactic apparatus, based on cartesian polar coordinate geometry, provides the "Grundriss" for this stereotactic endeavor (2).

An actual event is portrayed in Table 4–1 to familiarize the reader with the Zipro-T program. The program takes into account roentgenographic magnification where it has pertinence. In our practice it does not, and so we disregard these computations. It should be mentioned that all negative values are entered by pressing the (+/−) sign at the end of a numerical entry. Also, in order to prevent computer overrun (blinking of entry values), the target (X) and trephination (X) values must not be identical. Should this occur (although it very seldom does), adding, for example, 0.01 mm appeases the computer and allows smooth operation without sacrifice of accuracy. The remainder of the program is self-explanatory. To minimize electronic failure it is best to have the calculator fully charged or, preferably, connected to an outside electrical source.

Hence the Zipro-T program provides the surgeon with all the values necessary to reach an intracranial structure through a predetermined calvarial entry point. Thus in Table 4–1 the 146.21 mm in step 18 is the distance from the target to a designated point on the instrument arc. Step 19 (60.67°) provides the side-angle adjustment on the instrument bow. It is positive to the right, negative to the left. Step 20 (−79.83°) is the vertical angle—again positive forward, negative backward in regard to the stereotactic horizontal plane. The instrument block allows for additional adjustments with capabilities in both the horizontal (step 21) and vertical (step 22) planes. It should be noted that the vernier adjustments on the instrument block have both negative and positive values. Hence

Table 4–1 Sequential Zipro-T Program

Step	Procedure	Press		Display
1	Switch on calculator	–	–	0
2	Insert solid state softwear No. 1	CLR	–	1
3	Insert solid state softwear No. 2	2nd	–	2
4			A	10
5	X-ray magnification (lateral)	10	–	10
6	X-ray magnification (AP)	10	–	10
7	Target = X (e.g., 8.4 mm)	8.4	RS	8.4
8	Target = Y (e.g., 15.6 mm)	15.6	RS	15.6
9	Target X (e.g., 37 mm)	37	RS	37
10	Trephination = X (e.g., 38.4 mm)	38.4	RS	38.4
11	Trephination = Y (e.g., 0.0 mm)	0.0	RS	0.0
12	Trephination = Z (e.g., 82 mm)	82.0	RS	8.4 (TAX)
13	Check values (TAY)	RS	–	15.6
14	Check values (TAZ)	RS	–	37
15	Check values (TRX)	RS	–	38.4
16	Check values (TRY)	RS	–	0.0
17	Check values (TRZ)	RS	–	82
Computerized values				
18	Tumor depth from arc	RS	–	146.21
19	Side angle setting	B	–	60.67°
20	Horizontal angle setting	C	–	−79.83°
21	Vernier—horizontal	D	–	−3.19°
22	Vernier—vertical	E	–	−7.56°

TA = target. TR = trephination point.

with meticulous attention to detail, nothing should go wrong mathematically speaking. Yet translation of these data into a clinical setting is not always uneventful. For this reason the author has chosen selected clinical situations to illustrate surgical judgment in the light of stereotactic limitations.

Because all computerization must eventually be translated to specific adjustments on the stereotactic frame, it is appropriate to reestablish the ground rules. Hence, as shown in Figure 4–1, *A* refers to the distance from target to arc. *B* is the side angle on the instrument arc; it is positive to right, negative to left. *C* is the height angle, which is adjusted on the bow that supports the instrument arc; it is positive from the center of the stereotactic apparatus forward and negative below that. Figure 4–2 is a close-up view of the instrument block that displays the horizontal (*D*) and vertical (*E*) fine adjustments. All subsequent reference to the stereotactic parameters are referred to as described, i.e., *A, B, C, D,* and *E.*

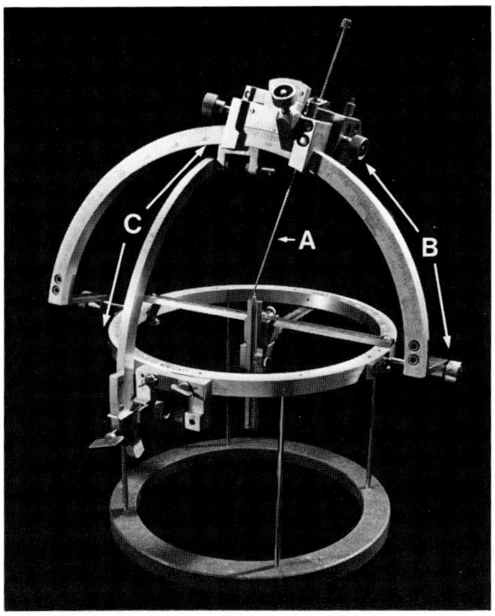

Figure 4–1 Stereotactic test phantom. *A* refers to the distance from the target to a designated point on the instrument arc. *B* indicates the horizontal angles of approach. Vertex is 90°; the angular readings are positive to the right and negative to the left, as indicated on the stereotactic bow. *C* designates the horizontal angle. It is positive toward the nose, negative down from the stereotactic horizontal midline.

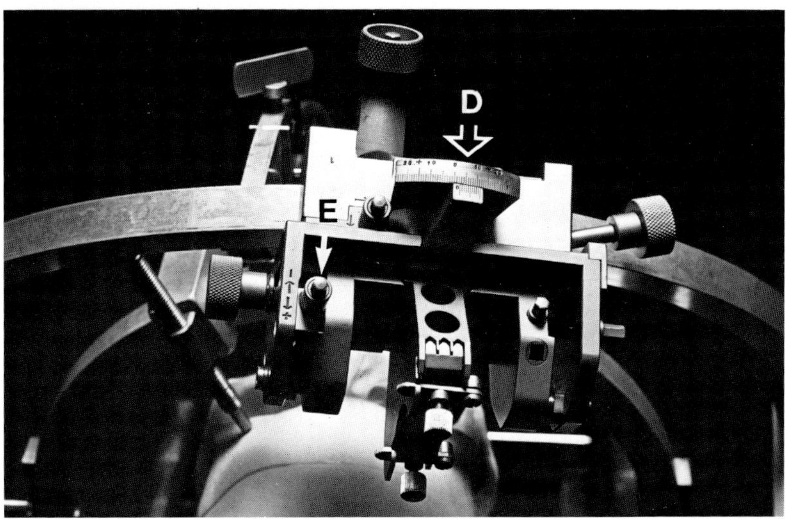

Figure 4–2 The instrument block is shown. *D* designates the horizontal and *E* the vertical vernier adjustments.

Frontal Lobe Lesions

Tumors which arise within the frontal lobe are probably the most amenable to stereotactic intervention because they offer low neuroanatomic risk combined with ease of surgical access. A stereotactic perspective is shown in Figure 4–3 to illustrate this point. It portrays how superbly adapted the equipment is to an approach to this part of the cerebral hemispheres. Computation of an approach to a frontal mass requires more cosmetic than neuroanatomic consideration. Hence, as shown in Figure 4–4, the trephination point chosen was at 78 mm, although the target

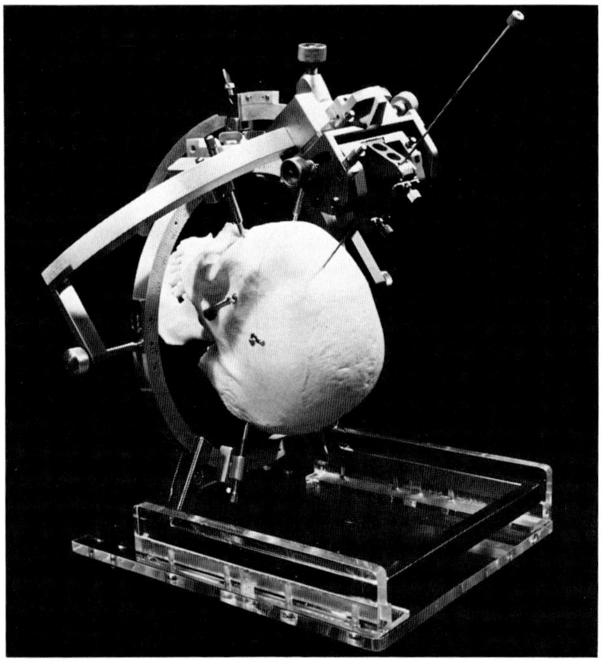

Figure 4–3 A surgical perspective of the anterior cerebral hemispheres is shown. From a stereotactic standpoint, this area of brain is mathematically and clinically ideally suited for stereotaxis.

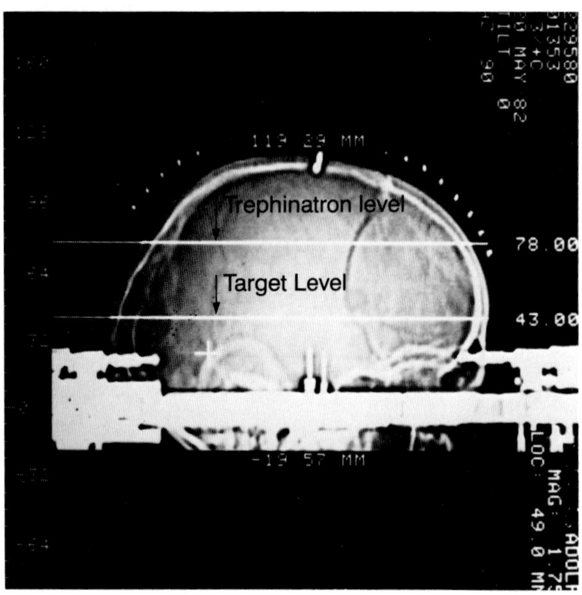

Figure 4–4 Although this lesion could have been approached by a trajectory calculated at the same level as the target plane, it was chosen to be 35 mm higher toward the vertex, mainly to accommodate cosmetic considerations.

level was at 43 mm. This was done primarily to avoid a surgical scar on the forehead. To demonstrate the computation of a trajectory to such a lesion, which serves both as a source of biopsy material and for placement of afterloading catheters for brachytherapy, the coordinates of the target and trephination points are depicted in Figure 4–5. The target is described by the following coordinate functions: X = 14.0, Y = 20.8, Z = 43. The trephination point (Figure 4–5B) is represented by: X = 53.2, Y = 54.0, and Z = 78. These coordinates compute to the following stereotactic settings: A = 159.94 mm, B = 56.19°, C = 51.57°, D = −5.39°, and E = 3.92°. The accuracy of such targeting is clinically acceptable, with the greatest error probably being caused by a bent cannula or imprecisely set angles rather than faulty computor data.

Posterior frontal lesions also present no special problems so long as they lie within the anterior two quadrants of the stereotactic CT scanner grid. A paraventricular lesion is shown in Figure 4–6A. Its target coordinates are: X = 14.8, Y = 5.2, Z = 57. A posterior frontal approach was chosen for the trephination point as depicted in Figure 4–6B. Its coordinates were as follows: X = 30.0, Y = 30.1, Z = 97. To reach this lesion, the following stereotactic settings were computed: A = 169.34 mm, B = 72.74°, C = 65.91°, D = −0.78°, E = 7.43°. These stereotactic computations were precise enough to allow biopsy of the lesion at 2-mm intervals three times.

Thalamic Lesions

If the patient's head is fixed in the middle of the base ring, it is not uncommon to find the lesion in question occupying both anterior and posterior stereotactic quadrants, as shown in Figure 4–7A. Its target coor-

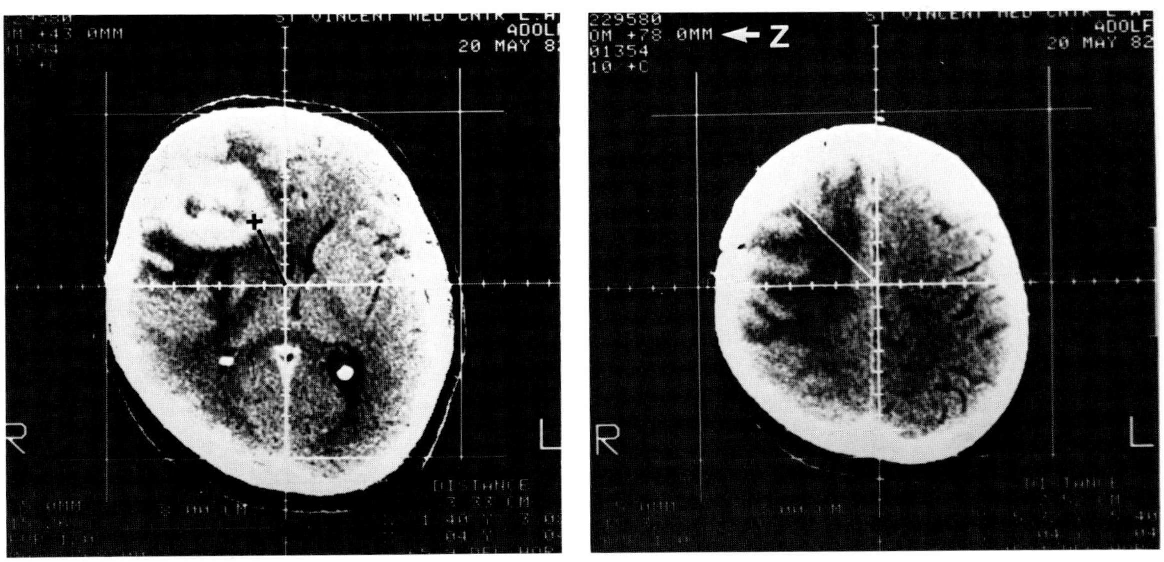

A B

Figure 4–5 **A:** How the target coordinates are read from the CT axial scan; X = 14.0, Y = 20.8, Z = 43. **B:** The chosen approach to the lesion in question. This, combined with the target data, should allow one to compute an approach trajectory.

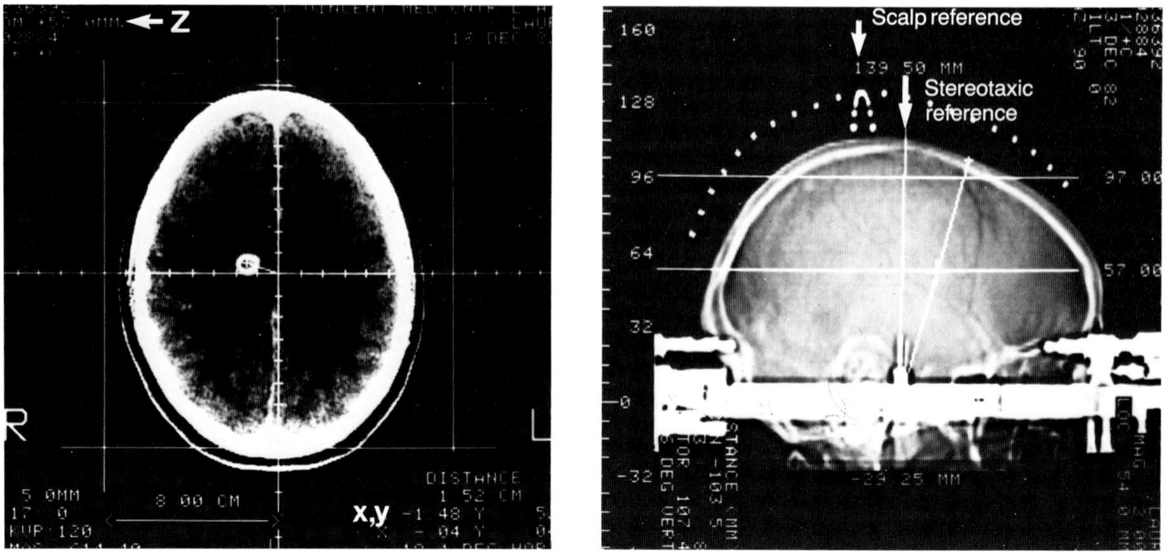

A B

Figure 4–6 **A:** A lesion lying in the right upper stereotactic quadrant is shown. **B:** Although stereotactically speaking the trajectory of approach is 3 cm forward, it is 5 cm as shown by the scalp reference matters.

dinate values are: X = 5.2, Y = −5.2, Z = 42. In an endeavor to avoid an approach to the lesion through the lateral ventricle, a reformat of the CT section was obtained (Figure 4–7B). Based on this, a trajectory was chosen by which to approach the lesion, missing the ventricular system yet passing through most of the lesion so as to allow multiple biopsies of it. Based on these neuroanatomic considerations, the following

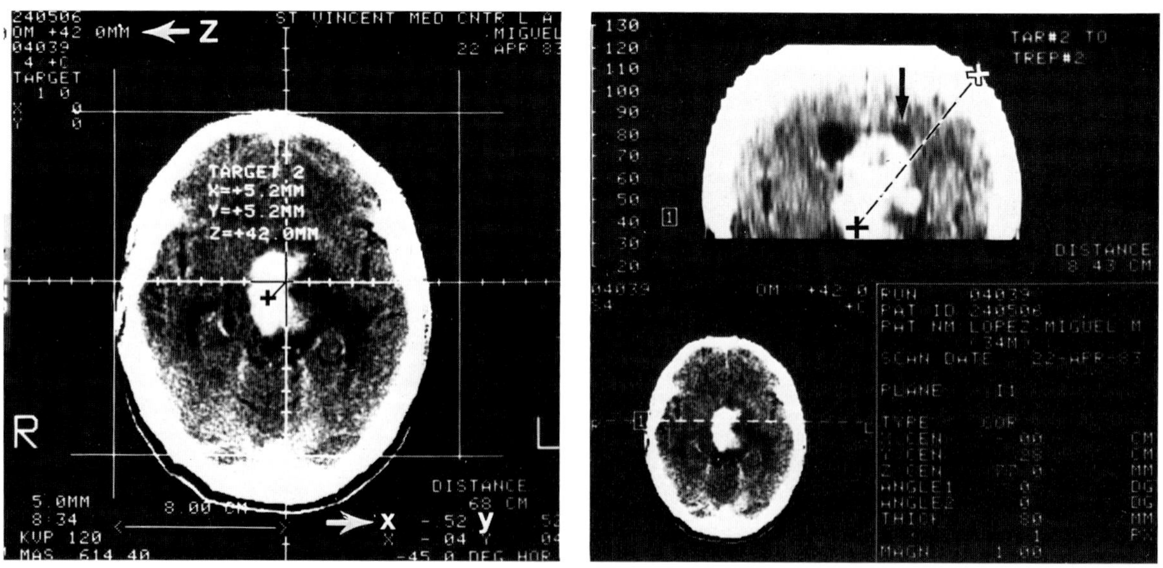

A B

Figure 4–7 **A:** Target coordinates of a thalamic mass are shown (X = 5.2, Y = −5.2, Z = 42). **B:** This coronal reformat was made in an endeavor to avoid entry of the lateral ventricle en route to the thalamic lesion. The *arrow* points to the elevated lateral ventricle. The trajectory from trephination to target point is shown.

trephination coordinates were derived: X = −40.4, Y = 14.0, Z = 107 (Figure 4–8). This yielded the following stereotactic data: A = 146.18 mm, B = −63.74°, C = 79.00°, D = 7.79°, and E = 4.52°. Serial biopsies along this trajectory established the diagnosis of grade II astrocytoma. This biopsy tract was then employed for placement of an afterloading catheter.

Such anterior lesions are easily represented on the test phantom. The problem arises when one tries to replicate the same geometric functions in the posterior quadrants of the stereotactic system. This is illustrated by another target that was chosen in the same patient just described. As shown in Figure 4–9, the target coordinates just fall into the posterior right quadrant. Their values were: X = 5.2, Y = −10.0, Z = 42. Because it is the endeavor of the surgeon to reach such a target parallel to the previously placed afterloading catheter, a trephination

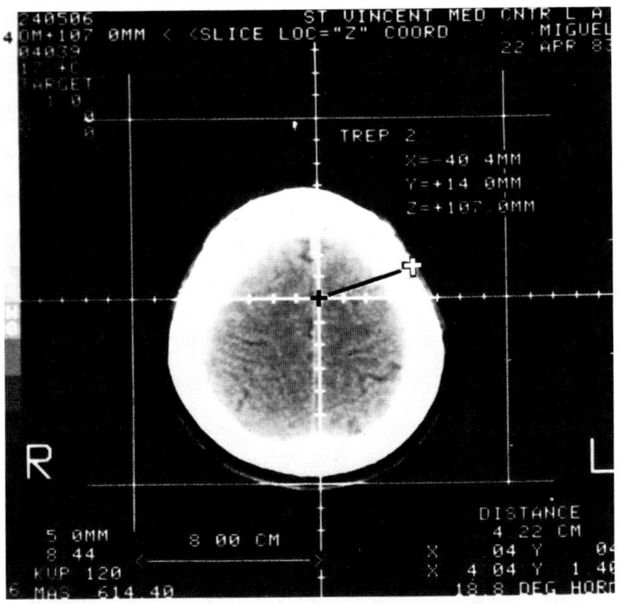

Figure 4–8 Typical trephination values are shown; X = −40.4, Y = 14.0, Z = 107.

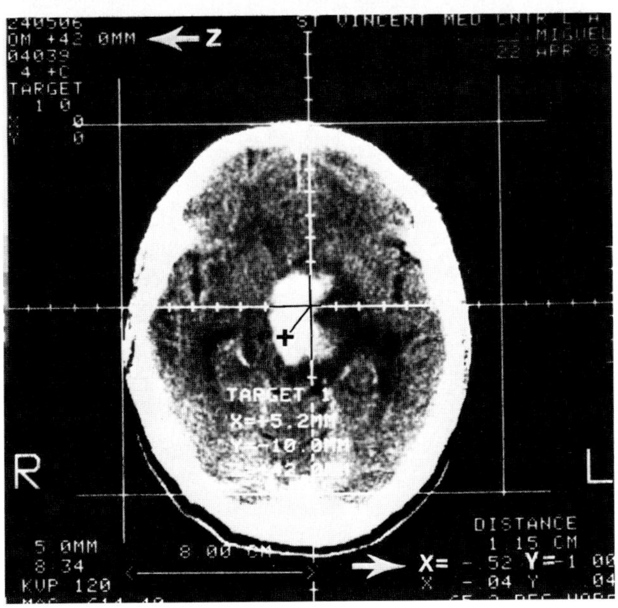

Figure 4–9 The target coordinates of this lesion fall into the posterior stereotactic quadrants. To represent them the test phantom must be turned 180°.

coordinate was selected which met this requirement, as shown in Figure 4–10. Thus this goal is achieved by enlarging the previously placed burr-hole several millimeters posteriorly. Based on these trephination values (X = −43.6, Y = 6.0, Z = 107), the stereotactic functions derived were as follows: A = 145.23 mm, B = −61.88°, C = 82.66°, D = +8.15°, and E = +5.24°. Mathematically all is well, but stereotactically the test phantom presents a problem. In order to represent these values, the phantom ring must be turned 180°, as described in Chapter 2. Moreover, it is sometimes impossible for lesions close to the midline to be represented on the test phantom because the Y axis bar impales on the instrument arc-supporting mount, as shown in Figure 4–11. Sometimes such an impasse is best resolved by estimating the Y axis in relation to the first trajectory, as was done in this case, although this is not ideal.

Brainstem and Pontine Lesions

To date the author has no personal experience with stereotactic biopsy of pontine tumors. To highlight the stereotactic principles involved, however, a hypodense pontine lesion is shown in Figure 4–12. Its target coordinates were X = −7.6, Y = −15.6, Z = 45. By turning the phantom 180° and making the appropriate adjustments, no problems should be encountered with the phantom representation of this lesion. The safest neuroanatomic approach is one that is lateral to the ventricular system and below the aqueduct of Sylvius, as shown in Figure 4–13. Although the base ring may be reverse-mounted to avoid artifacts, during CT scan-

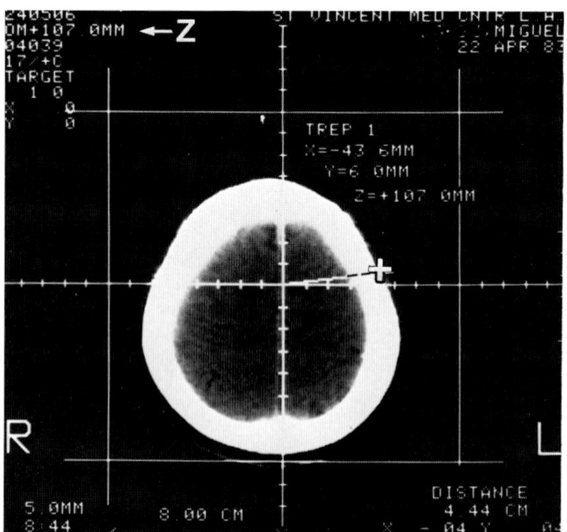

Figure 4–10 Because the calvarial entry for the second afterloading catheter must be parallel to the first, a slight posterior dislocation of the trephination satisfied this goal (compare with Figure 4–8).

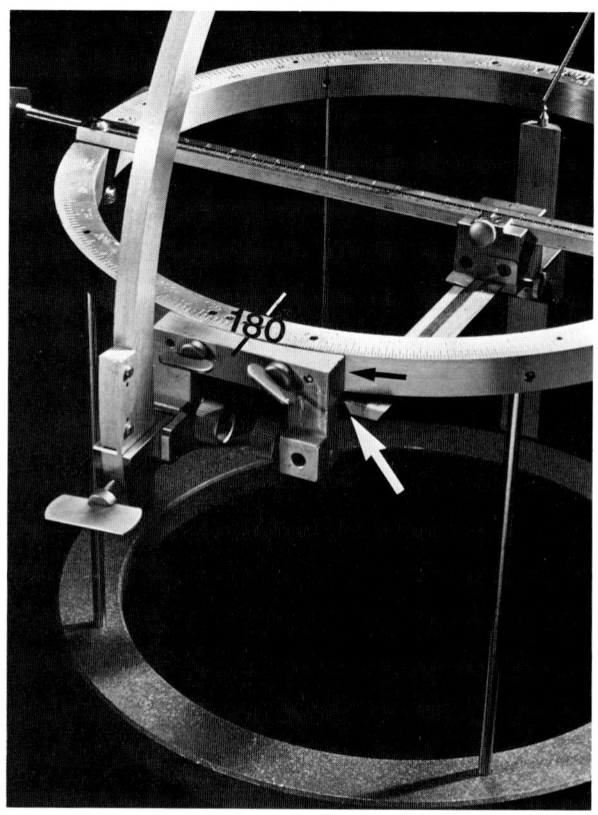

Figure 4–11 This illustrates an inherent but correctible problem in the test phantom. As the sagittal midline is approached, the clamp which anchors the instrument bow obstructs proper representation.

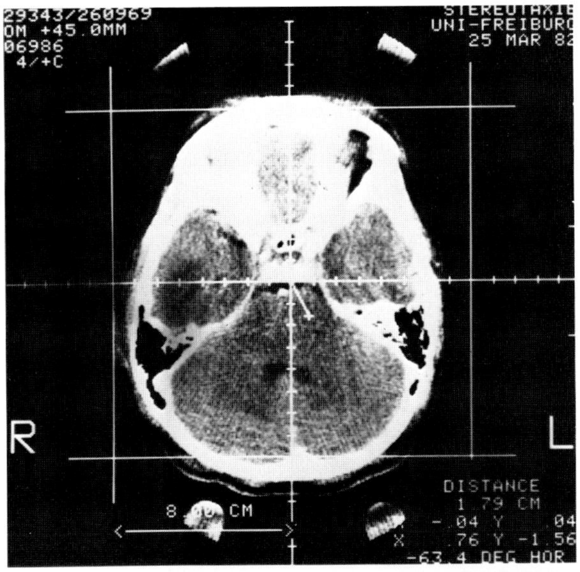

Figure 4–12 The target coordinates of an adolescent boy with neurologic signs pointing to a pontine lesion. Courtesy of Prof. F. Mundinger, University of Freiburg, West Germany.

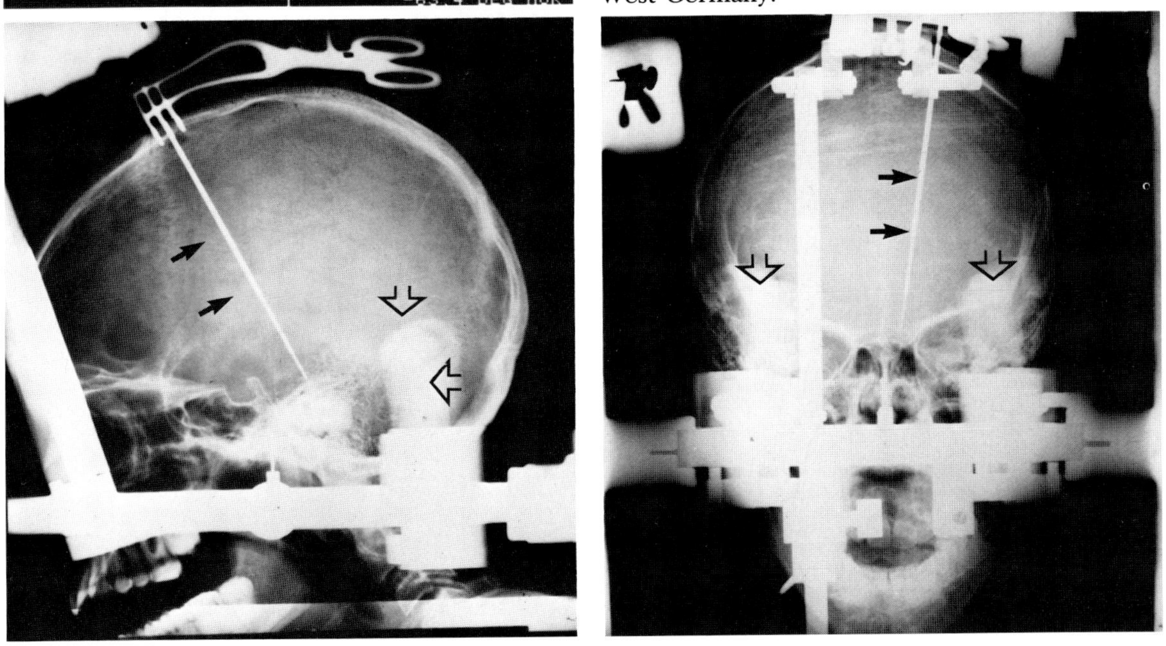

A **B**

Figure 4–13 **A:** Note that the biopsy targets traverse the parasagittal cerebral hemisphere in a trajectory that represents the shortest distance to the target in the pons. *Open arrows* point to a custom-made plastic pin mount. **B:** This illustrates an endeavor that avoids traversing the cerebral ventricular system. *Open arrows* point to custom-made plastic skeletal mounts.

ning it is simpler to displace the base ring by replacing the metallic commercially available skeletal pins with plastic ones (Figure 4–13A,B) on these special occasions. Small lesions in the brainstem are probably best treated by permanent implantation of the isotope rather than by brachytherapy. Curietherapy in this instance consisted of the placement of five 3.1-mm fragments of iridium-192 with a sum radioactivity of 1.258 mCi, calculated to deliver an accumulated dose of 12.000 cGy to a radius of 10 mm within the lesion.

Temporal Lobe Lesions

It is a foregone conclusion that to allow CT scanning of a temporal lobe mass the base ring must be mounted low enough. In order to highlight other stereotactic problems, a case in point is discussed.

A woman presented with a metastatic cerebral lesion from a small cell bronchogenic carcinoma. Its target coordinates were: X = 26.8, Y = 18.0, Z = 37 (Figure 4–14A). A trephination point was chosen 10 mm above (to vertex) the Z value for the target—not because this was clinically advantageous but because the stereotactic apparatus is not capable of accepting such stereotactic settings in the extreme lateral 20° of the system. To compensate for this handicap, a trajectory was chosen as shown in Figure 4–14B, with trephination coordinates shown on an axial CT section (Figure 4–14C). Thus the trephination coordinate became: X =

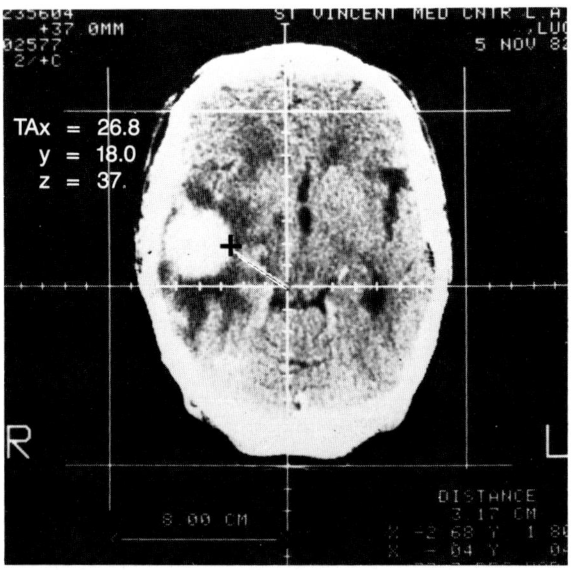

A

Figure 4–14 **A:** Coordinates for a target are shown (X = 26.8, Y = 18.0, Z = 37). **B:** A coronal reformat of the lesion in **A** is shown, emphasizing skeletal density. The *small arrow* points to the target and the *large arrow* to the coronal plane of the trephination point. **C:** Based on anatomic and CT reconstruction data, the following trephination coordinates were chosen: X = 67.6, Y = 20.4, Z = 47.

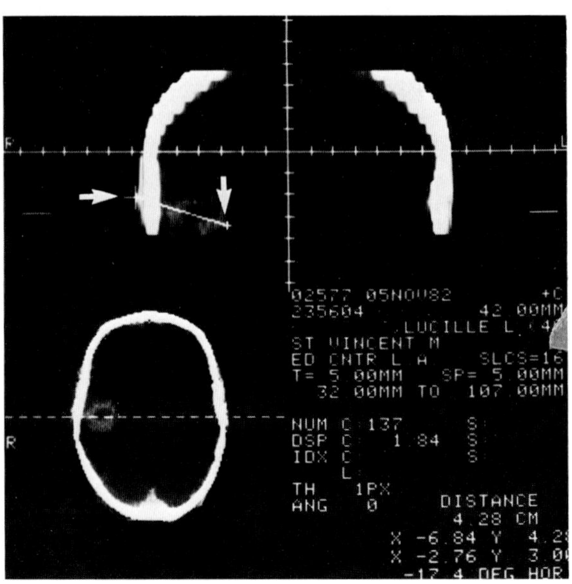

B

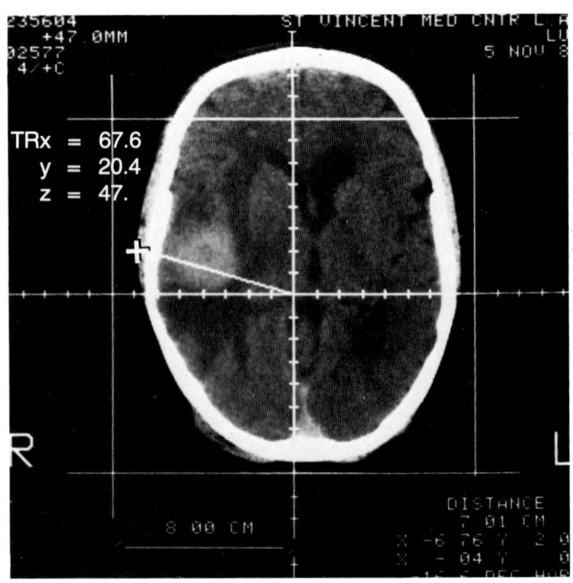

C

67.6, Y = 20.4, Z = 47. This yielded the following settings for the stereotactic frame: A = 153.13 mm, B = 23.71°, C = 70.11°, D = −9.64°, and E = −1.56°. Such a trajectory allowed histopathologic confirmation of the lesion and placement of afterloading catheters for interstitial irradiation. On the day of planned discharge from the hospital, the patient developed aortic thrombosis (see Chapter 7), accounting for one of the deaths in the series.

This illustration is included to point out that B = 23.71° constitutes essentially a limit to the lateral approach to cerebral lesions by this stereotactic apparatus. Hence practically speaking, the lateral approach angle is not 90° but, rather, about 75° from a sagittal midline. Only meticulous study of the stereotactic apparatus will make these comments pertinent; hopefully, however, they are a forewarning so that the reader will not duplicate previous errors.

Parietal Lobe Lesions

Tumors in the parietal brain lend themselves to easy stereotactic access and generally present no technical problem. The test phantom is turned 180° to allow display of the posterior two quadrants. Because parietal lesions are frequently subcortical, an approach that is as lateral as possible is surgically advisable in most instances. Hence with a lesion whose target coordinates were X = −38.8, Y = −1.2, Z = 53 (Figure 4–15A) the approach was chosen not because it represented the greatest dimension of the lesion but because it allowed an oblique trajectory through the lesion from a trephination point that was 10 mm higher (Figure 4–15B). Once again, this was done in order to work within the limitations of the equipment yet retain a lateral approach. This was expressed by the following trephination coordinate values: X = −68.4, Y = −30.0, Z = 63. Computation of these data yielded the following stereotactic parame-

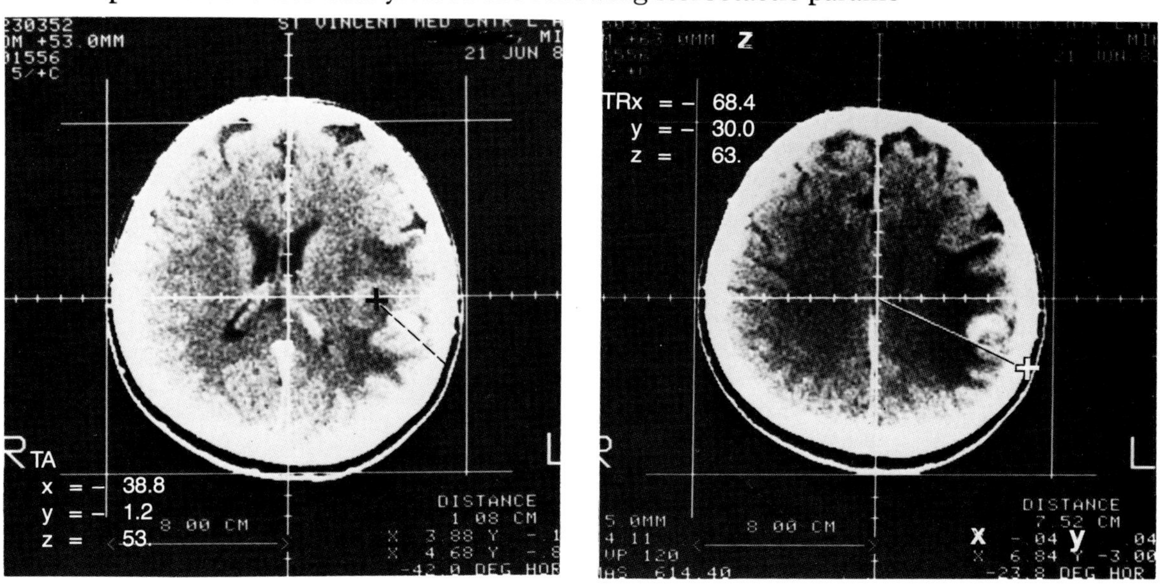

A B

Figure 4–15 **A:** The target coordinates of a lesion and the proposed approach trajectory are shown. **B:** The trephination coordinates to the target in **A** are illustrated.

ters: A = 161.68 mm, B = −43.42°, C = −40.55°, D = −0.38°, and E = −15.18°. This led to an uneventful surgical approach to the tumor.

Deeper lesions are probably best approached by a more parasagittal trajectory once it has been established that the lesion in question is beyond the major superficial cortical blood supply. In these instances angiography is often helpful when planning a surgical approach.

Infratrigonal Lesions

Infratrigonal temporoparietal lesions also mandate that one take into consideration neuroanatomic structure when plotting an approach to a target. The axial CT scans leave one with an illusion that a direct parasagittal trajectory to the lesion would accomplish the task most expeditiously, as shown in Figure 4–16A). Its target coordinates are: X = −19.6, Y = −50.0, Z = 37. Yet such a trajectory would pass through the trigone of

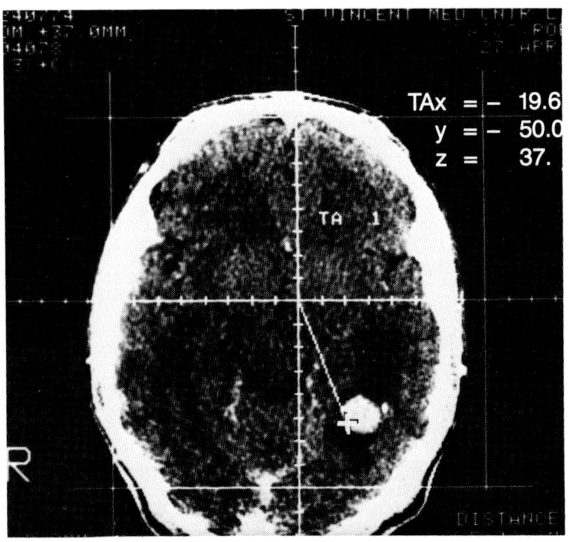

A

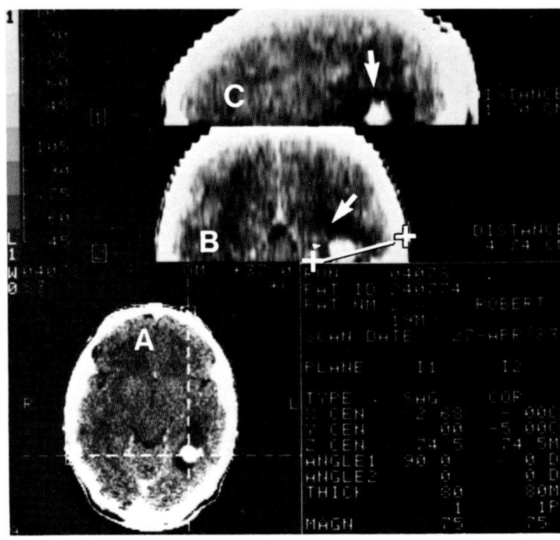

B

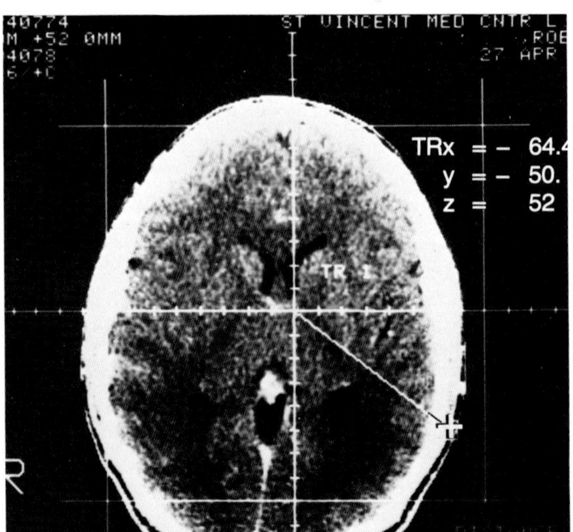

C

Figure 4–16 **A:** This lesion appears to be within reach via a parietal parasagittal approach. But where is the trigone? **B:** Coronal (*B*) and sagittal (*C*) reformats of the lesion in **A** are shown. The neoplasm displaces the ventricular trigone (*arrows*) upward and forward, and so the best approach to the lesion is a lateral one. **C:** Based on reformat data obtained from **B**, this trephination coordinate was decided on.

the ventricular system and possibly damage the choroid plexus within it. To avoid this potential complication a trajectory was chosen based in part on a reformat in both sagittal and coronal planes. Figure 4–16B clearly demonstrates that the trigone has been displaced both forward and upward by the underlying neoplasm, which was histopathologically verified to be a grade II astrocytoma in a 19-year-old patient with seizures who was suffering from von Recklinghausen's disease. Based on the reformat a lateral calvarial approach was undertaken (Figure 4–16C). The derived stereotactic values computed from these coordinates were: $A = 153.38$ mm, $B = -30.64°$, $C = -60.09°$, $D = 14.40°$, and $E = 9.00°$. As previously stated in this chapter, identical values for either X, Y, or Z do not compute; therefore because the Y values for both the target and the trephination point were identical in this instance, the latter value was changed to read −50.1 instead of −50.0. This slight difference satisfied the computer program and yielded the stereotactic settings desired.

Such minor license with input data does not compromise accuracy, as shown above, an important point to remember. Although two afterloading catheters were placed in this lesion, only the posterior trajectory was computed. The anterior catheter was simply placed parallel to the computed trajectory.

Corpus Callosum Lesions

To traverse one cerebral hemisphere and pass deeply into the other is a formidable undertaking even under stereotactic conditions. Such an endeavor is now described, having been undertaken only once to date. Although cerebral angiography is not essential in all instances, with corpus callosum lesions the course of the anterior cerebral arteries must be clearly defined before stereotactic intervention is undertaken.

A 60-year-old woman was referred after having received 50 Gy of teletherapy to an unverified intracranial mass; in spite of this, she continued to show progressive neurologic dysfunction. The target level CT scan (Figure 4–17A) depicts the dimensions of the lesion. Its target coordinates were: X = −22.0, Y = −10.8, Z = 50. To assist in planning a trajectory through the lesion that would provide tissue for histopathologic examination and drainage of a cyst content if present, as well as serving as a tract for placement of one of the afterloading catheters, reformating was essential (Figure 4–17B). Based on these data, the lesion was approached through the parietal calvarium, just 10 mm above the Z value of the target coordinates (Figure 4–17C). Their trephination coordinates were as follows: X = 69.2, Y = −26.8, Z = 60. Computation of these coordinates produced the following stereotactic values: $A = 107.58$ mm, $B = 25.56°$, $C = -57.42°$, $D = -14.97°$, $E = -4.99°$. Once histopathologic verification was made, the biopsy tract was used to insert the posterior afterloading catheter, with the anterior one being subsequently placed 15 mm anterior and parallel to it. The patient is alive and at home 10 months later, although the lesion proved to be a glioblastoma multiforme.

Occipital Lobe Lesions

With the base ring conventionally mounted to the skull, the lower 45° in the sagittal plane is stereotactically inaccessible (Figure 4–18), even if the base ring mount is reverse-mounted (as shown) to improve access

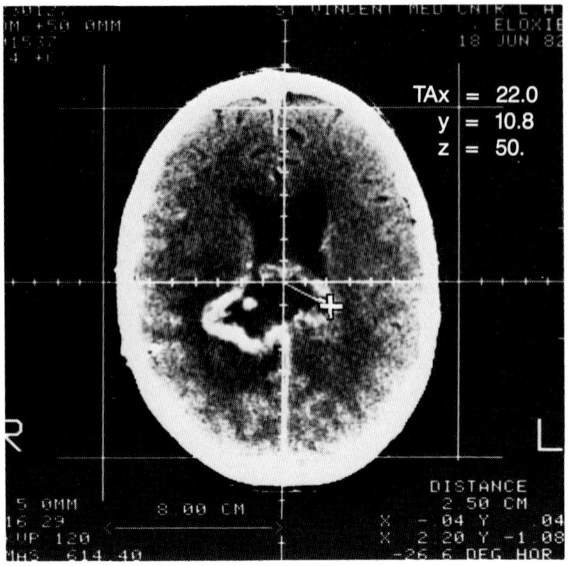

A

Figure 4–17 **A:** Target coordinates of a lesion. **B:** Coronal reformat of the lesion in **A**. The approach trajectory is indicated. **C:** Trephination coordinates to a transcallosal target.

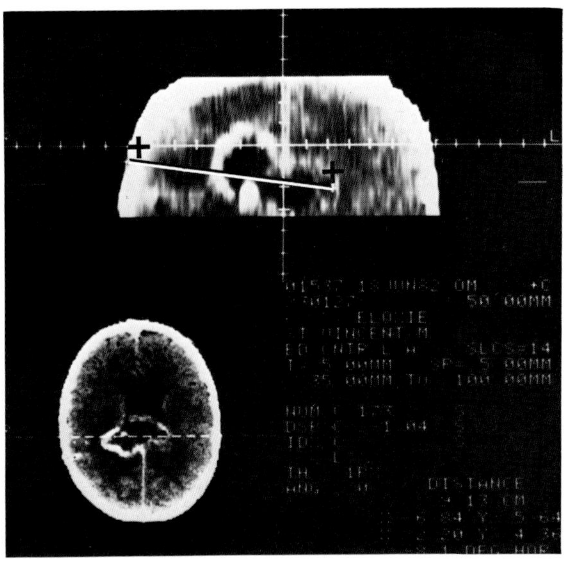

B

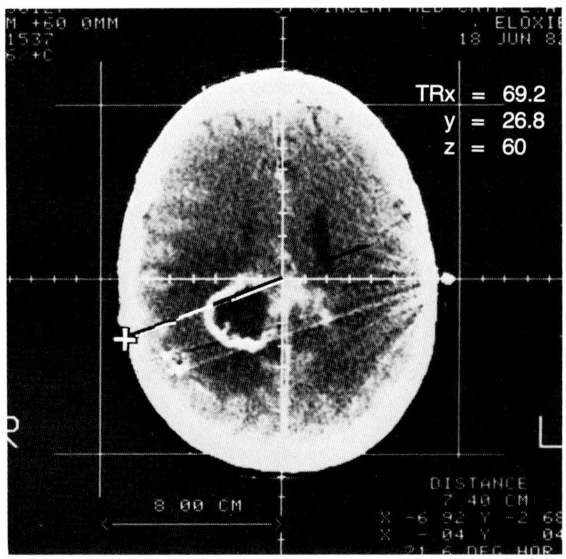

C

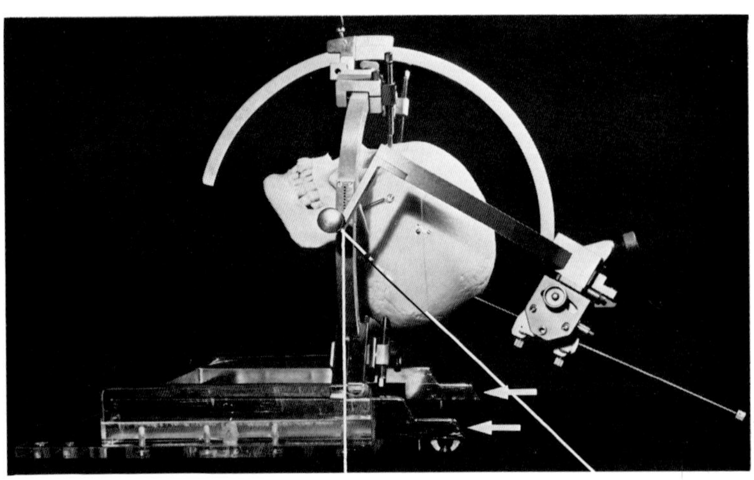

Figure 4–18 Note that the lower 45° of the sagittal plane is mechanically inaccessible. It goes without saying that even accessible occipital lesions are surgically cumbersome.

to the back of the head. It is an awkward task for the surgeon to work on an occipital lesion from a steep sagittal plane, even when the instrument block and cannula guide clear the physical obstacles. Figure 4–19A is a sagittal reformat of a mapped trajectory which was abandoned for a more lateral approach (Figure 4–19B) because the lateral approach was physically feasible whereas the parasagittal approach was stereotactically not to be accomplished because of equipment design limitations. Thus it is sometimes wise to compute more than one approach to an occipital lesion. This was done in a case of recurrent metastatic breast carcinoma (Figure 4–20). First a trajectory was decided on which went through the occipitoparietal parasagittal brain. Its target coordinates were: X = 17.2, Y = −42.0, Z = 42.(1). The chosen trephination coordinates were as follows: X = 33.2, Y = −55.6, Z = 62, which computed to the following stereotactic values: A = 173.79 mm, B = 61.69°, C = −52.13°, D = −5.32°, E = 2.99°.

It should be noted that apparently because Y and Z were both 42 mm the program would not compute until the Z value was altered to reflect a minor mathematical difference. An optional, extremely lateral trajectory was also computed based on another set of coordinates. Target coordinates were: X = 9.2, Y = −47.6, Z = 42. The trephination coordinates were: X = 52.4, Y = −48.2, Z = 42.05. It should again be observed that the Z values for the two coordinates were slightly altered intentionally, (because they were identical) so that the computer would accept the data input. The stereotactic settings obtained by this means were: A = 134.77 mm, B = 19.31°, C = −40.13°, D = −18.66°, E = −0.46°. Although a side angle of 19.31° is almost the ultimate limit of lateral excursion allowed by the instrument arc and bow, this trajectory made possible biopsy and subsequent placement of interstitial isotope implants. Had this not been stereotactically feasible, an optional approach was computed and on hand.

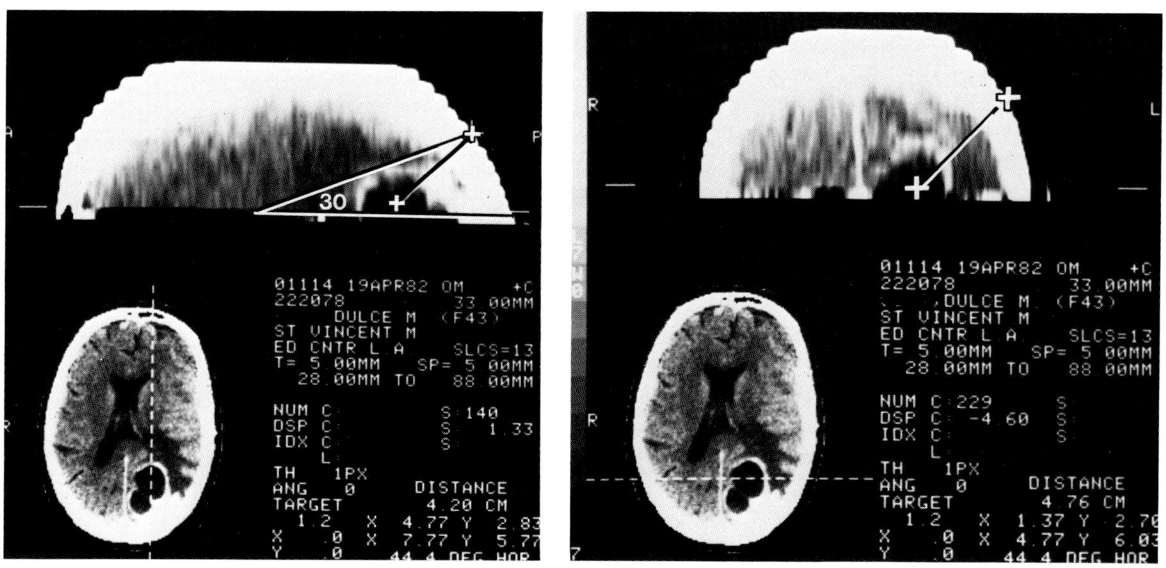

A B

Figure 4–19 **A:** A mathematically enticing approach is abandoned because it is stereotactically inaccessible. **B:** An optional lateral approach to the lesion shown in **A.**

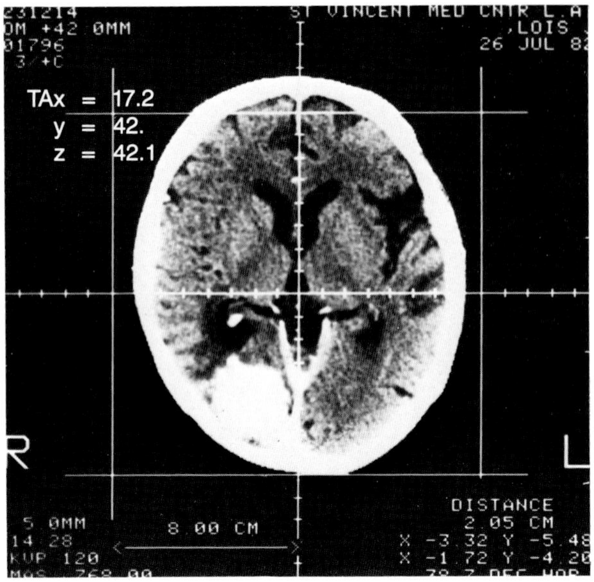

Figure 4–20 Metastatic occipital mass lesion.

It should be underscored that many of the problems associated with an occipital approach could be avoided if the patient were placed face down on the operating table. The occipital lobe then becomes the frontal lobe, stereotactically speaking; however, such an undertaking is extremely uncomfortable for the patient.

Cerebellar Lesions

The Riechert-Mundinger stereotactic apparatus, as it is commercially available today, is not well suited for stereotactic biopsy or curietherapy of posterior fossa lesions. The equipment is a kickback to the roentgen-guided stereotaxy era. Thus the available base ring mount for the GE-8800 CT scanner is bulky, is made of metal, and hence produces unacceptable diagnostic artifacts. Yet neither General Electric Corporation (Medical Systems Division, Milwaukee, Wisconsin) nor Fischer (F. L. Fischer, Hospital Equipment, Freiberg im Breisgau, West Germany) has made an overture to correct this impasse.

In spite of these handicaps, a stereotactic endeavor was undertaken in a woman with a recurrent metastatic cerebellar mass who suffered only from vestibular dysfunction and unilateral ataxia. The CT scan illustrates the dimensions and location of the lesion (Figure 4–21). Rather than perform a craniotomy, a decision was made to attempt stereotactic biopsy and brachytherapy. Under mild premedication the patient was CT-scanned and operated on face down, a position uncomfortable for the patient and foreign to the surgeon. Yet this was the only option open to the stereotactician. Commensurate with these limitations, a CT scan was made with the patient's base ring applied in a reversed position, pins pointing down, a technique described in Chapter 2. Although the neoplasm was not visible because of a metal artifact produced by the CT scanner base ring mount, enough skeletal anatomy was visualized to allow extrapolation of a trajectory through a lesion under acceptable

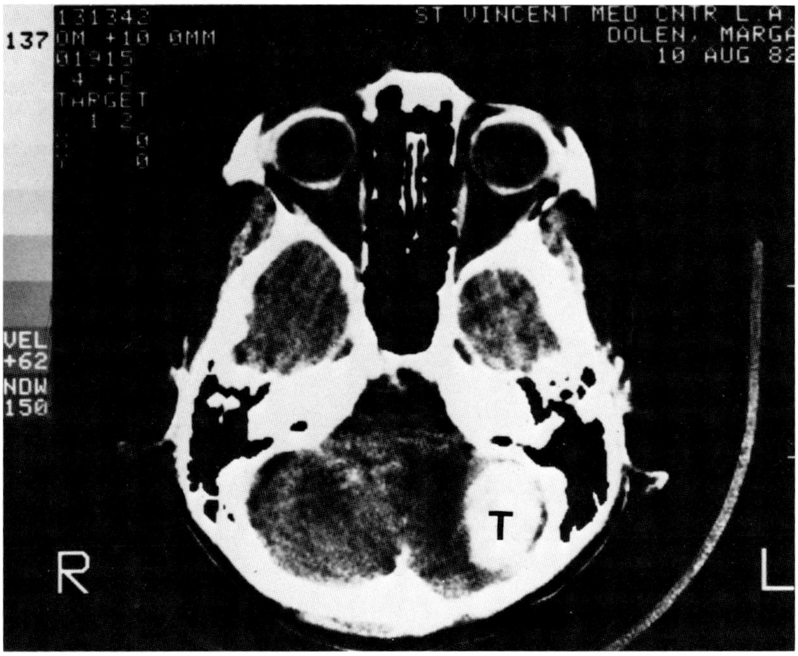

Figure 4–21 Metastatic cerebellar tumor from a bronchogenic carcinoma (*T*).

surgical circumstances. To accomplish this the unfortunate patient was destined to endure a face-down position during the entire endeavor. The target coordinates were X = −42.8, Y = 31.6, and Z = −95. Based on surgical and anatomic considerations, a decision was made to establish the follow-up values as trephination coordinates: X = −42.79, Y = 30.8, and Z = −100.0. Birg's (1) program for the TI-59 accepts these input data and derives meaningful stereotactic information, even if the stereotactic base ring is applied in a mirror image of normal. The computed values derived were: A = 213.50 mm, B = −77.58°, C = −85.27°, D = −7.48°, and E = 13.93°. Biopsy along the trajectory confirmed the presence of recurrent metastatic neoplasm. Brachytherapy has resulted in normal follow-up CT scans and produced a neurologically intact patient living in a fully independent fashion. In spite of the fact that the periphery of the lesion received 50 Gy, no neurologic misadventure ensued. By designing a sitting-position head fixation, an easier stereotactic approach to the posterior fossa may well be possible. A trend in this direction of equipment design is foreseen by the author.

Summary

The endeavor in this chapter was to present in greater detail the actual step-by-step surgical and stereotactic principles applied when arriving at a tumor site, taking into consideration important neuroanatomic facts in so doing. These steps may account in part for the extremely low complication rate encountered to date.

The calculations are offered in detail to assist the novice who might undertake this endeavor in a "cookbook" fashion. It is hoped the various limitations in equipment design have been sufficiently emphasized. The TI-59 computation program is expeditious and quite helpful; but as is apparent in this chapter, its "idiosyncrasies" must be understood.

References

1. Birg W, Klar M, Mundinger F: Programmierbare Taschenrechner bei stereotaktischen Hirnoperationen. Med Klin 72:135–136, 1977
2. Riechert T, Mundinger F: Beschreibung und Anwendung eines Zielgerätes für stereotaktische Hirnoperationen (Modell 2). Acta Neurochir (Wien) [Suppl 3], 308–337, 1956

5

Surgical Technique

Peter Dyck

Patient selection for short-term interstitial radiotherapy (brachytherapy) remains in a state of flux. No absolute guidelines have been established. Gutin et al. interstitially irradiated almost exclusively patients with end-stage disease in whom all "in vogue" therapy had failed (1). Hence their data provide no guidelines for patient selection. We have endeavored to modify these treatment guidelines.

There are credible data available to suggest that interstitial irradiation is equal, and probably far superior, to contemporary treatment modalities of intracranial tumors (1–4,8). Hence our own patient selection was based on tumor size and location as well as neurologic dysfunction rather than treatment failure in a conventional sense, although several patients with cerebral metastatic disease who had exhausted all conventional therapeutic means were included. Some presented with cerebral recurrence of neoplasm at surgical extirpation sites. In others the lesion had progressed in spite of teletherapy. In a few cases the metastatic lesions were in surgically inaccessible sites. All patients had one thing in common, however; they possessed a potential for useful survival.

Patients harboring low-grade astrocytomas often presented with minimal or no neurologic deficits, their medical attention having been heralded by an epileptic seizure or a lesser symptom, e.g., headache. Those patients harboring more malignant astrocytomas were included; even though they had neurologic deficits, there was potential for clinical improvement or stabilization of their neurologic illness. Among this group of malignant glioma patients, several had gone the full gamut of therapeutic endeavor—from craniotomy to teletherapy, to chemotherapy—without salutary effects.

Hence our current therapeutic leitmotif has been to accept patients for brachytherapy who possess, above all, a potential for useful survival; at the same time, though, we do not exclude all individuals with significant focal but manageable neurologic dysfunction at the time of evaluation.

Only in one instance was stereotactic biopsy not followed by interstitial irradiation, and this was because the lesion was not considered neoplastic enough to be irradiated. The case probably represented a very low-grade astrocytoma in a patient with von Recklinghausen's disease.

Patients with known cerebral metastatic lesions were clinically "staged" prior to acceptance into the treatment group. This helped exclude patients with a poor prognosis from our patient population.

Preoperative Preparation

The day before stereotactic surgery is undertaken, the scalp is cleansed with a bacteriostatic shampoo or soap on at least one occasion. The scalp is not shaven preoperatively.

Steroid therapy is initiated or continued in those patients who are already receiving it. Dexamethasone is the drug of choice in most instances. The dosage is titrated to facilitate improvement where indicated or stabilization of neurologic deficits when these are present.

Premedication

All stereotactic biopsies and placement of afterloading catheters are performed under the supervision of an anesthesiologist. Although the premedications vary emphasis is placed on the avoidance of oversedation. Prophylactic antibiotic therapy is initiated at the onset of stereotaxis as well.

Base Ring Fixation

The patient arrives in the operating room with only minor encumbrances. An electrocardiogram (ECG) monitor is then attached and an intravenous infusion line established.

Now, having transferred the patient to an operating table, intravenous infusion of iodine contrast material is begun in preparation for computerized tomography (CT) scanning. The nonshaved scalp is prepared with Betadine at sites of planned pin fixation. The scalp in these areas is then infiltrated with Buvocaine and epinephrine to prolong the regional anesthesia.

The base ring is securely fixed to the skull with metallic pins while it lies secured in a table mount (Figure 5–1). The base ring is placed as low as possible on the calvarium so as not to interfere with CT scanning through the lesion. Excessive neck flexion is avoided in order to prevent airway obstruction.

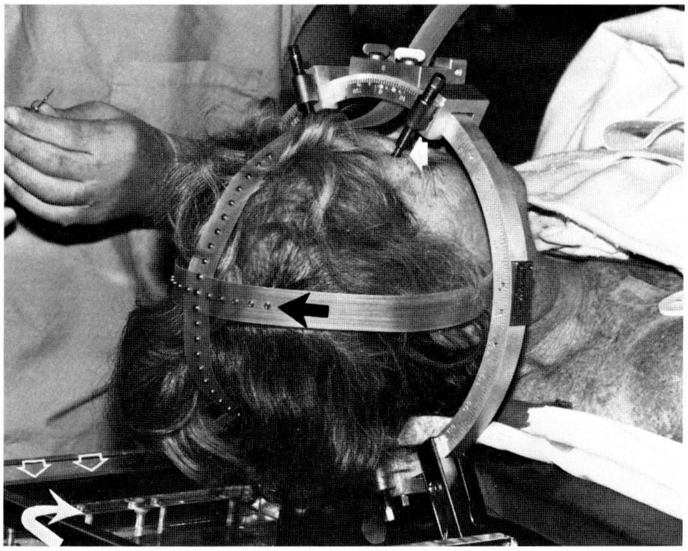

Figure 5–1 Patient has been placed firmly into the base ring employing premedication and regional anesthesia. Pin placement is as low as possible so as to expose maximal intracranial contents to CT (*white arrow*). The base ring mount (*open white arrows*) rests in a plastic table mounted holder (*curved arrow*). A scalp coordinate reference marker is shown (*black arrow*).

CT Scanner Suite

The patient arrives in the CT scanner suite from the operating theater with the base ring firmly attached to the calvarium and in the attendance of an anesthesiologist and a nurse (Figure 5–2). After transferring the patient onto the scanner table on an accompanying matt, the base ring is securely attached to the CT scanner mount (Figure 5–3). The ring is aligned, aided by provided etched markings. More-accurate calibration is then attained by a vertical and horizontal laser light source (Figure 5–4). This is done with the scanner table set at the 0 level. The scanner table may be raised or lowered electrically, but fine adjustment is also provided on the CT scanner mount.

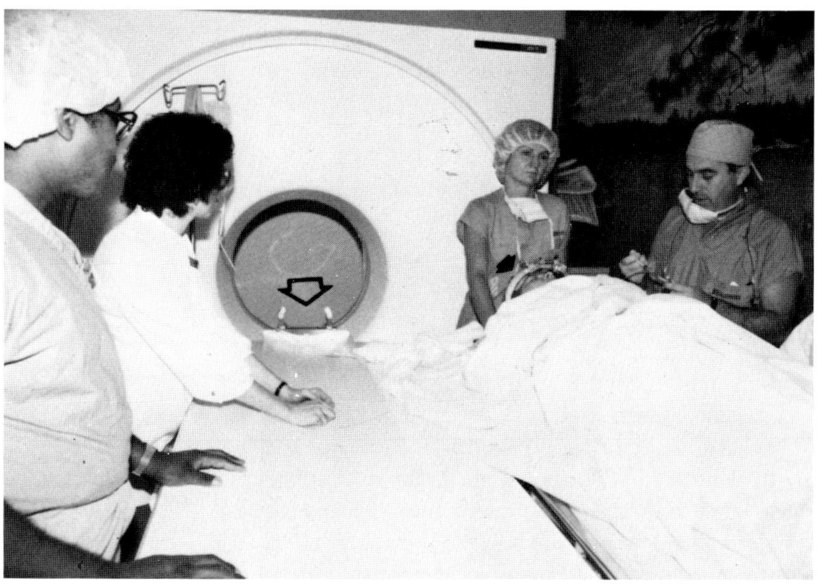

Figure 5–2 Patient with base ring arrives in the CT scanner suite attended by a nurse and the anesthetist. Note the base ring (*solid arrow*) and CT ring mount (*open arrow*).

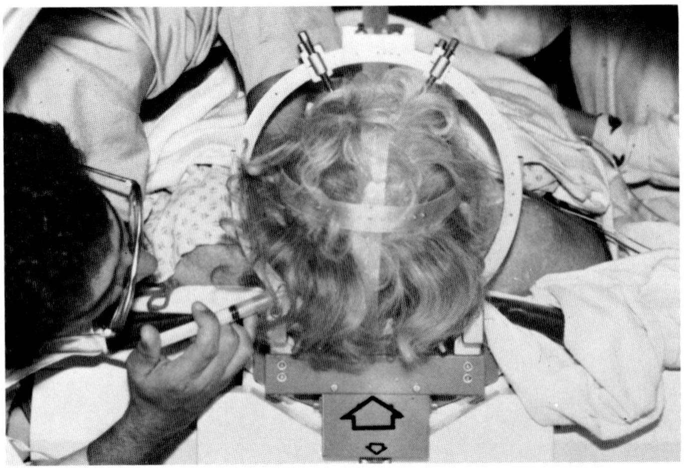

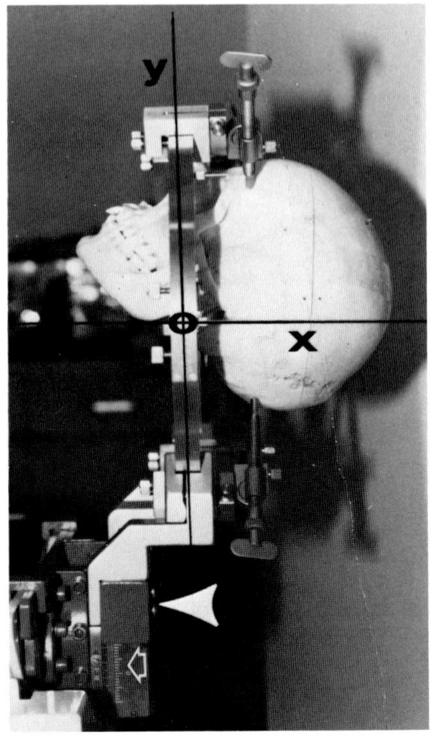

Figure 5–3 The base ring has been placed in the CT scanner mount (*large arrow*). A microdrive provides fine vertical alignment independent of the scanner table capabilities (*small arrow*). Additional local anesthesia may be infiltrated as needed.

Figure 5–4 This phantom test run illustrates the horizontal (x) and vertical (y) axis of the GE-T-8800 laser calibration capability. Note the unnecessarily bulky table mount (*white arrow*). Microdrive scale is shown (*open arrow*).

It goes without saying that the CT scanner gantry must be previously calibrated so that its center coincides with the center of the stereotactic ring. If this holds true, it is of no serious consequence where the head comes to rest within the base ring, at least mathematically speaking.

Axial scanning is then begun, usually at 5-mm intervals in the presence of larger lesions. Smaller cuts are obtained if the lesion is small.

At the completion of tomography, the patient is disengaged from the CT scanner mount and returned to the operating theater. In the meantime, the CT scanning data are assessed and the trajectory or trajectories are planned and the appropriate approach to the lesion is computed. The TI-59 hand-held calculator is employed for this purpose. This is described in greater detail in a subsequent chapter.

Surgical Preparation

The patient is comfortably repositioned on the operating table and the base ring once again mounted to the table mount. A limited area of scalp is shaved, as determined by the scalp markers previously shown. The scalp is then prepared for surgery, sprayed with an adhesive, and covered with a plastic drape (Figure 5–5). The patient is so draped as to leave the face exposed to allow verbal and visible contact (Figure 5–6).

The number of burrholes needed is determined by the size of the lesion and the treatment plan. Scalp infiltration with Buvocaine and epinephrine provides sufficient regional anesthesia when combined with adequate premedication in most adults. Children require general anesthe-

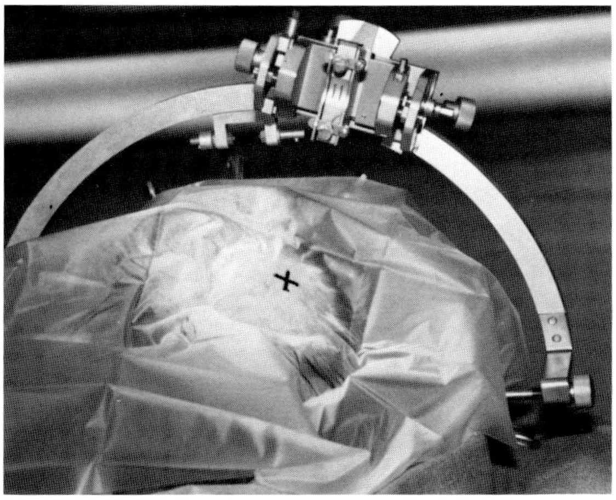

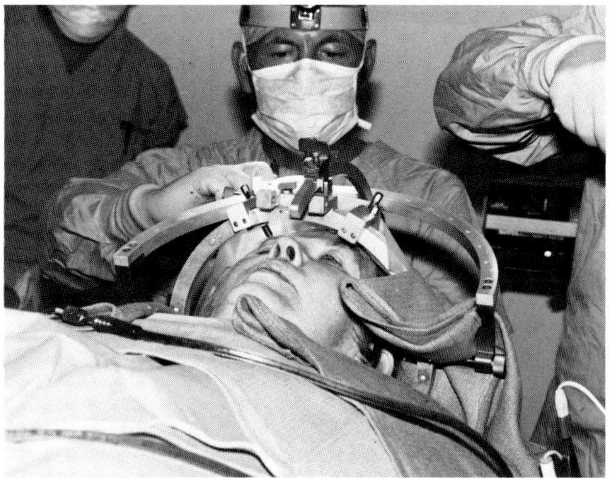

Figure 5–5 The head has been prepared for stereotactic surgical intervention. The *x* marks the calculated trephination point, which has been verified by the coordinate-adjusted instrument arc mounted to the base ring.

Figure 5–6 A sterile field is prepared, but the face is exposed to allow visible and verbal contact with the patient.

sia. If more than two afterloading catheter placements are contemplated, imaginative scalp incisions must be devised so as to avoid multiple stab wounds.

Phantom Calibration

Based on the target and trephination point(s) one chooses, it is possible to compute a surgical approach to any lesion in question. The phantom allows one to affirm these calculations before translating them to the patient (Figure 5–7). Practically speaking, the phantom also provides a platform to anchor the arc device and instrument block while the various calculated stereotactic angle settings are adjusted, making this important part of a surgical endeavor very convenient.

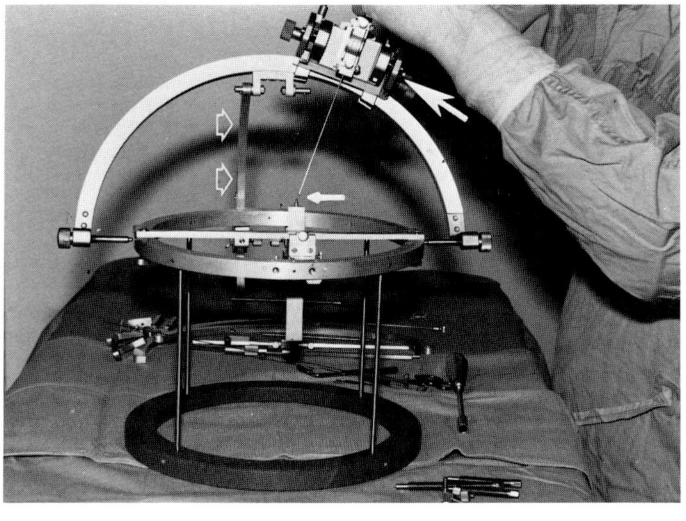

Figure 5–7 The phantom serves as a test platform for the calculated trajectory. The *small arrow* points to the XYZ coordinate functions of the target. The instrument block (*large arrow*) has the capability of allowing settings for all computerized functions but one, the horizontal plane of the trajectory. This is adjusted on a separate bow (*open arrows*).

Also, if one has no computer program for the stereotactic equipment but has the capacity to obtain the XYZ coordinates of a target, the lesion may be approached by randomly selecting an avenue of approach via clinical trial and error. Such an advance to the lesion is no less accurate than the computerized one. Yet computerization is valuable, and it represents the state of the art. It expedites the endeavor and is intriguing. Above all, it saves time.

Biopsy Technique

Retrieval of tissue for biopsy carries the greatest risk associated with stereotactic biopsy and brachytherapy of brain tumors. Hence it warrants more than a cursory discussion, even if the dissertation is based on a limited clinical trial. This appears in Chapter 6.

Specimen preservation and preparation of tissues for histopathologic examination are addressed under a separate heading. Emphasis is placed here on mechanical and surgical endeavors that yield the pathologist sufficient tissue to allow a conclusive diagnosis.

It has been our practice to establish a target that represents the most distal radius of the lesion away from the stereotactic instrument arc. Hence the tissue samples are recorded as: target −3 cm, −2 cm, etc. Such a technique facilitates a cross-sectional histopathologic examination of the lesion, with some tissue designated for rapid staining and other tissue preserved for paraffin mount techniques. Because tissue fragments are necessarily small, the procured specimens are handed personally to the pathologist in the operating room. This allows for expeditious processing of tissues and avoids desiccation of these mesoscopic specimens. Their preparation for appropriate histopathologic examination and staining is discussed in Chapter 6. It must be said, though, that cooperation between pathologist and surgeon is commendable and rewarding.

Afterloading Catheters

Keeping in mind the radiation properties of the selected radioisotope in this instance iridium-192, a placement plan for the afterloading catheter is constructed. As discussed in the chapter on radiotherapy, our general aim has been to deliver about 5,000 rads to the periphery of a lesion. It is our preliminary opinion that this can be accomplished without resorting to insertion of an unusually large number of afterloading catheters, hence avoiding the attendant risks.

Figure 5–8 illustrates placement of three afterloading catheters. The authors have placed as many as four, but in most instances two are sufficient to encompass the lesion for interstitial radiotherapy. Placement of a single afterloading catheter is limited to the treatment of small lesions. In these instances high-activity iodine-125 seems to be best suited, although its general unavailability and extremely high cost appear to outweigh its radiophysical advantages.

Once the afterloading catheters are in place, the stage is set for radiotherapeutic planning. In the meantime, "dummy seeds" are inserted into the afterloading catheters and the scalp is closed. The protruding afterloading catheters are secured in place by a Silastic cuff, as shown in Figure 5–9, or a silk tie that is anchored to the scalp on each side of it, thus preventing inadvertent extrication of the device (Figure 5–9).

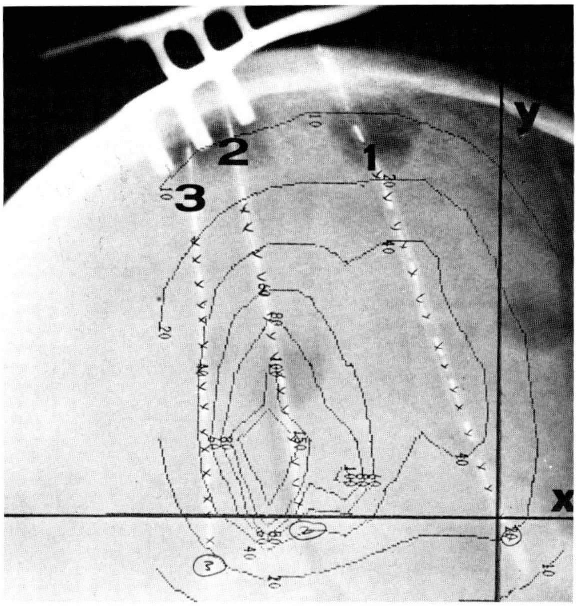

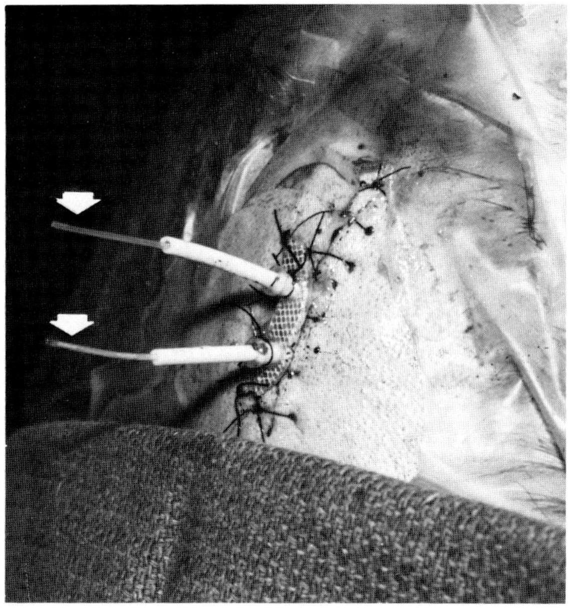

Figure 5–8 A lateral radiation dosimetry field is shown superimposed on a lateral skull x-ray. The XY reference coordinates are shown. After-loading catheters with dummy seeds in place are numbered front to back.

Figure 5–9 Protruding afterloading catheters formerly anchored to the scalp with a Silastic flange device are shown. "Dummy seeds" (*white arrows*) protrude.

Dosimetry Guidelines

The radiodensity of the barium-impregnated catheter and its calibration markings at 5-cm intervals serve as reference points for radiodosimetry calculations. This can be further enhanced by introducing the dummy seeds when reference roentgenograms are made in both the anteroposterior and lateral planes (Figure 5–10).

In our practice the radioactive source is inserted not during the time in the operating theater but later in the intensive care room. Antibiotic prophylaxis begins in the operating room and continues for the entire time the afterloading catheters remain in place. Standard nursing radiation precautions are employed at this time.

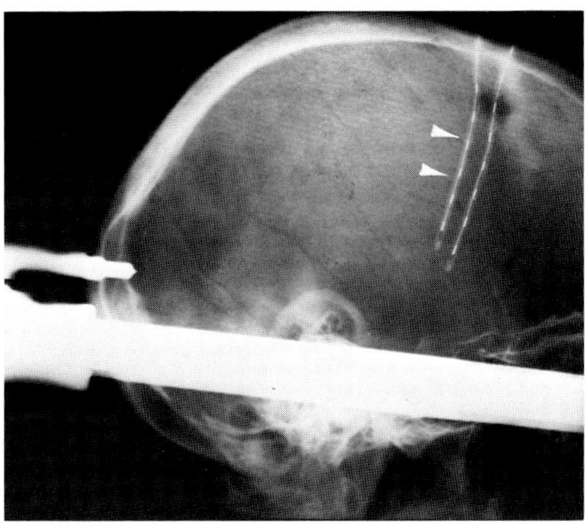

Figure 5–10 Intraoperative lateral roentgenogram. Its anteroposterior counterpart is also obtained. These then serve as a latticework on which the interstitial radiodosimetry is computed. *Arrowheads* point to the afterloading catheters. The "beading" is imparted by the "dummy seeds."

Complications

The immediate perioperative complications are equipment failure and intracranial hemorrhage. Loss of pin fixation because of faulty positioning or inadequate pin adjustment may force repetition of the entire localization sequence in the CT scanner suite. This should be an avoidable event.

Intracranial hemorrhage, on the other hand, is an ever-present danger. Because the patient is in verbal communication with the surgeon and anesthesiologist, however, subtle neurologic change may be detected early.

If hemorrhage occurs during biopsy, the surgical endeavor ceases until bleeding from the cannula stops. The commercially available metal cannula should eventually be replaced by an insulated one in order to facilitate unipolar thermocoagulation of the bleeding point, but this equipment is not yet available.

In one instance of significant parenchymal hemorrhage, the stereotactic cannula was replaced by the perforated Pudenz-Schulte ventricular shunt catheter (which we employ as an afterloading device) after bleeding from the cannula had stopped. An additional 20 ml of blood was passively evacuated, and within 5 min the patient returned to his preoperative mildly dysphasic state from a neurologic state that portended grave consequences. A CT scan performed the next day revealed no evidence of parenchymal hemorrhage (Figure 5–11).

In another instance, seemingly uneventful placement of an afterloading catheter produced a small parenchymal clot (Figure 5–12). No biopsy at the site was attempted. Self-limiting pneumocephalus has also been observed in three instances, with air outlining the frontal horns (Figure 5–13).

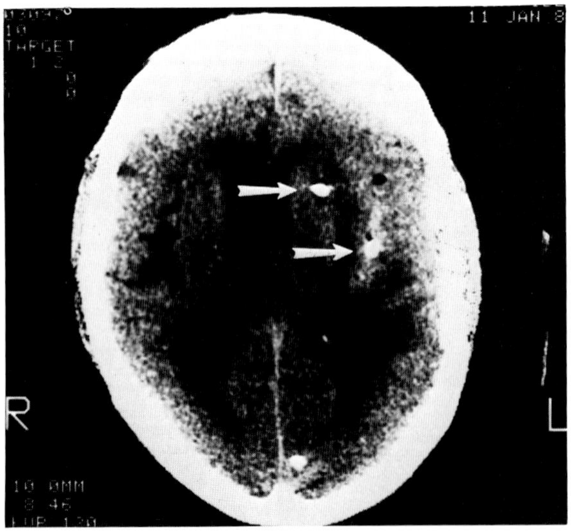

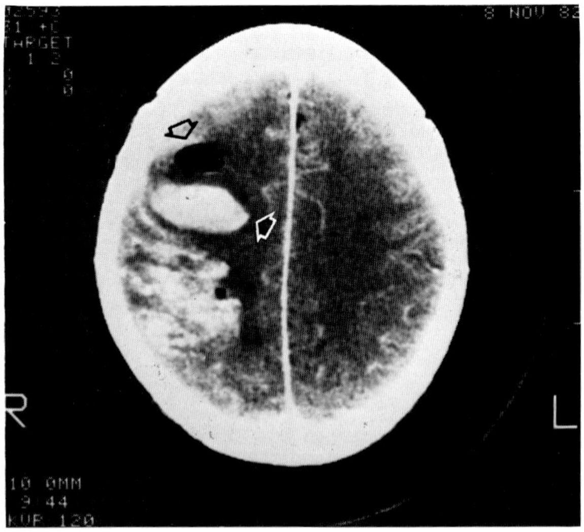

Figure 5–11 A nonenhanced CT scan was performed 1 day after stereotactic biopsy of a recurrent glioblastoma. Note that there is no evidence of hemorrhage around the anterior catheter (*upper arrow*). Only minor traces of parenchymal bleeding are evident around the posterior catheter (*lower arrow*).

Figure 5–12 Hemorrhage (*white arrow*) into a highly vascular glioma occurred at a site where no biopsies were made; only an afterloading catheter had been inserted. Air (*black arrow*) replaced some of the evacuated clot as the catheters are perforated.

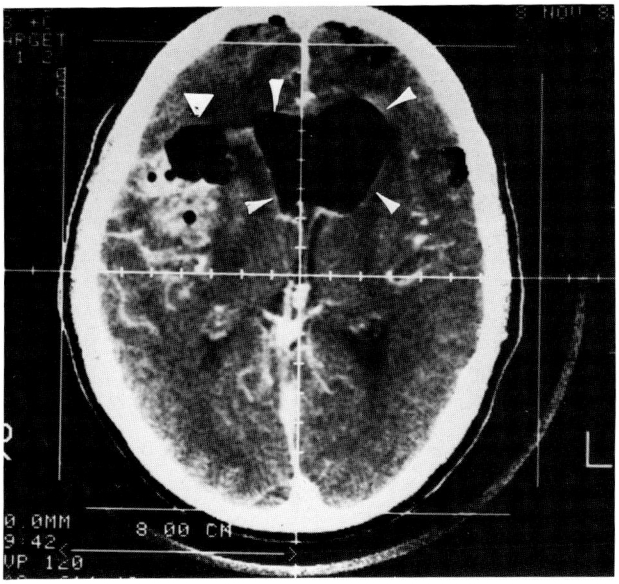

Figure 5–13 Same case as in Figure 5–12. Note that as the hematoma spontaneously evacuated the cavity was filled with air (*large arrowhead*), which upon rupture into the right frontal horn created a pneumoventriculogram (*small arrowheads*), as there was no ventricular obstruction absorbed spontaneously after reaching the surface of the brain.

Conclusion

A chronologic review of the surgical principles involved in stereotactic biopsy and planning of brachytherapy has been presented. With meticulous detail to all aspects of this dissertation, the reader should be left with one immutable fact: Parenchymal hemorrhage must be contended with at times. Ostertag et al. reported a mortality rate of 2.3% in an institution where many brainstem lesions are stereotactically biopsied and treated with interstitial irradiation (5). In 1981 Mundinger cited a 1.4% mortality rate caused by hemorrhage among 489 consecutively managed patients 1 year later in the same institution (3).

Sugita et al. reported no mortality after biopsy of 18 neoplasms in the vicinity of the third ventricle (7). Scarabin et al. have been equally fortunate, reporting no mortality during stereotactic biopsy of 200 supratentorial mass lesions (6).

The authors concur with Kelly (2) that refinement in interstitial radiotherapy has not reached its zenith. Stereotactic equipment modifications, to make it more compatible with CT scanning, is only in its infancy. Computerized tumor volume reconstruction and simulated three-dimensional dosimetric display cannot be far behind. Our own ability to now use radioisotopes with greater utility and the adaptations of others offer a never-ending vista for imaginative thoughts and improvement in technique in time to come.

References

1. Gutin PH, Phillips TL, Hosobushi Y, et al: Permanent and removable implants for brachytherapy of brain tumors. Int J Radiat Oncol Biol Phys 7:1371–1381, 1981
2. Kelly PJ: Future possibilities in stereotactic neurosurgery. Surg Neurol 19:4–9, 1983
3. Mundinger F: Die stereotaktische interstitielle Therapie nicht resezierbarer intrakranieller Tumoren mit Ir-193 und Jod-125. In: Kombinierte chirurgische

und radiologische Behandlung maligner Tumoren, edited by M Wannemacher, HW Schreiber, F Gauwerky. Urban & Schwarzenberg, Munich, 1981, pp 90–112
4. Mundinger F: Implantation of radioisotopes (curie-therapy). In: Sterotaxy of the Human Brain, edited by G Schaltenbrand, AE Walker. George Thieme Verlag, New York, 1982, pp 411–435
5. Ostertag CB, Mennel HD, Kiesling M: Stereotactic biopsy of brain tumors. Surg Neurol 14:275–283, 1980
6. Scarabin JM, Pocker J, Bruchner JM, et al: Stereotaxic exploration in 200 supratentorial brain tumors: its value in addition to computerized tomography. Neuroradiology 16:591–599, 1978
7. Sugita K, Mutsuga N, Takaokay, et al: Stereotaxic exploration of para-third ventricular tumors. Confin Neurol 37:156–159, 1975
8. Szikla G, Paragut JC: Irradiation interstitielle des gliomes. Neurochirurgie [Suppl 2], 21:187–228, 1975

6

Neuropathology of Stereotactic Biopsies

P. Gruskin
K. L. Saeger
J. N. Carberry

The smear technique for obtaining rapid diagnoses in neurosurgical procedures has been employed for approximately 50 years (2,8,9,21). Early techniques used supravital stains (8). With this method cells and their processes may be clearly defined and fine detail seen, features which otherwise are not appreciated if tissue has a fixation or freezing artifact. Although photographs may be taken, this method does not allow preservation of the specimen for future use. Permanently stained smears were used by Russell et al. (21), who modified a previous technique (7), Morris (16), and Jane and Bertrand (9). Russell (20) subsequently described additional experiences with this staining method. Present methods are modifications of these basic procedures.

Most pathologists, by virtue of their training, are more familiar and hence more confident when interpreting frozen sections or paraffin-mounted hematoxylin and eosin (H&E) stained tissue. There are, however, advantages to using the smear technique when tiny fragments of tissue obtained by stereotactic means are presented for examination.

The smear technique lends itself to rapid preparation and examination of tissues. It is particularly inviting when multiple small biopsies are submitted for microscopic examination. All of the tissue is examined, as opposed to a section at one level. Cytologic detail, cell processes, and some structural relationships (e.g., relations to vessels) can be appreciated. Although the fragments are small, often not more than 1 mm, they can be handled without great difficulty.

The interpretation of smear preparations requires experience on the part of the pathologist because of the small size of the biopsy material and the general unfamiliarity with the smear technique for diagnostic purposes.

Tissue smear preparations, however, have disadvantages. Soft tissue smears easily, but firm or rubbery tissues do not. It must also be remembered that a smear preparation may destroy tissue architecture. Smear preparations are variable in thickness so that cellularity may be more difficult to evaluate.

The smear technique does not supplant frozen section examinations, which remain useful in some instances. In fact, combined smear and frozen/paraffin sections should be used. Diagnostic tissue may be found only in the smear or the section material. Confirmation of one by the other may be important. The cell morphology of a smear often complements the cellular architecture of a tissue section.

Neuropathologic atlases and other publications illustrating brain smears are available, with discussion of differential diagnoses and the problems encountered (1,3,9,10,15,18–20). Adams et al. (1) have had a 20-year experience with this technique (8,000 biopsies) (*vide infra*) and Jane and Bertrand (9) 30 years' experience. In most instances the tissue was obtained at the time of craniotomy or by freehand biopsy of the lesion through a variable-sized surgical cranial defect.

As Ostertag et al. (17) demonstrated, recent techniques of stereotaxis integrated with localization by computerized tomography (CT) offers great improvement (*vide infra*). Conway (5) used stereotactic apparatus with radioisotopic and radiographic studies to obtain needle biopsy cores for paraffin section. Bosch's (4) stereotactic biopsies were aided by CT scan and angiography, but he preferred the spiral needle for biopsy rather than conventional aspiration needles.

Ostertag et al. (17) described the stereotactic biopsies of 302 patients with intracranial lesions. All tumors were examined by smear preparations (methylene blue) and then photographed for documentation (permanent record). Both cytologic and conventional histopathologic examination were attempted in 213 of the cases, and so correlation was possible. A broad classification divided the lesions into "gliomas" and "nonglial tumors." In the glioma group correlation was possible in 119 cases. The smear technique yielded 95% diagnostic accuracy as confirmed by histologic examination, whereas in the remaining 5% of cases significant diagnostic changes were necessary. Such changes included cytologic diagnoses of pilocytic astrocytoma to subsequent malignant astrocytoma, glioblastoma to metastatic carcinoma, astrocytoma to germinoma, and gliosis to pilocytic astrocytoma. In the second group, 14 cases (11.8%) of cytologic diagnoses could not be histologically confirmed and had to be amended. In 65 of the 213 cases (31%), although both smear and paraffin preparations were made the smear proved diagnostic and the paraffin section did not.

Adams et al. (1) discussed another large series examined by the smear technique. They emphasized that diagnostic accuracy is high in experienced hands. Over a period of 3 years 609 cases were so evaluated. Smears and subsequent paraffin sections were performed and compared, and in 93.6% the correct diagnosis was rendered on the smear. Diagnostic error was encountered in 6.4%, yet in most of the instances (4.6%) the error lay in an incorrect classification of malignant tumor and thus did not really affect the immediate neurosurgical management. In 1.8% the diagnostic error was significant; for example, a smear diagnosis of astrocytoma was actually fibrous meningioma, an infarct was actually anaplastic astrocytoma, gliosis was astrocytoma, pus was necrotic tumor, and finally, a smear diagnosis of astrocytoma was in reality Ammons horn. The authors retrospectively reviewed their 6.4% diagnostic errors and emphasized that with experience and more time to evaluate smears, diagnostic acumen in this group could be improved. It is noted that the biopsies in this series were not obtained with combined technique of CT scan and stereotaxis.

Prior publications (12,13) have discussed the reliability of the smear technique, but only over a 1 year period from the same series as above (Adams et al). The reported accuracy of smears was 94%.

Marshall et al. (14) advocated needle biopsy through a burrhole with a rapid smear technique in patients in whom craniotomy did not seem justified (e.g., malignant gliomas involving deep structures). In 60 cases of suspected malignant or inoperable gliomas, diagnosis was correctly made in 53 (88%) with the needle biopsy technique.

Liwnicz et al. (11) cytologically examined tissue obtained by aspiration from 84 intracranial lesions. In 66 cases cytologic and histologic diagnosis coincided, for a 92% correlation. The cytologic material was obtained with CT guidance through a twist drill orifice or via open craniotomy. CT-aided stereotaxy was not used. Comparisons could be made only with the open craniotomy material as obtaining aspirates through the drill orifice was the sole definitive diagnostic procedure in these cases. Except for two autopsy cases, verification of the aspirate-only material was based on therapeutic response and clinical course. Examples of the discrepancies included smear diagnosis of glioblastoma amended to melanoma, and "normal" central nervous system (CNS) tissue amended to metastatic carcinoma. Yet all in all, in only five of the 66 histologically verified cases (8%) was there a discrepancy between smear and final paraffin section diagnosis. Our discussion is based on experience with intracranial tissue obtained by CT-guided stereotactic means.

Stereotactic Brain Biopsies—Smear and Sectioning Techniques

The aim of stereotactic brain biopsy is to obtain histologic verification of the nature of the lesion while producing minimal injury to the surrounding structures. This becomes particularly important when multiple biopsies are obtained to delineate the extent of the lesion. Consequently the biopsy material, of necessity, is small, often not more than 0.5–1.0 mm. Such small biopsies reduce the chance of edema and hemorrhage. Handling such small specimens requires modification of technique, and smear preparations fulfill this need. Sufficient tissue is also obtained for both frozen section and paraffin mounts. We rely predominantly on the smear technique but also retain some tissue for paraffin sections. Our smear technique allows rapid intraoperative tissue confirmation of the pathologic process yet does not prevent safekeeping of the tissue for future reference.

The neuropathologist's role at the time of surgery is to: 1) confirm that the surgeon has indeed biopsied the lesion; 2) do this expeditiously;

3) prepare the material so that an adequate diagnosis may be rendered; and finally 4) preserve the tissue for future use.

It is not always essential to render a definitive diagnosis peroperatively. All smears and sections should be available within 24 hr. At our institution afterloading catheters are placed at the time of surgery, but the radioactive material may be inserted the following day. Should one not arrive at a definitive diagnosis after all the biopsy material is evaluated, the afterloading catheters may be withdrawn and interstitial radiotherapy abandoned or deferred.

One cannot overemphasize the need for cooperation between the pathologist and neurosurgeon. It is imperative that the pathologist be aware of the patient's clinical history, investigative studies, and operative findings. The pathologist should not attempt to interpret biopsy material without full knowledge of the case. McMenemey (15) believes that the pathologist should render an initial opinion based on the microscopic appearance of the tissue alone to reduce interpretive bias and then subsequently (during surgery) discuss the case with the neurosurgeon in order to reach a more definitive opinion.

At St. Vincent Medical Center we have adopted the smear and staining technique as routinely practiced in general pathology. This includes examination of tissue by smears and sections. The pathologist is present in the operating room at the time the biopsies are obtained and personally handles the tissue. A tray containing these items is available:

1. Coplin jar with 95% alcohol for immediate fixation of smears
2. Clean glass slides with frosted ends for labeling
3. Lens paper to wrap biopsy fragments designated for paraffin sections
4. Cassettes for wrapped biopsies
5. Container of formalin for cassettes with biopsies

Each slide is labeled in the operating room with the patient's name and depth of biopsy (see below). This prevents mislabeling. The smeared slides are immediately fixed in alcohol. The biopsy specimens are placed in labeled cassettes after being wrapped and then promptly immersed in formalin to prevent desiccation.

It is the neurosurgical practice here and abroad to designate a "target point." Hence specimens are labeled in reference to this target. A biopsy obtained 2 cm proximal to the target is labeled "target −2 cm" (T−2); and if biopsy is made 1 cm beyond the computerized target, it is designated as "target +1 cm" (T+1). Such technique allows histopathologic spatial reconstruction of the pathologic process.

The neurosurgeon obtains one or two biopsies from each level (e.g., T−1). The pathologist then endeavors to make both a smear preparation and a paraffin section from the material at each level. Smears are prepared by placing the tissue on a slide. The edge of another slide is held at approximately 30°, and the tissue is pulled away from the label across the first slide. If the tissue is firm, however, one may elect to make a squash or squeeze preparation. Material for a paraffin section is saved in formalin. Frozen sections may of course also be prepared. Only the most appropriate smears are immediately stained and the surgeon promptly informed of the cytologic findings. Remaining material may be prepared and examined later.

We have available a rapid blue staining technique (total time approximately 1 min) as well as a rapid H&E stain (total time approximately

4 min). A more formal H&E stain (10 min) is available, such as that ordinarily used in any pathology laboratory. All three of these staining methods may be employed in the examination of tissue smears or sections. One may employ Papanicolaou or other stains if so desired. Personal preference dictates staining time, techniques, and the agents used.

Microphotography is at our disposal and may be utilized at the pathologist's discretion. Although the rapid blue stain is often sufficient, the rapid H&E stain is more helpful under difficult circumstances. The rapid blue stain is not permanent. In order to retain the smear preparations stained with blue dye, we remove the coverslip, decolorize the smear with acid alcohol (95% alcohol to which a few drops of hydrochloric acid has been added), and then restain it with the rapid H&E stain or even the more time-consuming traditional H&E stain.

Staining Techniques

The various preparations are stained as follows, with the staining times being approximate):

1. Smear preparations
   a. Rapid blue stain (1 min)
   b. Rapid H&E stain (4 min)
   c. Standard H&E stain (10 min)
2. Frozen sections
   a. Rapid blue stain (1 min)
   b. Rapid H&E stain (4.5 min)
3. Paraffin sections
   a. Standard H&E stain (10 min)

Rapid Blue Staining Method

1. Flood smear with 95% alcohol for approximately 15–30 sec to fix material. Blow dry.
2. Cover material with blue stain (see next section, item 1) approximately 5–15 sec.
3. Dip slide into tap water to remove excess stain.
4. Place a few drops of mounting medium (we use Bruns medium—see next section, item 2) on the slide and add a coverslip.

Stains

1. *Rapid blue stain:* Methylene blue polychrome, Terry-Crystals. Chroma 1A446. Manufactured by Chroma-Gesellschaft, Schmid, GmbH and Company, Stuttgart-Untertürkheim, West Germany. (Distributed by Roboz Surgical Instrument Company, 1000 Connecticut Ave. N.W., Washington, DC 20036). *Content:* crystals 1 g, sodium bicarbonate 1 g, distilled water 100 ml. The stain works immediately, although there is better red and blue color differentiation after it ages 1–2 weeks. Without aging it is almost entirely a blue stain.

2. *Bruns medium:* dextrose 40 g, distilled water 140 ml, spirit of camphor 10 ml, and glycerin 10 ml. This makes approximately 160 ml of Bruns mounting medium; it is stable for 1 year.

Rapid H&E Stain (for Smears)

1. Fix smears immediately in 95% alcohol for 30 sec (may fix longer).
2. Rinse in tap water approximately 10–15 dips.
3. Place in Gill-2 hematoxylin for 1 min.
4. Rinse in tap water approximately 10–15 dips.
5. Place in eosin-Y for 30 sec.
6. Alcohol 95%, 10 dips.
7. Alcohol 100%, 10 dips.
8. Alcohol 100%, 10 dips.
9. Xylol 10 sec.
10. Second xylol 15 sec.
11. Coverslip using permount.
12. *For sections*
    a. Step 1 (fixation): 50% alcohol 30 sec, 70% alcohol 10 dips, and then 95% alcohol 10 dips.
    b. Step 3: hematoxylin 1.5 min.

Discussion

Interpreting neurosurgical biopsy material in general requires experience and caution. This is because of the inherent nature of the diseases that affect the nervous system, the sampling errors in biopsies, the limited size of biopsy material, and the similarity of reactive processes to neoplasm, e.g., gliosis and low-grade astrocytoma. It is well recognized that neoplasms, especially astrocytomas, may vary in different sites from low to high grade, so that biopsy of one area may lead to misinterpretation of the overall lesion. Reactive gliosis adjacent to infarct, hemorrhage, metastatic carcinoma, or an inflammatory process may be extremely difficult to discern from neoplasm.

Biopsy material obtained stereotactically has these problems in common in addition to others. Tissue obtained through a burrhole is small, adding to the pathologist's dilemma. The surgeon must biopsy an appropriate area in order to ensure a correct tissue diagnosis. Again, it is stressed that the pathologist and neurosurgeon must confer about the case. Knowledge of the clinical and other diagnostic data is essential. In instances where the patient received radiotherapy prior to biopsy, the pathologist's job is further complicated by histologic changes related to radiation.

We have encountered instances of metastatic carcinoma in one biopsy/smear and immediately adjacent encountered a gliotic reaction that was difficult to distinguish from a low-grade astrocytoma. Hence it is essential that all available tissue is carefully examined.

Tissue necrosis is another concern because necrosis in a glioma and a metastatic carcinoma may mimic one another. If necrotic tissue is obtained, the pathologist should request biopsy of a more viable lesion.

If sufficient tissue is obtained, some of it may be saved in glutaraldehyde for electron microscopy. More contemporary procedures (e.g., immunoperoxidase staining for glial fibrillary acid protein) may be useful, as are various histochemical studies. Tissue culture is possible.

Technical problems in smear preparation may also lead to errors. Thick smears always appear more cellular and "alarming." Some gliomas by nature are more rubbery and may not smear well. Such a specimen might be "squeezed" between slides.

One must also be familiar with the normal histology of the area being biopsied. Ammon's horn on smears may be confused with astrocytoma (1). The normal cell types present in aspirates of deep cerebrum are described with attention to features distinguishing them from neoplastic cells (6).

Inflammatory tissue reactions are another potential source of concern. Perivascular cuffing with lymphocytes and plasma cells may be seen in viral encephalitis but may also occur adjacent to primary and metastatic tumors or near a brain abscess. Culture examination is possible when needed.

It is not solely the experience of the pathologist which determines the diagnosis (or lack of it) rendered. The correct diagnosis is also contingent on the neurosurgeon providing representative tissue for examination. We have had cases where no definitive diagnosis could be rendered on the available biopsy material, even after consultation with an expert neuropathologist. Future repeat biopsy is sometimes necessary.

Case Discussion

To date we have endeavored to evaluate neuropathologically the first 20 cases where tissue was obtained by CT-guided stereotactic means. Other stereotactic brachytherapy has also been carried out but was based on previous tissue diagnoses. Eight of the 20 cases are illustrated and briefly discussed in Figures 6–1 through 6–25.

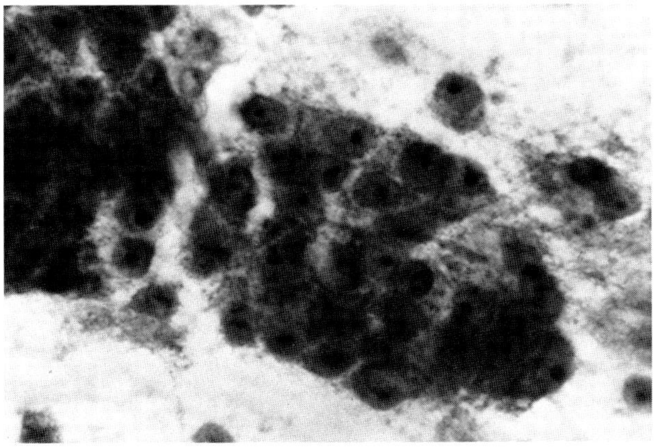

Figure 6–1 Metastatic adenocarcinoma from the lung to the cerebellum. The typical cohesive clustering of carcinomatous cells is seen. Unlike gliomas, these cells have a "honeycomb" appearance and prominent nucleoli. Blue-stained smear preparation, ×600.

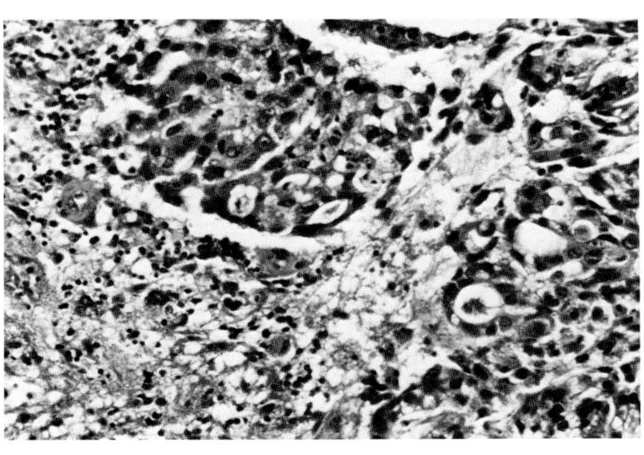

Figure 6–2 Same case as Figure 6–1. The gland formation is better appreciated in the section. H&E section, ×200.

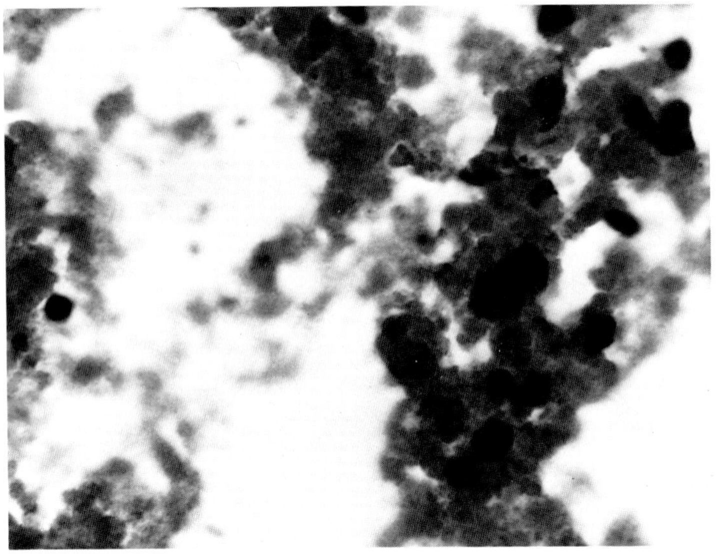

Figure 6–3 Metastatic adenocarcinoma from the rectum. A partially necrotic metastatic tumor as illustrated here may be difficult to separate from a necrotic primary tumor. H&E smear preparation, ×600.

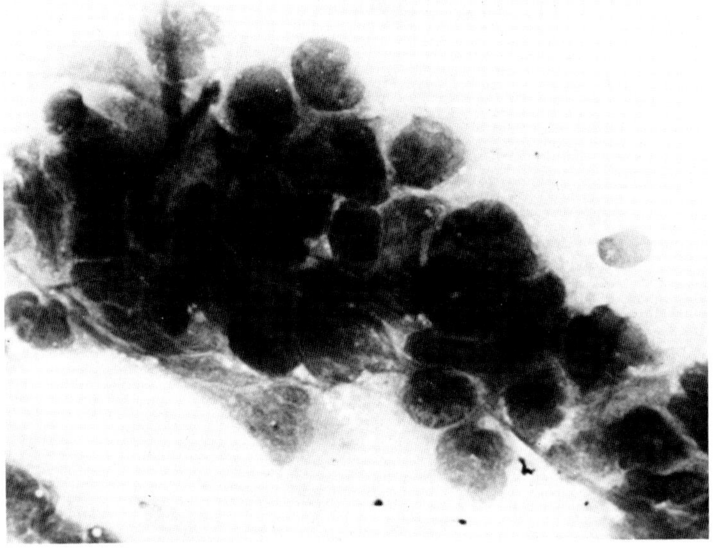

Figure 6–4 Same case as Figure 6–3. Another smear has a drying effect, yet the pattern is similar to that in the previous case (Figure 6–1) and can be recognized as carcinoma. Blue-stained smear preparation, ×600.

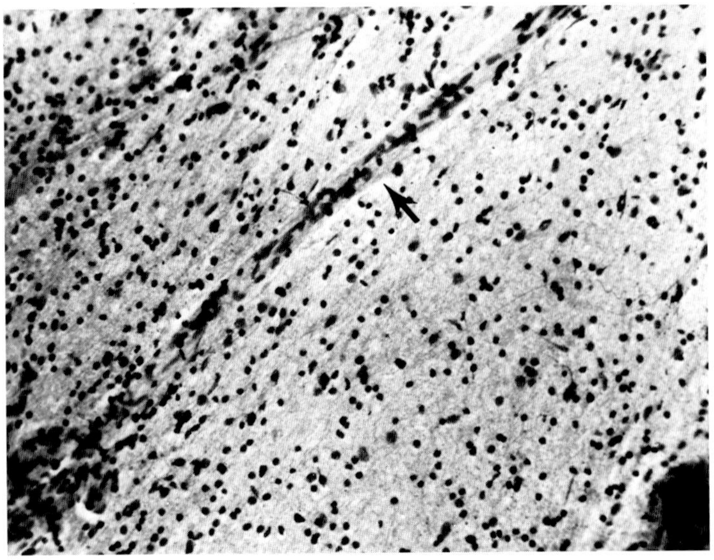

Figure 6–5 Same case as Figure 6–3. Vascular proliferation (*arrow*) and gliosis adjacent to metastatic carcinoma may mimic glioma. H&E smear preparation, ×200.

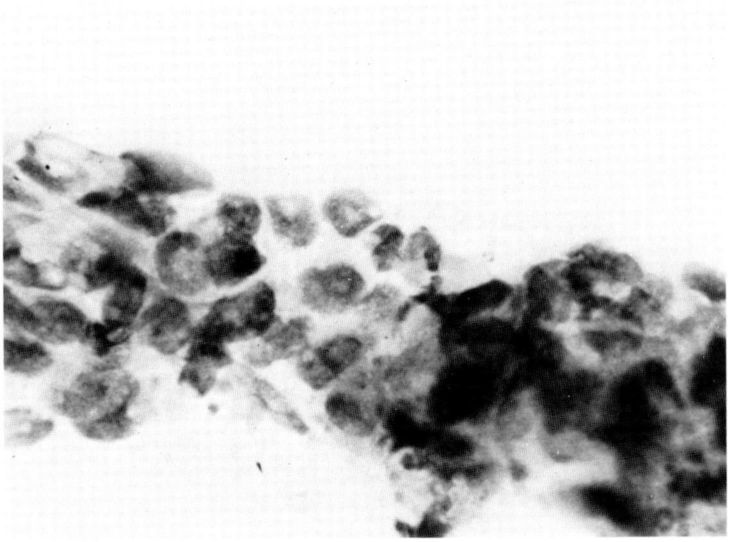

Figure 6–6 Brain with metastatic lung carcinoma. Partially necrotic and dried cells retain the pattern of metastatic carcinoma, although they are difficult to interpret as such. H&E smear preparation, ×600.

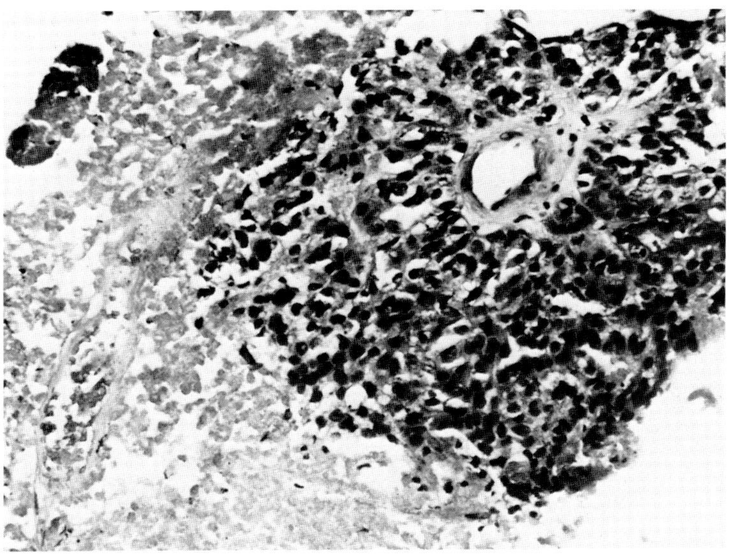

Figure 6–7 Same case as Figure 6–6. Cellular poorly differentiated carcinoma with necrosis. (Necrotic tumor is the pale-staining area at lower left.) H&E section, ×200.

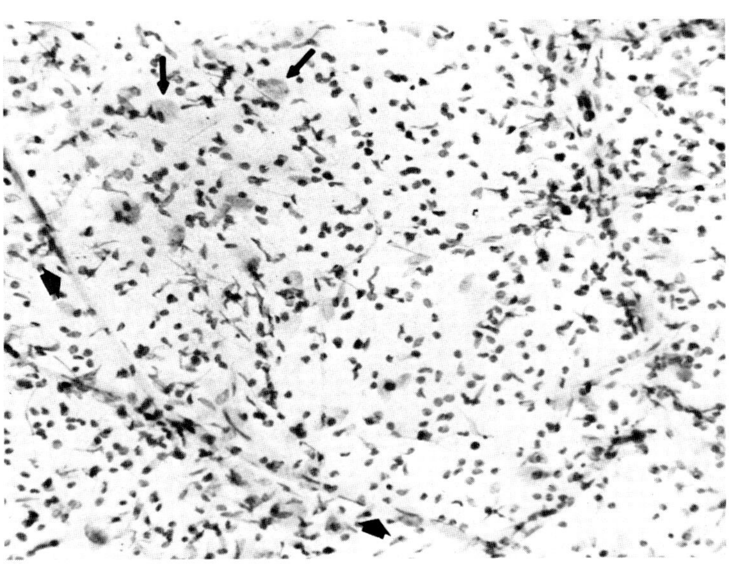

Figure 6–8 Same case as Figure 6–6. Again, as in the previous case (Figure 6–5), the cellular gliosis adjacent to the carcinoma resembles glioma. The polymorphous nature of the cell population with intervening neurons (*arrows*) favors a diagnosis of gliosis. Note the small vessels (*broad arrows*). H&E smear preparation, ×200.

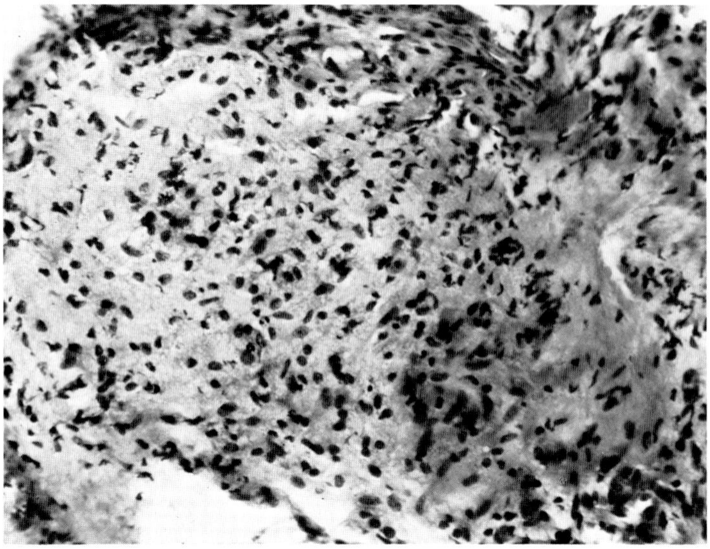

Figure 6–9 Same case as Figure 6–6. This section is suspicious for glioma but is actually reactive gliosis. H&E section, ×200.

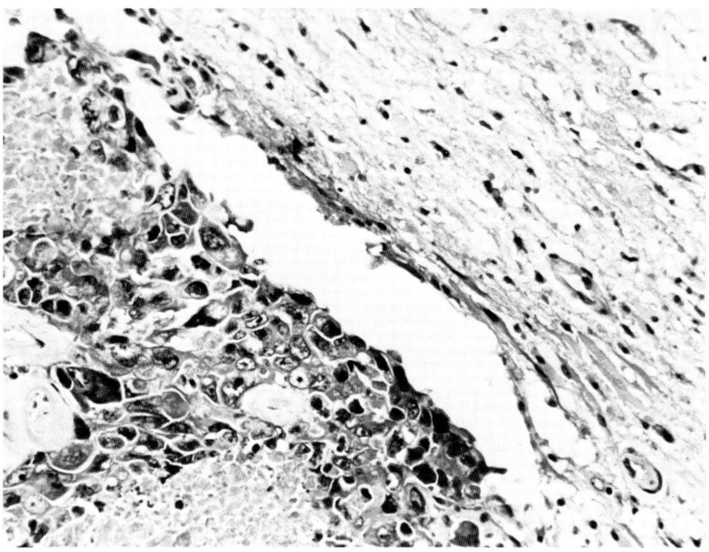

Figure 6–10 Same case as Figure 6–6. The patient received interstitial radiotherapy. Subsequently she hemorrhaged into the tumor and died. The epithelial nature of the carcinoma is more evident in this autopsy section of brain. The adjacent brain also exhibited gliosis. H&E section, ×200.

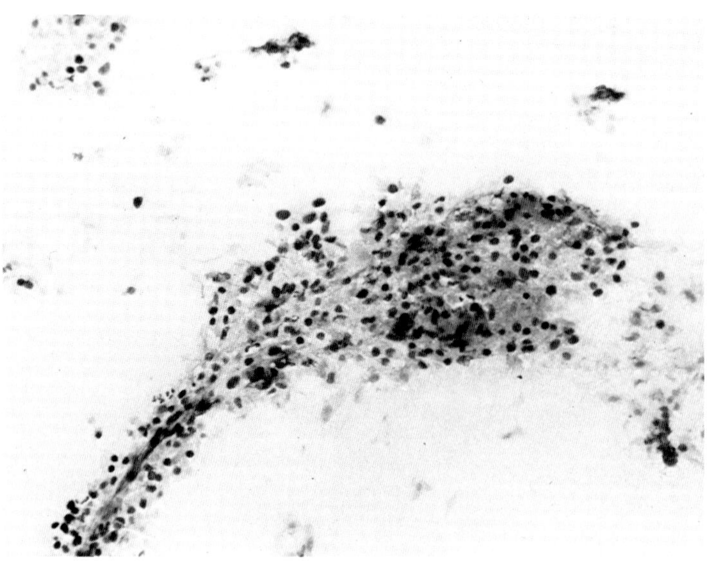

Figure 6–11 Metastatic adenocarcinoma from the cecum to the parietal lobe. This smear reveals moderately cellular partially necrotic tumor, but the diagnosis cannot be established with this material alone. H&E smear preparation, ×200.

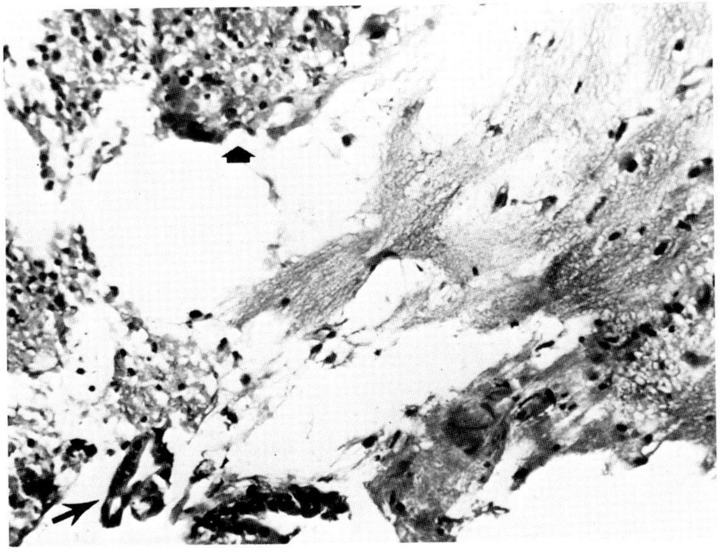

Figure 6–12 Same case as Figure 6–11. In this biopsy section the nature of the process is clarified. Gland formation typical of adenocarcinoma is seen focally (*arrow*) and is in contrast to the necrotic tumor (*broad arrow*). The multiple biopsy technique may be useful as in this instance. Of multiple biopsies, this was the only one with viable and diagnostic tumor. The tumor was compared to the original cecal lesion resected 1 year previously, and the two are identical. H&E section, ×200.

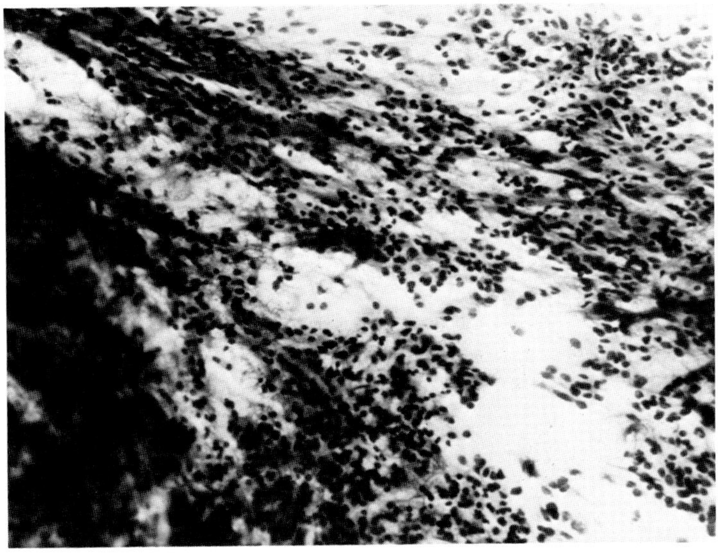

Figure 6–13 Fibrillary astrocytoma. This glioma is quite cellular with nuclear hyperchromatism. Blue-stained smear preparation, ×200.

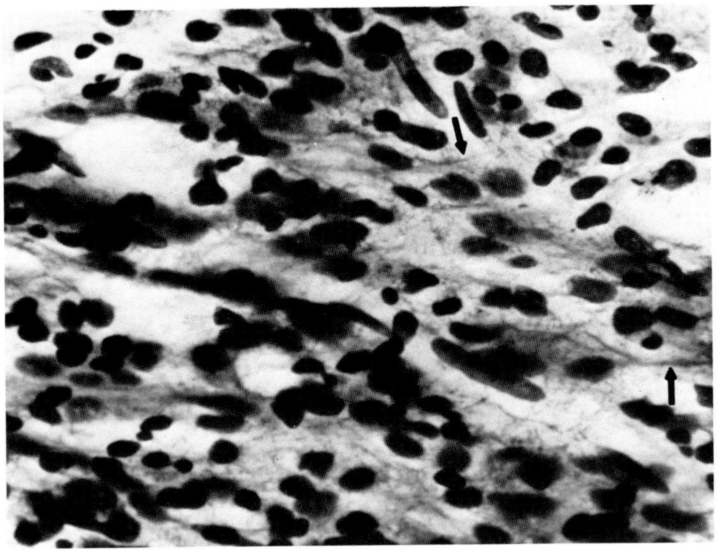

Figure 6–14 Same case as Figure 6–13. The fibrillary processes (*arrows*) can be better appreciated in smears than sections. Blue-stained smear preparation, ×600.

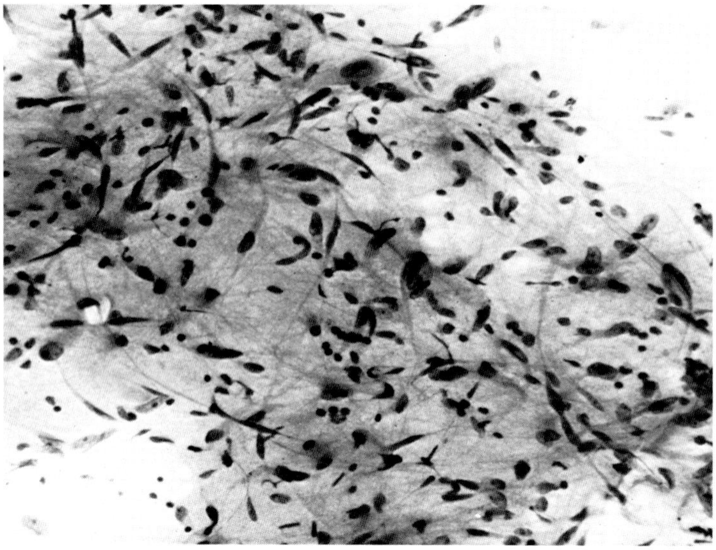

Figure 6–15 Glioma, probably grade II–III, in the parietal lobe. This is a moderately cellular lesion whose protoplasmic cell processes are clearly visible in the smear preparations. H&E smear preparation, ×200.

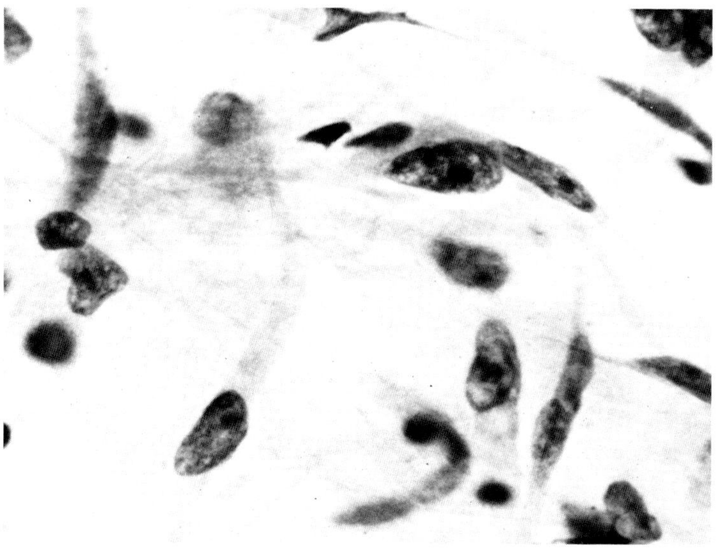

Figure 6–16 Same case as Figure 6–15. Higher-power photomicrograph demonstrating the protoplasmic cell processes. H&E smear preparation, ×600.

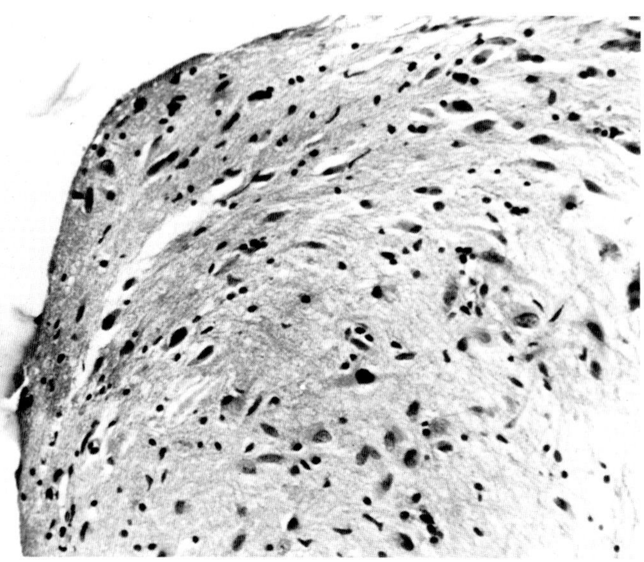

Figure 6–17 Same case as Figure 6–15. This biopsy section shows lower-grade glioma although it is suspected that a higher-grade lesion exists in this patient. H&E section, ×200.

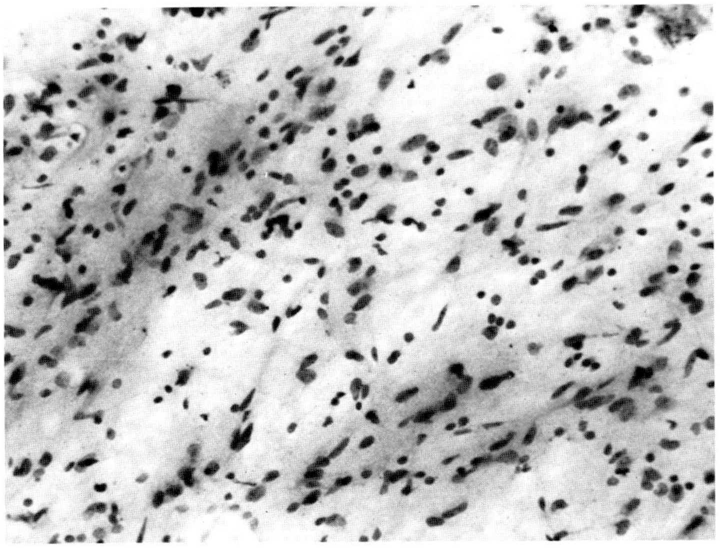

Figure 6–18 Astrocytoma, grade II. The lesion is moderately cellular and at this magnification resembles the gliosis seen in Figure 6–8. Blue-stained smear preparation, ×200.

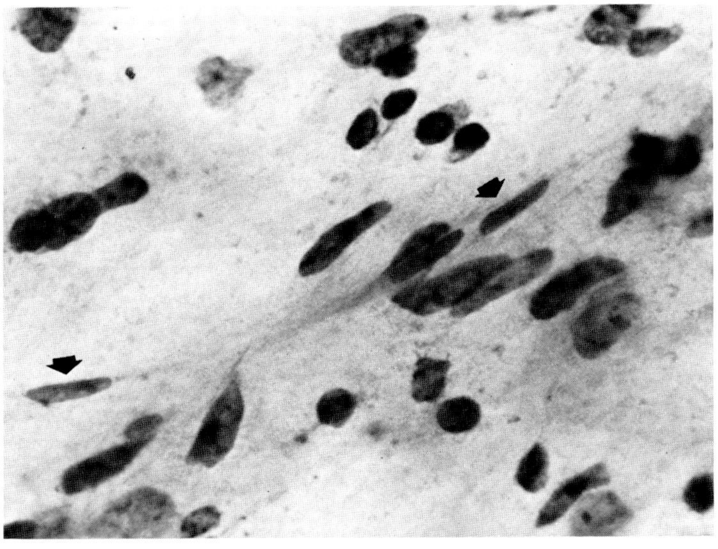

Figure 6–19 Same case as Figure 6–18. Higher power demonstrates the elongated, somewhat angulated nuclei with enlarged nucleoli. Endothelial cells of a small vessel are in the center (*arrows*). Blue-stained smear preparation, ×600.

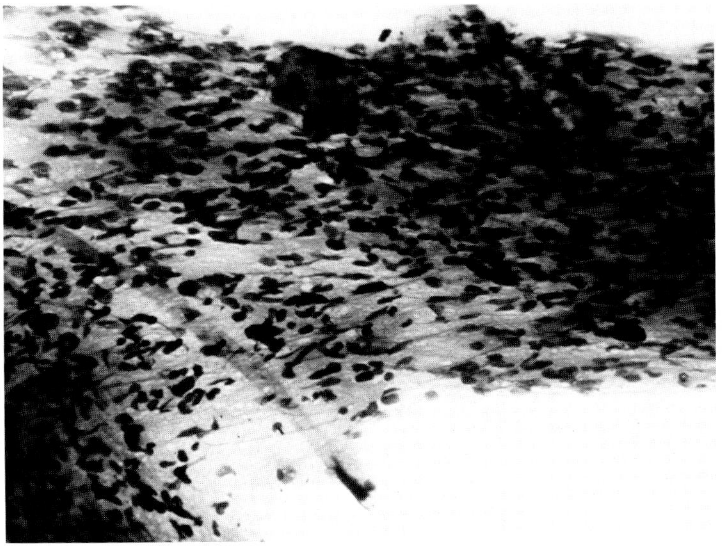

Figure 6–20 Glioma grade III (glioblastoma) in brain. This tumor is very cellular, more so than in the previous cases, and the appearance is not caused merely by the thickness of the smear. H&E smear preparation, ×200.

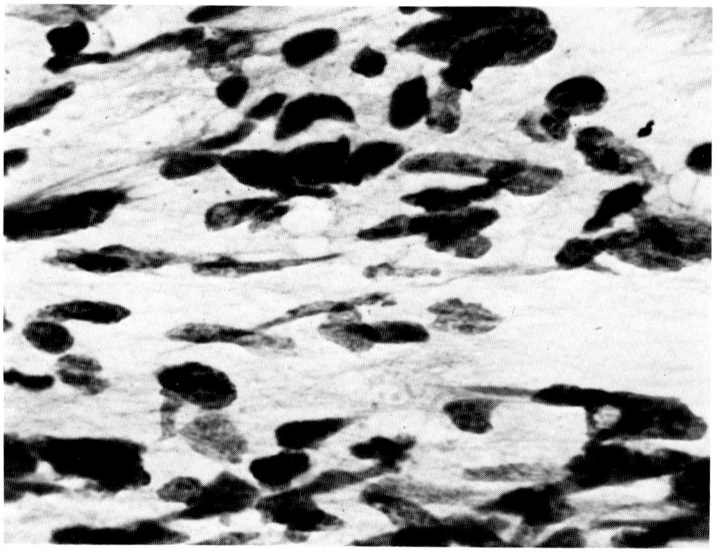

Figure 6–21 Same case as Figure 6–20. Higher power reveals irregular hyperchromatic nuclei. H&E smear preparation, ×600.

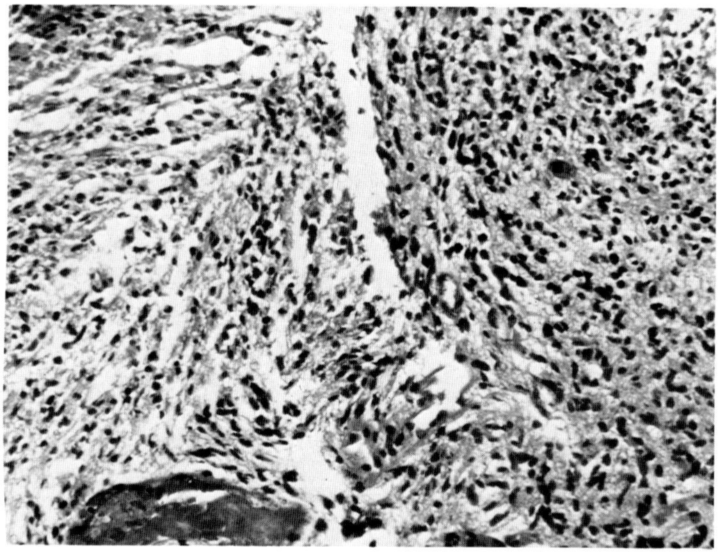

Figure 6–22 Same case as Figure 6–20. This biopsy section is typical of high-grade glioma with prominent cellularity and partial necrosis (*left half of figure*). A vessel (*lower left*) contains a thrombus. This tumor is not as pleomorphic as grade IV glioma (glioblastoma) and has less endothelial proliferation and no palisading. H&E section, ×200.

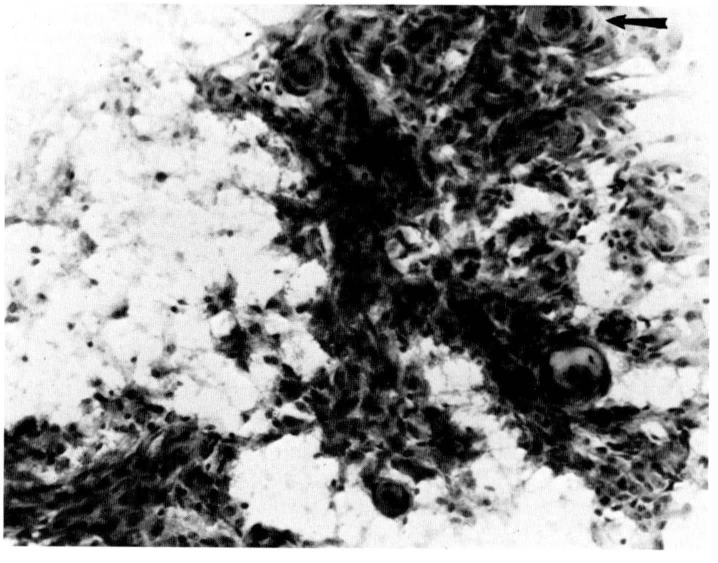

Figure 6–23 Frontal meningioma. The whorling pattern (*arrow*) typical of meningiomas is seen. Blue-stained smear preparation, ×200.

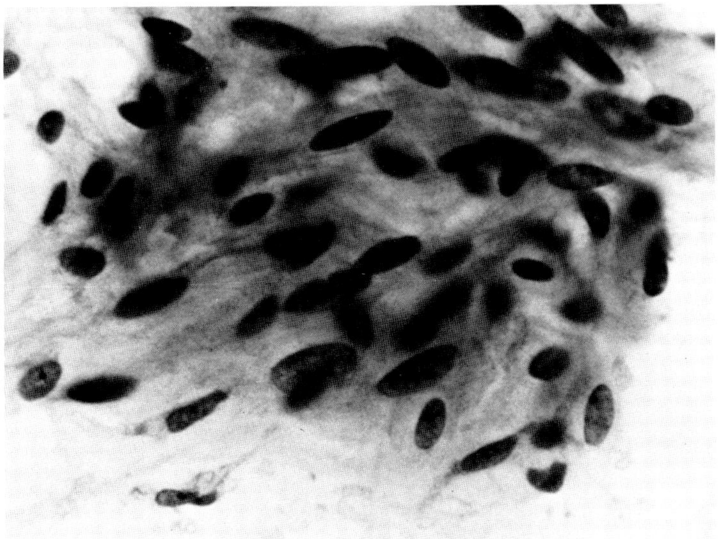

Figure 6–24 Same case as Figure 6–23. The nuclei are uniform and oval. Blue-stained smear preparation, ×600.

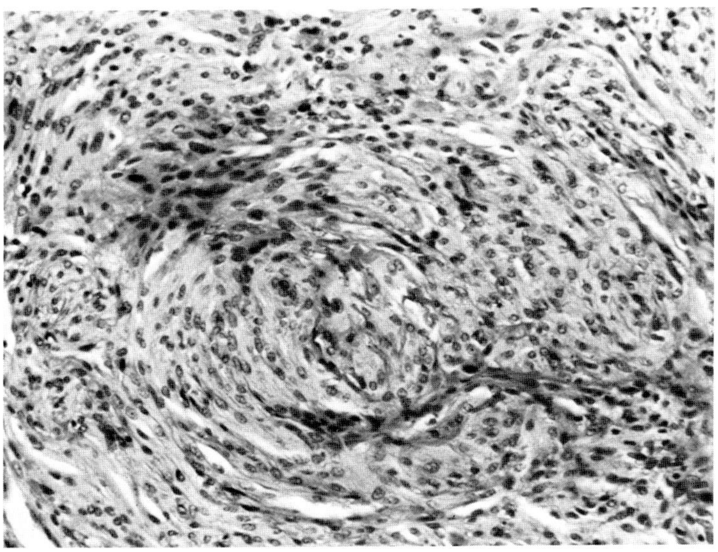

Figure 6–25 Same case as Figure 6–23. The cells are uniform without pleomorphism or mitotic figures. The whorling is characteristic. (Although the biopsies in this case were not obtained by stereotactic means, the smears were prepared with the same stereotactic technique.) H&E section, ×200.

Acknowledgments

The authors wish to thank our cytotechnologist Mary Levin for her assistance with the smear preparations, and our secretary Patricia Medina for typing the manuscript.

References

1. Adams JH, Graham DI, Doyle D: Brain Biopsy—The Smear Technique for Neurosurgical Biopsies. Lippincott, Philadelphia, 1981
2. Badt B: Mikroskopische Schnelldiagnose bei hirnchirurgischen Eingriffen. Z Neurochir 2:123–139, 1937
3. Barnard RO: Tumour biopsy in brain tumour. In: Handbook of Clinical Neurology, Vol 16: Tumors of the Brain and Skull, edited by PJ Vinkin, GW Bruyn. North Holland Elsevier, Amsterdam, 1975, pp 708–726
4. Bosch DA: Indications for stereotactic biopsy in brain tumors. Acta Neurochir (Wien) 54:167–179, 1980

5. Conway LW: Stereotaxic diagnosis and treatment of intracranial tumors including an initial experience with cryosurgery for pinealomas. J Neurosurg 38:453–460, 1973
6. Crain BJ, Bigner SH, Johnston WW: Fine needle aspiration biopsy of deep cerebrum. Acta Cytol (Baltimore) 26:772–778, 1982
7. Dudgeon LS, Patrick CV: A new method for the rapid microscopical diagnosis of tumours. Br J Surg 15:250–261, 1927–1928
8. Eisenhardt L, Cushing H: Diagnosis of intracranial tumors by supravital technique. Am J Pathol 6:541–552, 1930
9. Jane JA, Bertrand G: A cytological method for the diagnosis of tumors affecting the central nervous system. J Neuropathol Exp Neurol 21:400–409, 1962
10. Jane JA, Yashon D: Cytology of Tumors Affecting the Nervous System. Charles C Thomas, Springfield, Illinois, 1969
11. Liwnicz BH, Henderson KS, Masukawa T, et al: Needle aspiration cytology of intracranial lesions—a review of 84 cases. Acta Cytol (Baltimore): 779–786, 1982
12. Marshall LF, Adams H, Doyle D, et al: The histological accuracy of the smear technique for neurosurgical biopsies. J Neurosurg 39:82–88, 1973
13. Marshall LF, Jennett B: Smear biopsy in neurosurgical diagnosis. Arch Neurol 29:124–126, 1973
14. Marshall LF, Jennett B, Langfitt TW: Needle biopsy for the diagnosis of malignant glioma. JAMA 228:1417–1418, 1974
15. McMenemey WH: An appraisal of smear diagnosis in neurosurgery. Am J Clin Pathol 33:471–479, 1960
16. Morris AA: The use of the smear technique in the rapid histological diagnosis of tumors of the central nervous system: description of a new staining method. J Neurosurg 4:497–504, 1947
17. Ostertag CB, Mennel HD, Kiessling M: Stereotactic biopsy of brain tumors. Surg Neurol 14:275–283, 1980
18. Papo I, Colombo F: Possibilità e limiti dell'esame estemporaneo per schiacciamento e striscionella diagnosi peroperatoria dei tumori endocranici. Minerva Neurochir 3:134–147, 1959
19. Rubinstein LJ: Tumors of the Central Nervous System (Second Series, Fascicle 6). Armed Forces Institute of Pathology, Washington, DC, 1972
20. Russell DS: The wet film technique in neurosurgery. In: Recent Advances in Clinical Pathology, edited by SC Dyke, Churchill, London, 1947, pp 418–425
21. Russell DS, Krayenbühl H, Cairns H: The wet film technique in the histological diagnosis of intracranial tumors: a rapid method. J Pathol 45:501–505, 1937

7

Clinical Material

Peter Dyck

Our clinical experience with stereotactic biopsy and interstitial irradiation is limited. Although the number of cases now exceeds 20, the present observations are based on the first 20 consecutively treated patients. Table 7–1 summarizes the cases managed at the St. Vincent Medical Center from April to December 1982.

Age and Sex

There were six men and 14 women in the group. Their ages ranged from 30 to 78 years, the mean age being 56 years (the men averaged 54 years and the women 47 years). When metastatic lesions are excluded from consideration, the mean age of patients with grade I–II astrocytomas becomes 48 years and for those with glioblastoma 63 years. Thus 15 years separate the two groups. Because age itself is an important factor in survival of patients with astrocytoma (5), this must be kept in mind when assessing the results of brachytherapy. To date the data presented are not sufficient for statistical analysis.

Tumor Site

The location of a lesion is, functionally speaking, of paramount importance. Table 7–2 offers a breakdown of the 20 tumors; six were located in the frontal lobes, equally divided between right and left. The five

Table 7–1 Clinical Breakdown of the First 20 Consecutively Treated Patients By Age, Sex, Tumor Type, Tumor Site, Degree of Functional Disability and Clinical Outcome at Time of Evaluation

Stereotactic Data Sheet

Case	Age	Sex	Diagnosis	Lesion site	RX Date	Disability Scale	Comments
1-CJ	52	F	Metastasis	Parietal (L)	4–8–82	2	Seizures controlled
2-SD	43	F	Metastasis	Occipital (L)	4–19–82	2	2 more small lesions
3-HB	62	F	Astrocytoma-2	Frontal (R)	4–23–82	0	Seizures controlled
4-RD	48	F	Astrocytoma-2	Frontal (L)	4–23–82	0	Seizures controlled
5-MJ	41	M	Astrocytoma-2	Frontal (R)	4–30–82	0	Seizures controlled
6-GA	42	M	Astrocytoma-4	Frontal (R)	5–20–82	3	Stable deficit
7-BE	60	F	Astrocytoma-4	C-callosum	6–18–82	3	Improved
8-BN	68	F	Astrocytoma-3	Tempo-parietal (L)	6–21–82	1	Minimal aphasia
9-DS	69	F	Astrocytoma-4	Thalamic (L)	7–23–82	3	Stable hemiplegia
10-DL	46	F	Metastasis	Occipital (R)	7–26–82	Dead	Spinal metas. (4 mos)
11-ND	70	M	Astrocytoma-4	Frontal (L)	7–30–82	3	Stable deficit
12-DM	70	F	Metastasis	Cerebellar (L)	8–16–82	1	Symptom free, retired
13-AR	60	M	Metastasis	Fronto-parietal (L)	9–1–82	4	Static hemiplegia
14-VC	68	F	Astrocytoma-4	Fronto-parietal (L)	9–17–82	2	Lives with family
15-RT	30	F	Astrocytoma-1	Occipital (R)	9–22–82	0	Mild hemiparesis
16-SM	50	F	Astrocytoma-4	Panhemisphere (L)	9–28–82	Dead	Died 6 wks later
17-SA	78	F	Astrocytoma-4	Tempo-parietal (L)	10–6–82	2	Aphasia resolved, home
18-CG	47	M	Astrocytoma-2	Frontal (L)	10–11–81	0	Working
19-MA	61	M	Astrocytoma-2	Panhemisphere (R)	11–3–82	4	Alert-hemiplegic
20-WL	59	F	Metastasis	Temporal (R)	11–5–81	Dead	Aortic thrombosis

parietal lesions all occupied the dominant hemisphere. There was a single right temporal metastatic mass. Three lesions were in the ocupital lobe. The corpus callosum and the left thalamus were the sites of two glioblastomas. A recurrent bronchogenic carcinoma occupied the cerebellopontine angle on one occasion, though having arisen within the cerebellum. Finally, there were two cases of panhemispheric glioma where biopsy confirmation of the nature of the lesion was preeminent and attempted brachytherapy a secondary consideration.

Tumor Size

Next to patient age, tumor size is probably the single most important determinant of therapeutic outcome and hence "useful survival," in contrast to survival as a whole. Mundinger and Weigel proposed that any lesion greater than 150 gr. of tumor bulk is probably not amenable to interstitial radiotherapy (4). There were two glioblastomas and three metastatic lesions that approached or exceeded this limit. In spite of this, in one instance the cystic lesion was stereotactically drained and the patient neurologically improved (Figure 7–1). In the others, progression of deficits was held in abeyance, although there was no great functional improvement.

In the remainder of cases the tumor volume was not sufficient to cause extensive destruction or deformation of brain and hence lent itself more favorably to brachytherapy.

Table 7–2 Classification of the Cerebral Neoplasm By Site of Involvement

Frontal (R-3, L-3)	6
Parietal (R-0, L-5)	5
Temporal (R-1, L-0)	1
Occipital (R-2, L-1)	3
Thalamic (R)	1
C-callosal	1
Panhemispheric (R-1, L-1)	2
Cerebellar	1
Total	20

Table 7–3 Adaptation of Seiler's Performance Evaluation Important in Determining "Useful Survival."

0	Fully employable
1	Employable part-time
2	Unemployable but independent
3	Partially independent (50% in bed)
4	Bed-ridden

(Rolf W. Seiler: Late results of multimodality therapy of high-grade supratentorial astrocytomas. Surg Neurol 15:88–91, 1980).

Performance Index

Seiler proposed his own version of the Karnofsky scale (6). In it there are five categories which range from total independence and minimal neurologic abnormality to complete dependence (Table 7–3). Our patients were categorized in accordance with Seiler's scale, as indicated in Table 7–1.

Tumor Type

From a histopathologic standpoint, there were 13 astrocytomas in the group, ranging through the entire spectrum of Kernohan's classification. Five of these were grade I–II lesions; the remaining eight were more

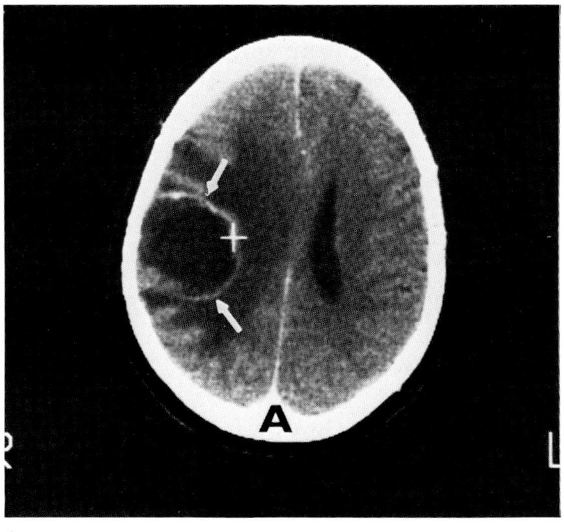

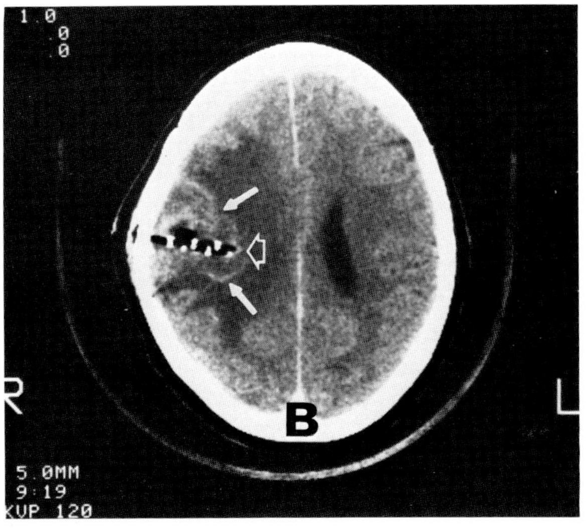

A B

Figure 7–1 CT scans obtained on the day of stereotaxis and one day following. **A:** The arrows outline the contrast enchanced perimeter of a metastatic mass with a hypodense center. **B:** After draining 10 ml from the neoplastic cyst, the enhancing periphery of the neoplasm is shown hugging the two after-loading catheters (*open arrow*). Although it is not apparent in this axial view, the afterloading catheters were separated by 1.5 cm in the Z-plane.

malignant and were classified as grade III–IV. The seven metastatic lesions were from primaries in the lung, breast, and gut, in that order of frequency.

In 17 cases the correct tissue diagnosis was made peroperatively on a stained smear or squeeze preparation alone. A hematoxylin and eosin (H&E) stained paraffin mount was necessary in the remaining three instances (see Chapter 6).

Patient Selection

Our small group of patients has served as a basis for establishing selection guidelines for the future, rather than as a proposed group for brachytherapy. For this reason some discussion is imperative. From a standpoint of neurologic deficit, the group was heterogeneous. The grade II astrocytoma patients in all but one instance were neurologically intact and presented with only a seizure disorder. Tissue diagnosis was made stereotactically in all but one instance (case 5) where previous craniotomy had established the diagnosis and stereotactic biopsy at the time of brachytherapy only reconfirmed it. The only case of grade I astrocytoma presented, ironically, with slowly progressive pyramidal signs. A previous craniotomy with excision of a contralateral temporal pole astrocytoma 6 years earlier and two large café au lait spots made a diagnosis of von Recklinghausen's disease highly likely.

The eight patients with grade III–IV astrocytoma had variable neurologic dysfunction and duration of illness. One patient presented with a subtle expressive aphasia, progressive over 2 months. Another patient with similar speech dysfunction was hospitalized after a grand mal seizure. It is of interest to note that this woman had had a seizure 1 year previously but a negative CT scan of the brain.

There were three failures of surgical debulking procedures and postoperative teletherapy. The patient with the corpus callosum glioblastoma was externally irradiated without tissue diagnosis because the lesion had been deemed surgically inaccessible. The patient with the thalamic lesion was hemiparetic but was able to live at home.

The cases of single metastases to brain all represented failures of tele- and chemotherapy and in some instances of surgical debulking procedures. All of these patients were considered to have a reasonable life expectancy under the circumstances and were not seriously encumbered by metastatic disease elsewhere. All but one lived at home with their families but were partially disabled from a neurologic standpoint. All were receiving glucocorticoid therapy in varying dosages, as mandated by symptoms or signs, at the time of their evaluation for stereotaxis and brachytherapy.

The two instances of what was essentially a panhemispheric lesion were included in the group with the understanding that biopsy confirmation of the pathologic process—not great expectations from brachytherapy—was the reason for their inclusion. One of these patients died 6 weeks later, the other remains alive but disabled by a dense hemiplegia.

Among the entire group, none of the astrocytoma patients had received chemotherapy, although glucocorticoids were palliatively administered to three prior to evaluation for stereotaxis.

There were three patients with papilledema but none with impending or portended neurologic decompensation. In two of three patients in whom previous craniotomy had been performed several months earlier, it was the family's request not to entertain further surgical reduction of tumor bulk.

Our group of patients differs greatly from that reported by Guten et al. (2) in that their diagnoses do not represent end-stage central nervous system (CNS) disease and invariable failure of "in vogue" therapy, before being treated with brachytherapy.

Surgical Complications and Deaths

In view of hemopoietic suppression, infection ranks high as a complication of irradiation and chemotherapy. This applies to minor surgical procedures, e.g., burrhole placement for stereotaxis and brachytherapy (2). Fortunately, no instance of local or more extensive infection was encountered in our small group. Antibiotic prophylaxis was employed in all instances, and the exteriorized afterloading catheters were protected by an antibiotic ointment. Parenteral antibiotics were discontinued 1 day after retrieval of the implanted catheters.

Neurologic deficit was aggravated in one instance. Although usually parenchymal hemorrhage is caused by vessel laceration at the time of biopsy, we produced a 2.5-cm hematoma where no biopsy was taken—only an afterloading catheter was placed into a highly vascular tumor, resulting in aggravation of the neurologic deficit (case 19).

Because standard ventricular shunt catheters (Heyer-Schulte) have been employed in most instances, cerebritic infection has remained a concern—although none has yet been encountered. It is plausible that local ionizing radiation may be intense enough to hinder local bacterial replication.

Death was recorded in three instances, but in only one case was it due to a cerebral cause (case 16). This patient died at home 6 weeks after stereotactic biopsy of her lesion and having received 4,700 rads to the periphery of the frontotemporal mass. Additional teletherapy was deemed inadvisable in view of the patient's poor functional state.

The other two deaths comprised metastatic lesions. One patient died as a result of terminal pneumonia and respiratory compromise from spinal metastases, although ironically the recurrent occipital lesion disappeared within 3 months after brachytherapy (Figure 7–2).

The other patient's demise was heralded by aortic thrombosis, which caused paraplegia and ischemic gangrene of the entire left lower limb prior to death. At autopsy the brachytherapeutically treated temporal lobe lesion was almost entirely replaced by clot, commensurate with the patient's agonal alteration in the conscious state.

CT Findings After Brachytherapy

Computerized tomography (CT) of the brain has introduced a new dimension to the scrutiny of radiotherapy. In the past the greatest diagnostic reliance was placed on neurologic function. However, this parameter is now receiving serious competition from CT scans of the brain, even though this diagnostic modality raises as many questions as it solves.

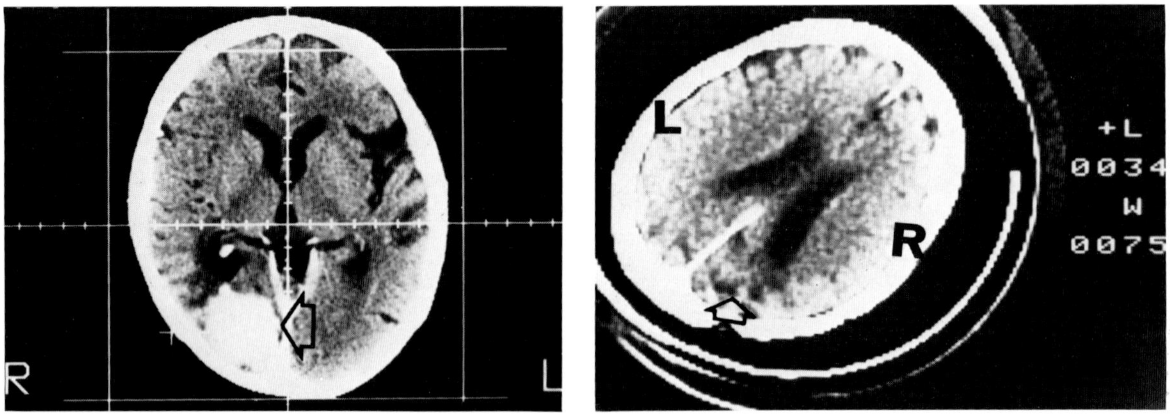

A B

Figure 7–2 Recurrent metastatic mass lesion from carcinoma of breast (Case 10 in Figure 1–1). The top CT scan shows a significant contrast enhanced mass (*open arrow*). The patient was a failure of tele and chemotherapy. The lower CT scan was obtained 3 months later. Note the resolution of the lesion after brachytherapy with Ir-192.

No prognostically favorable innuendo is offered here, only some clinical observations. Figure 7–3 illustrates that after brachytherapy to a metastatic lesion evidence of a residual lesion may completely disappear within a short time. Yet in other instances, a glioma is replaced 6 months later by a cystic, necrotic tumor residue (Figure 7–4). The low-grade astrocytomas remain hypodense silhouettes of their former selves at this point.

Commensurate with neurologic stabilization if not improvement, CT scans of nine patients showed a reduction in abnormality if not complete resolution. In one instance of metastatic disease complicated by

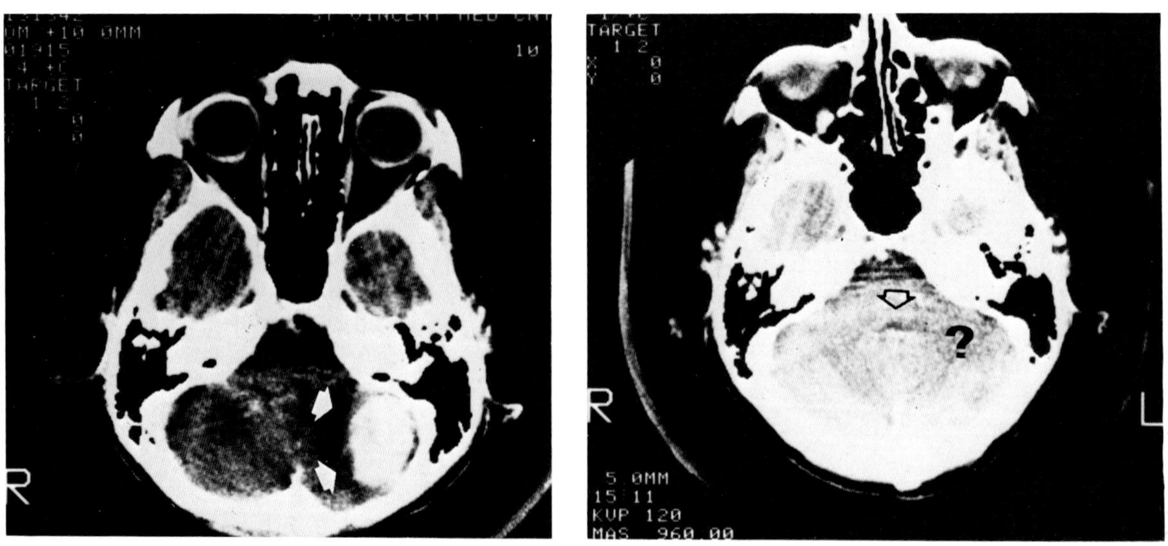

A B

Figure 7–3 Metastatic bronchogenic carcinoma is shown in the left cerebellopontine angle (*white arrows*). The lower CT scan was obtained 5 months later. There is no evidence of a posterior fossa mass and peri-tumoral edema has resolved. The 4th ventricle is located midline (*open arrow*) and the patient has had no ill-effects from 5000 rads delivered to the periphery of the lesion.

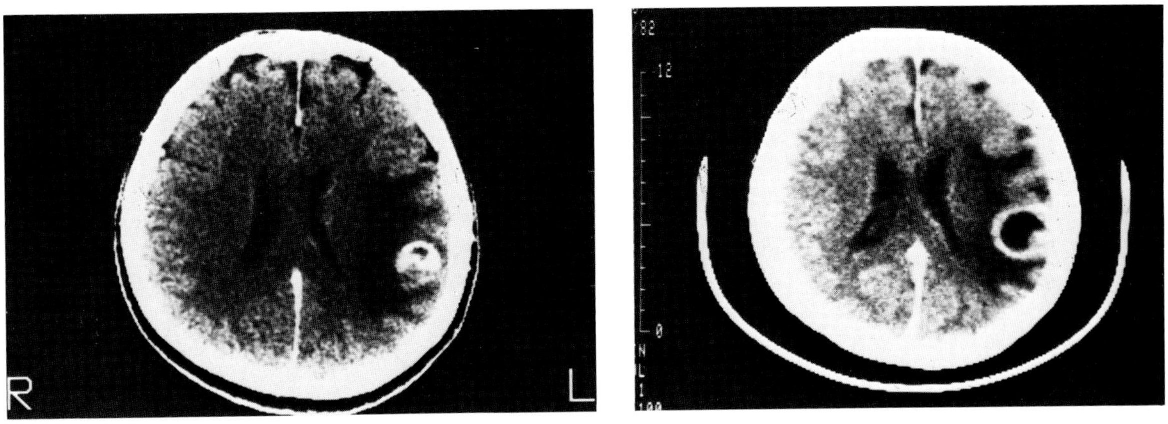

A B

Figure 7–4 Case 8: A 68-year-old woman presents with a progressive receptive aphasia. The top CT scan was obtained just prior to stereotaxic biopsy and brachytherapy. The bottom CT scan, 6 months later, shows no progression of the lesion and only a cystic radionecrotic mass.

the appearance of additional cerebral lesions, the originally interstitially treated lesion also showed enlargement 8 months after brachytherapy. Another patient with a frontal glioma manifested definite extension of the lesion across the corpus callosum 6 months later, although there was little neurologic change aside from steroid dependence.

Time is required to correlate the CT findings with the neuropathology. To date, CT findings of radionecrosis within a neoplasm cannot be confidently distinguished from residual tumor without biopsy corroboration.

What CT suggests in our small group of patients over a dismally short follow-up period is that interstitially irradiated tumors often become smaller or disappear; they seldom enlarge. This favors a longer symptomstatic interval and hence prolongs useful survival. Time will teach us more.

Conclusion

A small group of patients treated prospectively with brachytherapy are presented. Although the follow-up interval is short, the trend suggests that brachytherapy deserves further study. The optimism expressed by Mundinger (3,4), Szikla (7,8), and others (1,2) warrants careful scrutiny.

References

1. Bernstein M, Gutin PH: Interstitial irradiation of brain tumors: a review. Neurosurgery 9:741–750, 1981
2. Gutin PH, Phillips TL, Hosobushi Y, et al: Permanent and removable implants for brachytherapy of brain tumors. Int J Radiat Oncol Biol Phys 7:1371–1381, 1981
3. Mundinger F: Implantation of radioisotopes (curie-therapy). In: Stereotaxy of the Human Brain, edited by G Schaltenbrand, AE Walker. George Thieme Verlag, New York, 1982, pp 410–435
4. Mundinger F, Weigel K: Personal communication, November 1982

5. Scanlon PW, Taylor WF: Radiotherapy of intracranial astrocytomas: analysis of 417 cases treated from 1960 through 1969. Neurosurgery 5:301–307, 1979
6. Seiler R: Die Undifferenzierten Astrozytome des Grosshirns: Eine Übersicht der aktuellen Therapiemöglichkeiten. Springer-Verlag, New York, 1982, pp 13, 27
7. Szikla G (ed): Stereotactic Cerebral Irradiation (Proceedings of the INSERM Symposium on Stereotactic Irradiation). Elsevier-North Holland Biomedical Press, Amsterdam, 1979
8. Szikla G: Stereotactic Symposium, Buffalo, New York, May 1982

8 Radiotherapy of Brain Tumors

Armand Bouzaglou

Of the leading causes of death in the United States, cancer ranks second only to heart disease. Statistics reveal that 396,992 patients died of cancer in 1978. Of these cancers, 10,800 were listed as arising within the brain and central nervous system (CNS) (245). Incidence estimates based on rates from the National Cancer Institute (NCI) SEER program reveal that 855,000 invasive cancers will be seen in 1983 and of those 12,600 will arise in the brain and CNS (178).

A number of sources have revealed an autopsy incidence of primary brain tumors of 1–2% (215,217), of which approximately 50% are gliomas (48,115). Over 55% of gliomas are grade III–IV (Kernohan classification) lesions, and 20% are grade I–II. The incidence of brain tumors for all ages is estimated to be 4.2–5.4/100,000 population (124,178,245).

Even though these tumors remain localized to the cranial vault in the majority of cases, this has not led to a greater survival rate in the more aggressive lesions (72,137,179,238). The traditional treatment of gliomas is surgery followed by external beam irradiation. The extent of surgery depends primarily on the location of the tumor because this affects the surgical mortality (49,91,264). Gliomas arising in silent areas (e.g., the predominant frontal lobe) can be aggressively resected (202,275), whereas lesions localized to cortical areas (e.g., the motor strip and brainstem) may be able to tolerate only a biopsy (29,39,156,265). Even radical surgery (e.g., lobectomy or hemispherectomy) has led to disappointing results as these tumors show areas of "skip" dissemination or crossover by invading the corpus callosum.

Jelsma and Bucy (106,107) found that extensive resection, when feasible, doubled the 6-month survival rate compared to that after partial resection. Roth and Elvidge (211) reported an 11.5-month average survival in 236 patients undergoing extensive resection as compared to an 8.4-month survival in 163 patients undergoing partial resection only. More recently, Weir (280) reported no substantial difference in survival rates in patients undergoing complete versus partial removal.

Series of untreated gliomas are difficult to find. However, Ley et al. (137) in 1962 reported on 39 patients who did not undergo surgery because of poor medical risks; 90% of their patients died within 6 months of onset of their symptoms. Frankel and German (72) in 1958 reviewed 219 patients with glioblastoma multiforme undergoing surgery alone and found a 30% 6-month survival rate versus an 8% 1-year survival rate. Walker et al. (274) in 1978 reported a 3% 1-year survival rate in patients undergoing surgery alone and a 16% survival rate at 6 months.

The role of surgery has come under considerable scrutiny. In an earlier series an operative mortality rate of 20–40% was reported for the presteroid era decreasing to the present level of 1–3% during the poststeroid era. Indeed, what is the actual benefit of surgical intervention in these patients? Data from series of untreated patients reveal life expectancies of 2–4 months (137,263,264).

Apart from the immediate relief of dangerous intracranial pressure, a debate remains as to the exact value of extensive surgery in the gliomas, particularly the high-grade lesions. The median survival after surgery alone was found to be 30 weeks in a recent review by Yung et al. (287) and 14 weeks in the series by Walker et al. (276).

These observations are not meant to belittle the considerable advances made in the neurosurgical treatment of brain tumors during the past few decades. They point out, however, that the prognosis in these tumors is greatly dependent on multiple variables, e.g., the age of the patient, the location of the tumor, the initial performance status (112), and finally the tumor's histopathologic grade (Table 8–1).

Teletherapy

Technique

It is an undeniable fact that postoperative irradiation definitely improves the survival rate in gliomas (1,2,47,61,66,67,105,190,197). The cooperative clinical trial reported by Walker et al. (274) revealed an increased median survival of 150% in patients undergoing irradiation. The effectiveness of radiation therapy in primary brain tumors can no longer be discounted. There is now a wealth of reports in the literature regarding its effectiveness in brain tumors (106,203,204,211,226,228,243,248,261). The major radiotherapeutic technique in the United States until recently has been the use of external beam irradiation with beam energies in the range of less than 1 MeV. Most of these beams were in the range of 250–300 KVP. These were the standard by which all external radiation treatment was evaluated for many years. They were soon replaced by megavoltage units starting with the cobalt-60 machine and followed by the linear accelerator. The range of energy of these machines varies between 1.3 MeV gamma rays for cobalt-60 to 4–20 MeV x-rays for the

Table 8–1 Karnofsky Performance Status Scale

Condition	%
Normal; no complaints, no evidence of disease	100
Able to carry on normal activity; minor signs or symptoms of disease	90
Normal activity with effort; some signs or symptoms of disease	80
Cares for self; unable to carry on normal activity or to do active work	70
Requires occasional assistance but is able to care for most personal needs	60
Requires considerable assistance and frequent medical care	50
Disabled, requires special care and assistance	40
Severely disabled; hospitalization indicated although death not imminent	30
Hospitalization necessary; very sick; active supportive treatment necessary	20
Moribund, fatal processes progressing rapidly	10
Dead	0

linear accelerator. These more energic beams allow the radiation oncologist more latitude in sparing the skin, delivering a greater dose to the tumor-bearing site. The critical difference between normal brain tissue and tumor lies in the relative radiosensitivity and repair of the two tissues.

The present approach to radiation therapy is based on the following principles:

1. The greater the radiation dose, the greater the likelihood that a large fraction of tumor cells will be destroyed or rendered unable to divide at the time of their reproduction.
2. There is a limit to the total dose that one is able to deliver with external radiation because of the large incidence of radionecrosis with doses greater than 6,000 rads.
3. There will still be an unpredictable number of tumors which do not respond even with maximal doses of external radiation.

Obviously, it is impossible to irradiate an intracranial tumor effectively without at the same time irradiating the adjacent normal brain tissues. The relative radiobiologic tolerance of the latter areas varies considerably, and this may depend on a host of factors, ranging from their relative involvement by microscopic disease to their state of oxygenation.

Our discussion of external beam irradiation is not meant to be all-inclusive. However, suffice it to state that the effectiveness of these various beams depends on a number of factors, including the following: 1) The percentage depth dose, which depends primarily on the energy of the radiation, is important. 2) The skin-sparing effect of the supervoltage radiation is quite important in these patients as the whole scalp is within the treated field. 3) The importance of megavoltage radiation therapy in brain tumors is marked because the effect on bone absorption is minimized, leading to a reduced incidence of delayed necrosis.

The major steps in planning any course of teletherapy are as follows: 1) tumor localization and assessment of the volume of tissue to be irradiated; 2) selection of the radiation quality and treatment machine; 3) choice of treatment portals and beam-shaping devices; 4) choice of daily fraction dose and total tumor dose; and 5) evaluation of treatment dosimetry and calculation of daily treatment time. The first step in planning is the accurate localization of the tumor within the cranial cavity. Obviously, clinical data as well as diagnostic information have been obtained by the time the radiation oncologist evaluates the patient. The site and extent of the tumor is assessed from prior radioisotope scan(s), angiography, or computerized axial tomograms (CT scans). If the patient is seen postoperatively, the operative findings are to be added to the diagnostic ones. The histologic findings also determine the treatment portals and the total dose to be received by the tumor.

After the tumor has been located, an outline of the skull is made through the center of the tumor (Figures 8–1 and 8–2). This outline is then transferred on a sheet of paper, and vital structures taken from relevant atlases are drawn onto it. Once the treatment machine has been selected, most commonly a cobalt-60 beam unit or a linear accelerator, the choice of dose and dose-time relationship is decided on. Gliomas are fairly radioresistant tumors and as such require a minimum of 5,000 rads for adequate control. Two major factors limit the radiocurability of brain tumors: 1) the inherent radiosensitivity of the gliomas; and 2) the relative radiation tolerance of the supporting glial cells and vasculature within the surrounding normal brain tissue. The frontal, temporal, and occipital lobes seem to tolerate irradiation better than the spinal cord and brainstem (49,121,263,264). The radiotolerance of these various areas depends on the volume of tissue irradiated, the dose given, whether the brain tissue has been previously injured, and if any chemotherapeutic agents were given. Smaller fields, in general, can tolerate higher doses. (224) Because these tumors infiltrate widely into the surrounding brain tissue, large treatment fields are generally selected.

Megavoltage radiation is the most common modality used today. It has the advantages of a small penumbra, a short-treatment time because of the high output of these machines, and good percentage depth dose with better absorption of energy at greater depths. This is usually deliv-

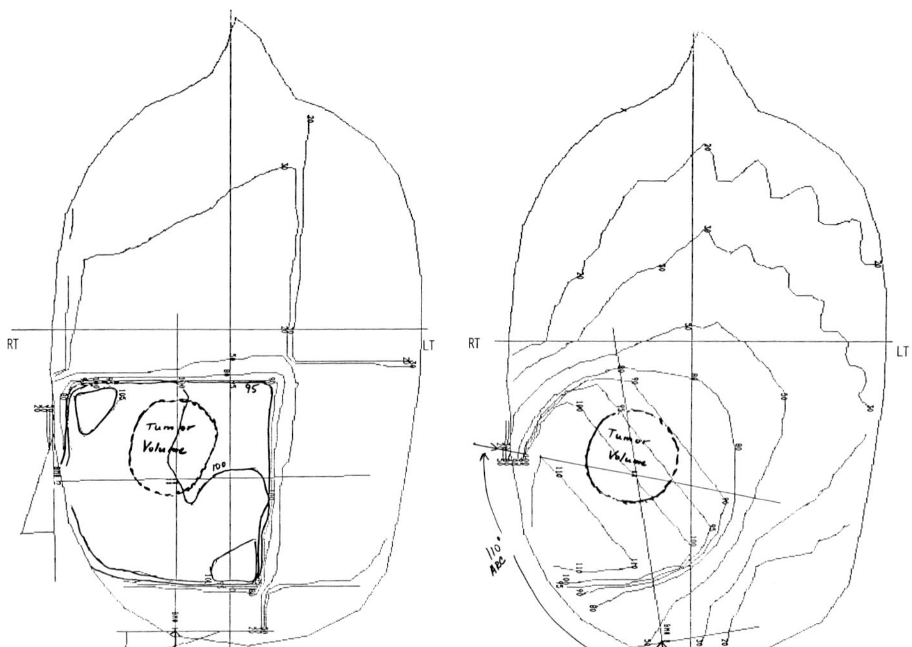

Figures 8–1 and **8–2** Outlines of a skull with the tumor localized (from CT scan data) prior to initiating external irradiation. Localization of tumor prior to therapy allows for precise and adequate dose distribution.

ered by parallel opposing lateral beams. It is then followed by a boost field to the area of the primary tumor with some margins added. Care is taken so that no "hot" or "cold" spots develop within the treatment field arrangement. The entire treatment volume must receive an adequate and uniform radiation dose. Because the skull has a curved surface, the incident radiation beam does not strike a flat surface. This presents a field obliquity, requiring a beam-shaping device to eliminate dosimetric distortions (Figure 8–3).

Results of Teletherapy—General Groupings

Extensive analysis of the result of external beam irradiation have been reported by Bouchard and his colleagues from the Montreal Neurological Institute (19–21). They irradiated incompletely resected gliomas (biopsy proved) in patients considered suitable for craniotomy and surgical removal and those presenting with tumor masses growing in the pons or brainstem. Bilaterally opposing field techniques were used in their patients with additional posterior or superior portals as required by the location of the tumor. A total of 449 patients were reported initially: 176 with glioblastomas, 123 with astrocytomas (grade I–II), and 40 with unclassified gliomas. The results revealed a 1-year survival rate of 44% in glioblastoma patients, 86% for those with astrocytomas, and 71% in patients with unclassified gliomas. The respective 3-year survival rates were as follows: 13%, 65%, and 48%. This is to be contrasted to the following 5-year survival rates of 7%, 52%, and 30% in each of those categories.

Various other authors have reported on their experience with these

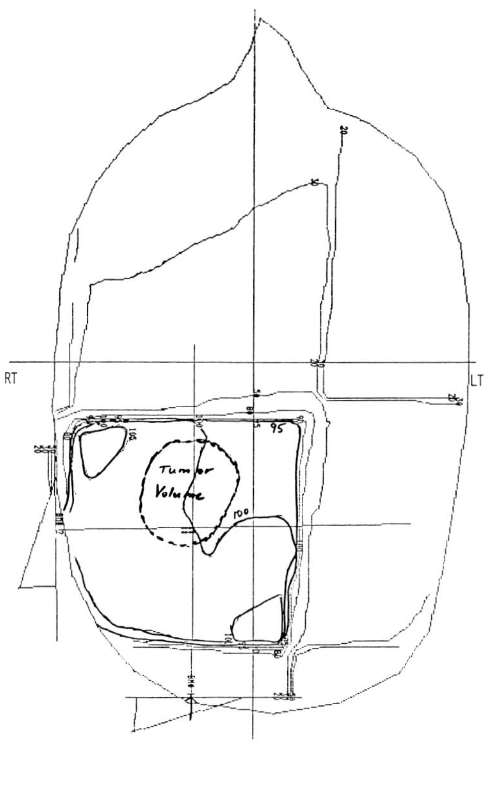

Figure 8–3 Right occipital lobe mass treated with 45° wedges. The tumor volume is delineated. All of the tumor is within the 95% isodose curve. No high-dose or low-dose areas appear within the treated volume.

tumors. Levy and Elvidge (136) reported on grade I–II gliomas. A 5-year survival rate was 26% in 42 patients treated by surgery alone compared to a 36% 5-year survival rate in patients undergoing surgery and irradiation. Kramer (119) in 1973 reported on grade III and IV gliomas receiving 6,000 rads to the whole brain and showed a 1-year survival rate of 35% versus 15% in grade III versus grade IV lesions with surgery and irradiation as compared to 22% and 0% at 5 years in patients with grade III versus grade IV lesions undergoing resection and irradiation, respectively. Stage and Stein (248) showed a 1-year survival rate of 14% versus 41% in patients undergoing surgery versus the combined modality as compared to a 2-year survival rate of 8% versus 6%. Most recently the Brain Tumor Study Group has shown that in patients receiving a minimum tumor dose of 5,000 rads of whole brain irradiation the median survival time was 40 weeks for patients undergoing irradiation and surgery versus 15 weeks for patients undergoing surgery alone (274).

Roth and Elvidge (211) reported on 100 patients undergoing surgery alone in glioblastoma multiforme. The 1- and 5-year survival rates were 14% and 2%, respectively. A group of 114 patients undergoing surgery and irradiation showed 35% and 6% 1-year and 5-year survival rates, respectively.

Shryver et al. (231) in 1976 reported on 48 patients with grade III and IV astrocytomas receiving surgery and irradiation. The 1- and 3-year survival rates were 44% and 33%, respectively.

Various techniques have been used to treat gliomas. The most common one is to irradiate the whole brain with a dose fraction of 150–200 rads/day to 5,000 rads in 5 weeks with a boost of 1,500–2,000 rads in 1.5–2 weeks to the tumor-bearing area. Large fields, including the middle cranial fossa, are favored because recurrence at the margin of smaller fields has been shown to occur with glioblastoma multiforme (221,266). Parallel opposed portals only or the three-portal technique are quite adequate for deep or centrally located tumors. Small and well-circumscribed tumors, more peripherally located, can be well suited for wedge filter pair arrangements (Figs. 8–4 and 8–5).

Most radiation therapists are in agreement that generous portals are required in the higher-grade lesions (19,20,43,136,222,224,240,278). However, the optimum dose required to fully control these tumors have not been fully established (150,222,223,278). Kramer et al. (122) postulated a 5% risk of brain damage with the above-mentioned regimen. Mundinger's data suggest an upper limit of 7,000 rads tumor dose to be delivered in 7 weeks.

Results of Teletherapy—By Tumor Grade

Grades III and IV

Sheline et al. (242) reported on selected data from the literature, analyzing the importance of the tumor grade of malignant gliomas to the survival rate. For prognostic purposes, they segregated the gliomas into three groups. Their first group included tumors classified as grade 3 astrocytomas, malignant astrocytomas, or anaplastic astrocytomas. The pooled data reviewed revealed a 1-year weighted average survival rate of 40% with postoperative irradiation versus 12% with resection alone. At 3 years the survival rate was 27% versus 7%, and by 5 years the corresponding figures were 16% versus 3%. The second group consisted of grade IV astrocytomas or glioblastoma multiforme. The pooled average

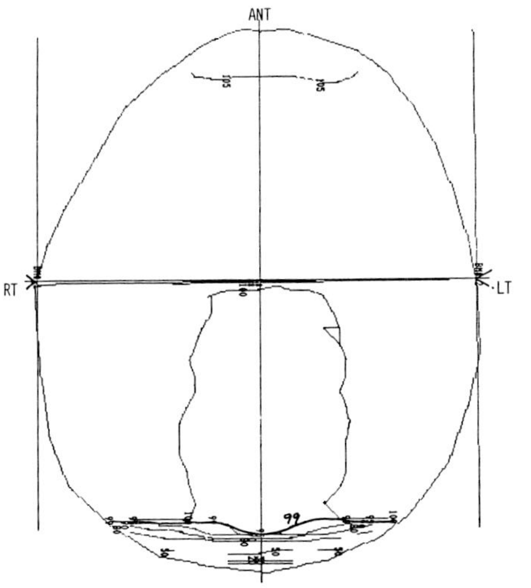

Figure 8–4 Whole brain irradiation. Right and left lateral portals are shown. The isodose curve is as expected from such a setup.

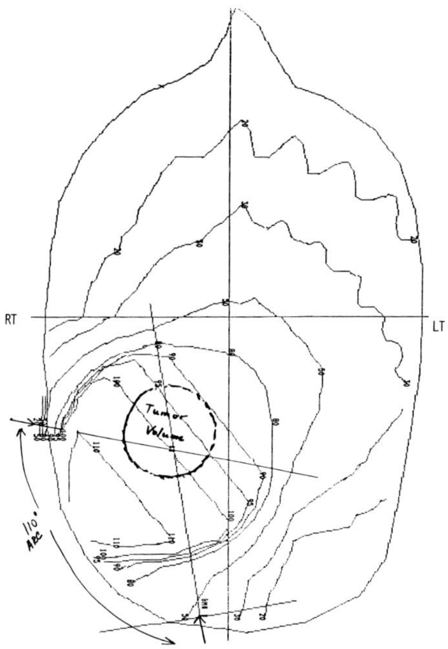

Figure 8–5 Right occipital tumor mass treated with a 110° arc. Most of the tumor volume is encompassed within the 90% isodose curve. There are no unacceptable high-dose (hot spots) or low-dose (cold spots) areas.

1-year survival rate was 24% in the combined group versus 8% in the resected group only. The respective figures at 3 years were 6% versus 0%. There were no survivors at 5 years in either group. The following studies delineate not only the prognostic evaluation in the various histologic groups but also attempt to describe the "ideal" time-dose-volume relationships in the treatment of gliomas.

Rutten et al. (218) reported on the results of postoperative irradiation in patients with grade II, III, and IV gliomas. A total of 142 patients were studied retrospectively; 74 patients had grade IV astrocytoma, 41 had grade III lesions, and 27 had grade II lesions. All patients had previously undergone partial tumor resection. Parallel opposing fields or wedge pairs were used to treat the majority of the patients with a midline dose of 4,000 rads (40 Gy) in 4 weeks with a boost of 1,000–1,500 rads to the site of the primary tumor through right-angled wedge fields or weighted parallel fields. The survival rate for patients with grade IV lesions was 33% at 1 year and 6.9% at 3 years. The 5-year survival rate for those with grade II lesions was 44%, and 26% for those with grade III lesions. Of the grade IV patients, 79% had a Karnofsky scale greater than 70, whereas 95% and 80% of the grade II and III patients had a Karnofsky scale of more than 70.

The results of this study (218) indicate that postoperative radiation therapy improves the survival rate for patients with incompletely resected intracranial gliomas. In addition, Rutten et al. recommend that in view of these results grade II, III, and IV gliomas should be analyzed separately in regard to their prognosis after therapy. Their recommendations have been repeatedly reasserted in other series, i.e., that histologic grade is the most important prognostic factor and that grade III gliomas are associated with a better survival rate than grade IV lesions when postoperative irradiation is undertaken.

Walker et al. (278) analyzed the dose-effect relationship in malignant gliomas. A total of 621 patients gathered from three successive protocols between 1966 and 1975 were the source of their data. Doses ranging from less than 4,500 rads up to 6,000 rads were utilized in those studies. The entire cranial contents were irradiated through parallel opposing lateral portals at daily midplane doses of 170–200 rads. The great majority of their patients (86%) had a diagnosis of glioblastoma multiforme. The initial performance status (Karnofsky) was close to 70. A direct relationship between doses of 5,000–6,000 rads and an increased survival rate was found in those patients. A median survival of 18 weeks was found in patients not undergoing radiation therapy compared to 13.5, 28.0, 36, and 42 weeks for patients receiving less than 4,500, 5,000, 5,500, and 6,000 rads, respectively. Whether this dose-effect relationship holds true for grade III gliomas remains to be seen as most of their patients clearly had grade IV lesions.

Salazar et al. (224) reported on 28 patients with glioblastoma multiforme receiving high-dose radiation at greater than 6,000 rads (median tumor dose of 7,000 rads). There were more survivors at 1 year (64% versus 46%) with this high-dose regimen than with those given a standard dose of 5,000–6,000 rads. The median survival of 50 weeks in the high-dose group contrasts with the 34 weeks' survival in the standard-dose group.

Five autopsies were performed among the high-dose group of 18 patients. No gross evidence of necrosis was observed from 5 to 54 months in those patients. Microscopic studies to evaluate vascular and neuronal changes were not described, however. Of significance is the fact that all patients had recurrence of their tumors even with doses of 6,000–8,000 rads.

Salazar et al. (222) took the dose-effect analysis relationship a step further when in 1979 they reported on 41 patients with grade III tumors and 59 patients with grade IV tumors receing 5,000 rads or more postoperatively. They divided their patients into four groups: 28 patients received doses of 7,000–8,000 rads, 27 patients received doses of 5,000–6,500 rads, and 34 patients received more conventional doses of 5,000–5,500 rads.

The median survival rate in 22 patients with grade IV lesions receiving more than 7,000 rads was 56 weeks; it was 42 weeks in 15 patients receiving up to 6,500 rads and 30 weeks in 16 patients receiving up to 5,500 rads. These differences disappeared at 2 years, when the survival curves became similar for all dose groups.

The survival rate per dose group with grade III lesions was found to be 204 weeks in patients receiving more than 7,000 rads, 82 weeks in patients receiving up to 6,500 rads, and 43 weeks in patients receiving up to 5,500 rads, again with a disappearance of these differences at 4 years. By 19 months 90% of recurrences were detected in the grade IV lesions; this is in contrast to a value of 80% at 3.5 years for grade III lesions.

Salazar et al. concluded that doses as high as 8,000 rads were unable to "cure" more patients with the grade IV gliomas. Furthermore, 93% (26/28) of patients showed recurrence of their lesions with demonstrable viable tumor cells in 10 of those patients who underwent an autopsy. Necrosis was seen at the periphery of recurrent tumors in their patients and included vascular changes, e.g., thickening and hyalinization, as well as homogenization and necrosis of blood vessel walls. The parenchyma showed evidence of local areas of hemorrhage, coagulation necrosis, reactive glioma, and local areas of demyelinization.

In view of these findings, these authors acknowledged that use of very high doses should be explored only in younger patients with grade III lesions in whom a sustained and significant increase in median survival rate could be expected. However, they cautioned against a possible increase in radiation-induced normal brain necrosis, which would then negate the favorable effect of these high doses.

Walker et al. (271,276,277) reported on the Brain Tumor Study group analysis of a prospective, randomized study (BSTG 72–01) designed to compare radiation therapy alone, carmustine (BCNU) plus radiation, semustine (MeCCNU) alone, and semustine plus radiation. A total tumor dose of 6,000 rads with 170–200 rads daily fraction was delivered to the whole brain by parallel opposed portals using megavoltage equipment. A total of 467 patients were randomized to the above regimen, 84% of whom were classified as having glioblastoma multiforme and 10% as having malignant astrocytoma (grade III). A median initial performance status of 60% (Karnofsky scale) was obtained. The median survival in the MeCCNU group alone was 24 weeks, compared to 42 weeks in the MeCCNU plus postoperative irradiation group, 36 weeks in the radiotherapy group, and 51 weeks in the BCNU plus irradiation group. Their study supports the position that radiotherapy is beneficial in the treatment of malignant gliomas. The question of the efficacy of nitrosoureas in combination with radiation treatment in these lesions, however, could not be fully answered. Their statistical findings did not indicate a significant improvement over irradiation alone.

Grades I and II

Sheline et al. (239–241) described the survival rate data of relatively well differentiated astrocytomas (grades I and II) as reported by various authors. Bouchard (19) reported on 123 patients with grade I and II supratentorial astrocytomas located primarily in the frontal lobes in the great majority. Of the 105 patients evaluated for lesions at those sites, 49% survived 5 years and 64% survived 3 years. Their patients received 5,000–6,000 rads delivered with the use of cobalt-60 irradiation. They compared their results to those of 42 patients undergoing surgery alone, as reported by Levy and Elvidge (136), whose series showed a 3-year survival rate of 52% and a 5-year survival of 26%. Bouchard et al. concluded that supratentorial grade I and II astrocytomas respond best to surgical resection followed by external beam x-irradiation. This improvement in survival rate is best seen after the third year of treatment.

Fazekas (69) compared survival data of patients with grade I and II astrocytomas undergoing postresection irradiation with those undergoing partial resection alone. The majority of their patients (82% of 68 patients) had grade II lesions, the remaining 12 patients having grade I lesions. A 5-year survival rate of 41% was obtained in 32 patients undergoing partial resection with adjuvant irradiation; this is in contrast to a 13% 5-year survival rate in 15 patients undergoing partial excision alone. However, a 90% 5-year survival was found among patients with completely excised lesions. Of interest was the disappointing finding of a 20% 5-year survival rate in their 12 patients with grade I lesions, pointing out the necessity for adequate doses of radiation even in this subset. The 10-year survival data revealed a 28% rate in the combined modality group versus 25% in the resection-only group; this seems to indicate that the majority of these lesions are not cured by the treatment but are rather effectively palliated.

Leibel et al. (132) presented a retrospective review of 147 patients with low-grade astrocytomas treated at the University of California at San Francisco between 1942 and 1967. The astrocytomas were classified into fibrous (diffuse, pilocytic, gemistocytic) and protoplasmic groups. These tumors correspond to the Kernohan classification of astrocytomas grade I and II. The usual tumor dose after surgical resection was 5,000–5,500 rads delivered at 180 rads daily fraction. There were 108 patients with incompletely resected lesions, 71 of whom underwent postoperative irradiation. The 5-year survival rate for all patients treated with surgery alone was 41% compared to 46% for those undergoing surgery plus postoperative irradiation. However, for incompletely resected lesions these rates were 19% and 46%, respectively, at 5 years for the surgery group versus the surgery plus irradiation group. Six of their patients with incomplete resection and postoperative irradiation survived at 20 years.

Leibel et al. concluded that irradiation significantly delayed death and led to a greater survival rate. The most common tumor was the fibrillary type (91%). Of the tumors, 74% were considered to be grade I lesions and 26% grade II lesions. Because their series consisted predominantly of the fibrillary type of astrocytoma, it is notable that the 5-year survival rate in the irradiated patients was 50% compared to only 13% in the incompletely excised series. The increase in survival rate was also significant in both groups, with 5-year survival rates of 58% and 23% in the irradiated group with grade I and II lesions compared to 25% and 0%, respectively, in the surgery-only group.

Side Effects of Teletherapy

Of interest is the more recent analysis of the late results of therapy for high-grade astrocytomas by Seiler et al. (233–235). Fifty-one patients with Kernohan grades III and IV supratentorial astrocytomas were analyzed. Cobalt-60 irradiation was utilized to deliver a tumor dose of 5,000 rads to the whole brain after surgical excision. A boost dose was delivered to give a total dose of 6,800 rads. The median survival rate was 56 weeks for 20 patients undergoing irradiation and chemotherapy (CCNU, bleomycin, procarbazine) versus 51 weeks for 32 patients receiving postoperative radiation therapy alone. Fourteen of 51 patients (27%) were still alive 30 months postoperatively. However, six of the 14 long-term survivors showed a slowly deteriorating neurologic status consisting of a progressive psychoorganic syndrome and signs of increased intracranial pressure. Serial CT scans revealed evidence of cortical atrophy or hydrocephalus secondary to cerebral atrophy (Figures 8–4 through 8–6A,B, 8–7). Those changes were thought to be secondary to radiation damage potentiated by chemotherapy.

Marks and Gado (148) noted a lesser incidence of hydrocephalus as a result of cerebral atrophy in patients receiving less than whole-brain irradiation as determined by serial CT studies. They concluded that limited external beam irradiation to gliomas should be reevaluated. In the light of such extensive and comprehensive data, the next steps were to combine surgery and external beam irradiation with other modalities in the hope of further increasing the overall survival rate.

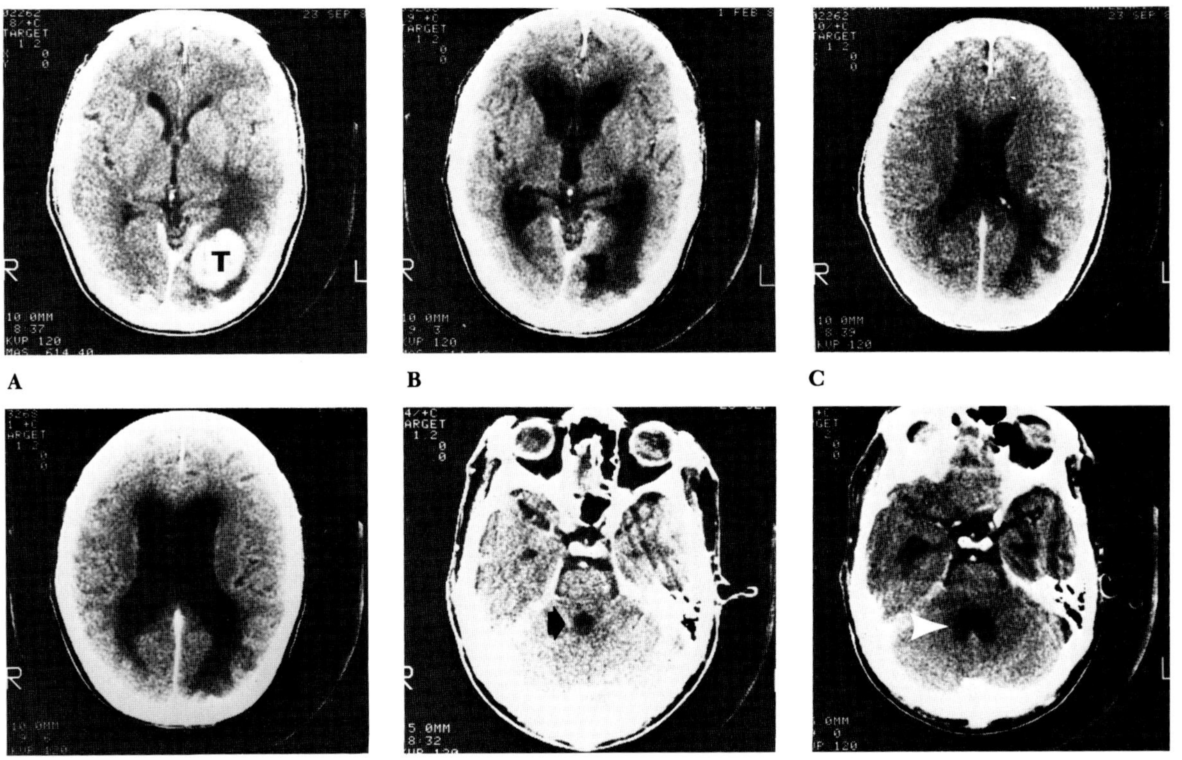

A B C D E F

Figure 8–6 Brain tolerance to teletherapy. **A:** Left occipital tumor mass, metastatic. Tumor stain has disappeared from September to February (a 5-month period). There is peritumoral edema. **B:** Bilateral ventricular enlargement is evident with white matter edema after a tumor dose of 3,000 rads in 10 fractions. **C:** Peritumoral edema over the left occipital area. **D:** Diminished brain density on CT scan, diminishing peritumor edema, and developing hydrocephalus consistent with an atrophic pattern. **E:** Edema in the left occipital white matter. **F:** Fourth ventricular enlargement from September to February occurred after a total tumor dose of 3,000 rads in 10 fractions.

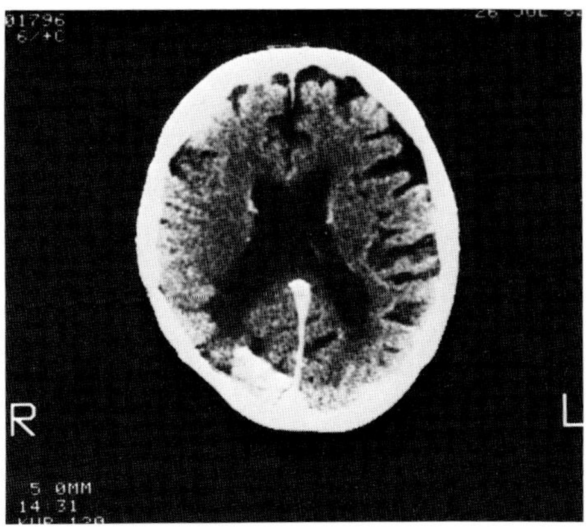

Figure 8–7 Ventricular enlargement (bilateral) and cortical atrophy associated with sulci enlargement in the left hemisphere after a course of external beam irradiation to a total tumor dose of 5,000 rads.

Other Investigational Approaches

Considerable efforts have been made by investigators to search for new avenues of approach. Optimal dose-response range and unconventional fractionations have been tried. These approaches, however, have not yielded definite improvement in terms of length of remission or tolerance in various studies (14,43,246,262). Radiosensitizers in various forms have also been tried. These include the nitrofuran derivatives, e.g., metronidazole and misonidazole (6,267), hyperbaric oxygenation (37,80), the halogenated thymidine analogues, e.g., 5-bromodeoxyuridine (BUdR) (55), and most recently hyperthermia. Unfortunately, no statistically significant conclusions could be drawn from these studies either. Finally high-LET (linear energy transfer) radiation in the form of fast neutrons and negative pi-mesons have been under way for the last few years (129). It is still too early to evaluate the data; furthermore, these techniques require highly complex and difficult-to-duplicate installations.

The particular dilemma confronting the physician in the treatment of gliomas consists of being able to deliver a high radiation dose to the tumor-bearing site while at the same time preserving the vitality of normal brain tissue. This dilemma has been resolved at other tumor sites where a large localized dose of radiation has been required for cure. This occurs with head and neck neoplasms where the combination of external radiation and interstitial implantation has led to greater local control rates while at the same time sparing normal tissue. This situation is repeated in prostatic, breast, and gynecologic implants as well.

Before we review the recent data on stereotactic brain implantation, a basic review of the radiation tolerance of brain tissue and the radiobiology of tumors in general and gliomas in particular is necessary.

Radiation Tolerance of Brain Tissue

The response of brain tissue to ionizing radiation has been extensively studied and described in a wide body of literature. The functional cell of the brain is the neuron. Because the biologic effects of radiation therapy depend on the mitotic death of proliferating cells and because the neuron is a nonproliferating cell, the efficacy of ionizing radiation may be secondary to its action on the vascular cell compartment and the supporting glial cells. Neurons are nonreverting postmitotic cells, and therefore a mechanism other than DNA-synthetic or mitosis-connected damage needs to be invoked. Moreover, it is difficult to assess early histopathologic effects of irradiation on CNS tissues because the direct injury response of the supporting tissues evolves over many weeks, and some of the symptoms may have been brought on by the neoplasm per se, as well as by the effects of surgical manipulation.

Acute Reaction

Most of the early responses to irradiation of brain tissues have been studied through the use of single nonclinical high-dose exposures in a variety of animals (32–34,40,104,121,122). This effect, however, probably does not apply to clinical doses of fractionated irradiation as delivered in a therapeutic setting.

Acute Reaction

An acute reaction in a nonclinical setting was reported by Quinlan and Michaelson (201). They delivered single doses in excess of 10,000 rads to a dog's whole brain, which led to immediate convulsions and death within 2 hr.

Gregersen et al. (82) also reported on single-dose exposure in dogs with doses ranging from 2,000 to 5,000 rads to the whole brain. Little change in water content or electrolyte balance was noted, implying that edema and increased water content of the brain as described in other studies are probably not caused by irradiation per se but probably result from an interplay of surgery, irradiation, and tumor.

After a single exposure of several thousand rads, as occurs in radiation accidents, there is a prompt clinical reaction, with a fatal outcome occurring within hours. The following events have been held responsible. A direct pathophysiological effect on all neural and glial elements leads to cystic liquefaction and cavitation. This acute response is essentially an autolytic response mediated by the release and activation of lysozomal enzymes. Microvascular damage also occurs, leading to endothelial swelling and increased permeability of the vessels. Perivascular edema develops with the transudation of protein-rich fluids. Finally, extravasation of leukocytes and erythrocytes occur with rupture of the vessels as a last event. Fibrinoid necrosis of the vessels is noted, and arterioles and small arteries become occluded with evidence of ischemic necrosis of large areas of parenchyma (288).

The clinical picture could then consist of drowsiness, listlessness, and apathy caused by nonbacterial inflammatory foci associated with vasculitis and encephalitis. These symptoms are then followed by generalized seizures and death.

The acute changes observed after conventional doses of radiation, however, are different from these extreme situations. Young et al. (286) gave whole-brain radiation using dose fractions of 750 rads. A complication rate of 49% was incurred in the high dose fractions compared to a more modest 15% complication incidence in patients receiving the more conventional dose fraction of 200 rads. Those complications consisted of nausea, vomiting and headaches and also more ominously cerebral herniation in 6 of thier patients.

Caveness and colleagues (32–35) demonstrated the dose-dependency effects on delayed cerebral changes in monkey brains. Single-dose fractions varying between 1,000 and 2,000 rads were delivered to monkey brain with increasing damage being inflicted with the larger fractions. The damage was expressed as cerebral edema, dilated ventricular systems, and scattered focal white matter lesions consisting of minute areas of necrosis, which later coalesced into larger zones of necrosis and ultimately showed confluent necrosis. Early delayed reactions in monkeys are usually transient and appear a few weeks to a few months after irradiation. This syndrome has been less well recognized in humans.

Transient Delayed Reaction

As early as 1934 Scholz and Hsu (230) recognized two phases of delayed radiation reactions of the CNS. Transient delayed reactions are known to occur within a few weeks to months after irradiation to the spinal cord. This has been described as Lhermitte's syndrome and consists of paresthesias on forward neck flexion, particularly in the lower extremities (109). Patchy foci of demyelination may appear within weeks to a few months after irradiation at therapeutic levels. These areas of demyelination are first seen in the white matter because of damage to the supporting glial cells. Axons degenerate with time and may indeed progress to necrosis. This syndrome has been associated with temporary demyelination of sensory neurons in the irradiated segments of the spinal cord (14,15,108).

Lampert and Davis (128) described similar intracranial processes in two patients. One patient, undergoing orthovoltage irradiation for a carcinoma of the tonsil, died 3 months after treatment. Autopsy findings revealed areas of punched-out demyelination in the lower pons and upper medulla with pronounced microglial and astrocytic proliferation. Similar findings were described in the second patient. Druckmann et al. (57) also described a transient syndrome consisting of somnolence within 6–8 weeks after irradiation in 3% of children treated for trichophytosis of the scalp.

Boldrey and Sheline (18) reported on the appearance of transient symptoms during the first 10 weeks after completion of external irradiation. The symptoms consisted of lassitude, drowsiness, difficulty in reading, and increased seizure frequency, as well as nystagmus, vertigo, ataxia, nausea, vomiting, and headaches. These side effects appeared with tumor doses in the clinical range of 5,000 rads.

Late Delayed Reaction

Of a more sinister impact is the late delayed reaction (10,24,53,-58,68,79,86,142,146,149,155,268,269). This occurs several months to years after the initial exposure to radiation. Numerous cases have been reported in the world literature (15,16,27,120–122,138,139,195). Sheline et al. (239,241,244) reported on more than 100 cases in the literature. The incidence of a late delayed reaction among irradiated patients ranges from 0.5% to 25% (54). Cerebral radionecrosis occurred in patients treated not only for brain tumors but also for pituitary lesions (adenomas, craniopharyngiomas) and skin cancer. It appears that in the majority of cases these reactions are progressive, dose-related, and irreversible, leading to a fatal outcome (244). The hypothalamus and white matter are more radiosensitive than the cortical areas (52,126).

The pathology of late radiation effects depends mainly on the severity of the vascular damage. Zonal ischemia with progressive demyelination and necrosis occurs secondary to this compromised vascular barrier with separation of the brain parenchyma from the vessels. A zone of well-demarcated focus of central necrosis associated with a zone of demyelination with astrocytic and microglial proliferation is the final pathway. During this chronic phase the above-mentioned changes extend beyond the field of irradiation (138).

In 1972 Kramer et al. (122) discussed 57 cases of biopsy-documented brain necrosis. In only five cases did the tumor dose consist of less than 7,000 rads. The time interval to onset of symptoms peaked between 1 and 3 years after irradiation.

Marks et al. (147) in 1981 reported on seven of 139 patients who received 4,500 rads or more total dose treated with 4 MeV x-rays. All of these patients had pathologically demonstrated evidence of necrosis, four without residual tumor and three with minimal residual tumor. The median time to the development of necrosis was 14 months, with the risk of necrosis increasing from 1,630 to 1,730 normal standard dose (NSD). The NSD was calculated as follows: total dose = NSD $\times N^{24} \times T^{11}$ where N is the number of fractions and T is the time in days. In their analysis a threshold dose of 5,400 rads in 30 fractions over 42 days was not found to be associated with radionecrosis in the brain (64,186) (Figure 8–8).

Mundinger et al. (165,167,172,173) reported a necrosis incidence of 4% for their irradiated population of 259 patients (10 patients). With the advent of stereotactic biopsy of these lesions, this rate may increase because these patients can now be evaluated sooner.

Burger et al. (27) in 1979 evaluated a series of 25 patients with malignant glioma treated by various modalities (MeCCNU, external irradiation, and nitrosoureas). Five patients received chemotherapy alone, six patients external radiation alone (3,600–6,000 rads), 14 patients radiation and chemotherapy or high-dose steroids. The findings indicated evidence of extensive coagulation necrosis of both vessels and parenchyma in the irradiated patients. The white matter surrounding the tumor bed frequently contained vessels with fibrinoid necrosis as well as perivascular pallor and chronic inflammation. This finding continues to confirm the known predilection of radionecrosis for white matter. They also found astrogliosis and demyelinization in the degenerated white matter. There were four cases of radiation necrosis among 17 patients who received 5,000–6,000 rads. Radiation necrosis is difficult to diagnose clinically premortem because it can mimic recurrent neoplasm clinically as well as radiologically, as determined by CT scan or brain scan. Stereotactic biopsy may be necessary for its diagnosis. It is well known that cerebral edema may potentiate the effects of radiation. Because none of their patients receiving high-dose steroids developed radiation necrosis, their finding raises the possibility of protective effects by steroids against radiation necrosis possibly by stabilization of the basement membranes without activation of lysosomal enzymes.

Three of the four cases of radiation necrosis occurred in the combined-modality group (radiation plus chemotherapy). Severe reactive gliosis, spongiosis, and selective loss of myelin as well as multiple foci of coagulation necrosis were observed. Radiation effects resulted in extensive coagulation necrosis, vascular thickening, perivascular fibrosis, calcium deposition, fibrin exudation, telangiectasis, and perivascular chronic inflammatory cell deposits.

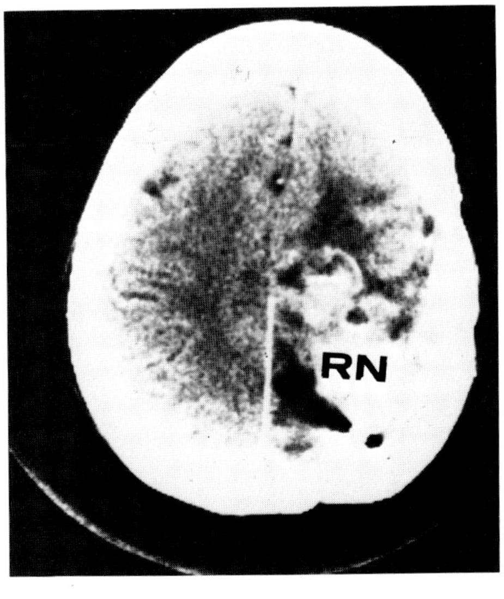

Figure 8–8 There is an increase in stain and white matter edema here with little mass effect consistent with radiation necrosis (*RN*).

Not only does radiation by itself cause the above-mentioned effects, but the combination of external irradiation and chemotherapy seems to potentiate them. Phillips and Fu (196) quantified those combined reactions. Their report deals mainly with the synergistic effect of methotrexate and irradiation. Leukoencephalopathy and necrotizing encephalopathy were described when methotrexate was combined with doses of radiation ranging from 2,400 to 6,000 rads.

Breuer et al. (22) described discrete, multifocal pontine lesions in patients receiving external beam irradiation to the whole brain in conjunction with methotrexate. These lesions consisted of loss of myelin and axons with multiple axonal swellings.

Burger et al. (27) reported on the morphologic effects of irradiation for intracranial gliomas. Two of their groups received chemotherapy plus external radiation. Conspicuous changes in the white matter consisted of extensive coagulative necrosis and telangiectasis. Four patients developed radiation necrosis of the brain surrounding the tumor site. Three of those patients received radiation plus chemotherapy. Although not fully indicative of a synergistic effect, these findings do suggest potentiation of the radiation effects by the chemotherapeutic agents.

Wilson et al. (276,284) reported on morphologic changes associated with combined BCNU and radiation therapy in patients with glioblastoma multiforme. Cell size, mitosis, and vascular alterations were described in three groups of patients: 1) six patients receiving BCNU plus radiation; 2) 11 patients undergoing irradiation; and 3) nine patients treated with surgery alone. A statistically significant increase in the incidence of giant and monstrous cells was found in the first two groups and particularly so in the subset of patients receiving both BCNU and radiation therapy. These data support the premise that the changes are secondary to therapy. However, some tumor cells apparently did not show any response to these regimens.

Radiobiology of Brain Tumors

Response of Microcirculation

The crucial assumption that the CNS is relatively resistant to irradiation has often led to the delivery of high doses to the entire brain. However, reports of radionecrosis appeared in the literature as early as 1945, and the vulnerability of brain tissues has actively studied since then. It seems from multiple pathologic analyses that the microcirculation is the primary site of radiation damage with secondary changes occurring in glial and neuronal elements.

The capillary endothelial cell particularly has been implicated as the basic target cell leading to delayed CNS damage by ionizing radiation (155,207). As more and more cells of the vascular compartment are damaged, the neuronal elements dependent on these endothelial cells lose their nutritional supply. With time, a pattern of vascular and parenchymal changes develop consistent with a picture of radiation necrosis. However, there remains a dearth of information regarding these vascular changes at the ultrastructural level. Llena et al. (141) and Matsumura et al. (154) described widened perivascular spaces containing a variety of abnormal material ranging from fibrin, collagen fibers, and plasma. Endothelial cell proliferations with increased cytoplasmic organelles and intraluminal unfoldings were observed.

Glial cells and vascular endothelium replicate slowly. For such a cell renewal system, radiation injury is a function of the total radiation dose as well as the fraction size and duration of treatment.

Cell Survival Curves

The clinical changes described rest on an extensive foundation of cellular radiobiology. This foundation begins with the important body of literature describing the cell survival curves. The latter have been reported on numerous cell lines, the most common being HeLa cells derived from a human cervical carcinoma line, mouse L-cells derived from mouse connective tissue, hamster cell lines from lung or ovary of a newborn Chinese hamster, and kidney cells of human origin (8,42,-63,198) (Figure 8–9). The important characteristics of a radiation cell survival curve consist of two parameters: 1) the slope of the straight portion of the curve (D_o), indicating the radiosensitivity of the cell population; and 2) the extrapolation number (N). D_o is defined as the dose required to reduce the tumor cell population by a factor of 0.37 or $1/E$. N is defined as the point at which the straight portion of the curve,

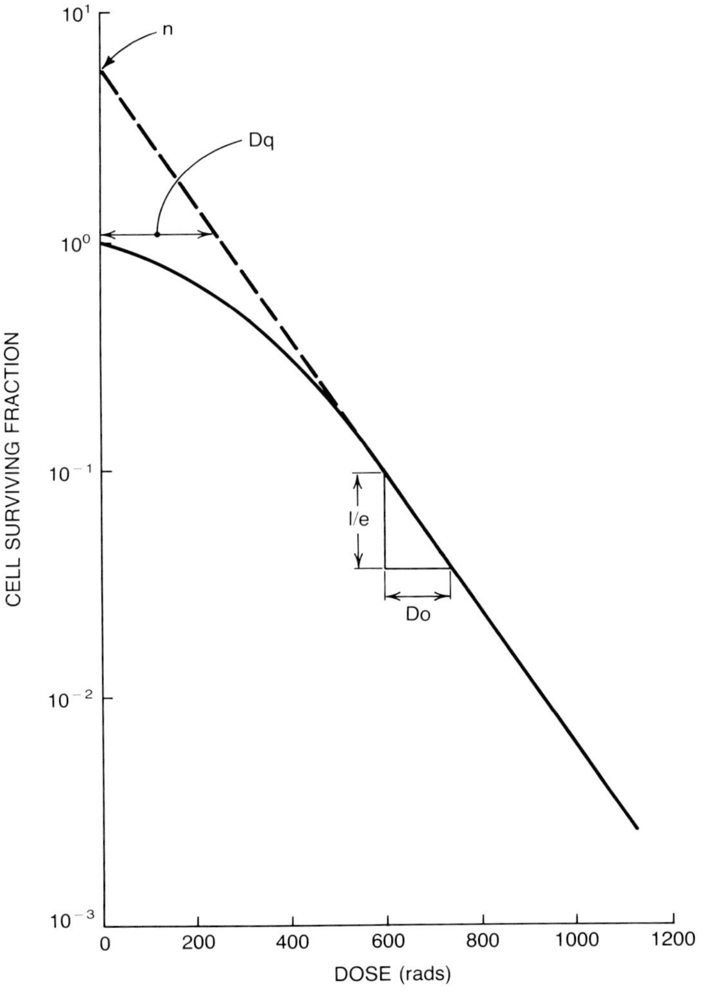

Figure 8–9 Typical survival curve for a mammalian cell exposed to radiation. Dose is plotted on a linear scale. The fraction of surviving cells is plotted on a logarithmic scale. Radiosensitivity is described by D_o, the slope of the final straight portion of the curve. D_q is a measure of the extent of repair of sublethal damage. N is also a measure of the extent of the initial shoulder D_q. All three parameters are related by the following equation: loge $N = D_q/D_o$.

when extrapolated back to zero, intersects the surviving fraction axis. This number N is a measure of the extent of the initial shoulder found in these curves. The shoulder can also be described by the quasithreshold dose D_q, which is the dose at which the extrapolated straight portion of the dose-response curve intersects the dose axis. D_q is also a measure of the dose lost when the radiation exposure is divided into two fractions separated by a time interval. The two dose fractions, however, are not as effective as the sum of the doses delivered in a single fraction.

Cell survival studies in brain tumors have been reported by Rosenblum et al. (212), including one in which a rapidly growing transplanted rat astrocytoma was treated with BCNU. At the LD_{10} dose, the cell survival decreased to a value of 10^{-3}. This type of study is important for demonstrating that cell survival data can be measured in experimental brain tumors.

Dose Rate Effect

A body of experimental data has also shed a good deal of information on what is commonly referred to as the four Rs of radiobiology: 1) repair of sublethal damage; 2) redistribution of cells within the cell cycle; 3) repopulation of cells following a treatment; and 4) reoxygenation. *Repair* of sublethal damage was extensively described by Elkind and co-workers (63,63). This concept describes the decreased effectiveness of a radiation dose when delivered in multiple fractions rather than as a single exposure. This occurs because sublethal damage may be repaired during the interval between fractions so long as the time interval exceeds 6 hr (251). *Redistribution* refers to the rearrangement of the surviving cells in various phases of the mitotic cycle. Irradiation of a typical mixed population with individual cells at the stages of the generation cycle tends to synchronize the whole population. *Repopulation* describes the process of repeated division of surviving cells necessary to repair cell losses. *Reoxygenation* describes the process by which hypoxic cells become oxygenated after a dose of radiation.

A wide range of radiation dose rates has been employed in clinical radiotherapy, ranging from high dose rates of 1,000 rads/min to 10–20 rads/hr (25,84). Brachytherapy utilizes dose rates in the 30–200 rads/hr range. Continuous low-dose irradiation as delivered by brachytherapy is thought to represent a situation of an infinite number of small fractions. It is a well known fact in clinical radiotherapy that normal cells need to repair themselves in order for the patient to withstand a treatment regimen. This is accomplished by delivering a series of fractions. However, tumor cells given sublethal doses are damaged but not killed and may then be able to repair themselves. The width of the shoulder (D_q) of the survival curves represents this amount of sublethal repair damage, which varies with the type of radiation used and the level of hypoxia. Multifraction regimens allow for a greater cell kill of tumors because hypoxia does not protect these cells.

The principal dose rate effect in clinical radiotherapy occurs between 1 and 100 rads/min. However, as the dose rate is reduced, more and more sublethal damage may be repaired. At a dose below 1 rad/min, all sublethal damage is repaired and the cell-killing effect is due only to nonrepairable damage, and this level becomes a function of dose per cell cycle.

The usual dose rates in brachytherapy are above 30 rads/hr, a dose rate sufficient to inhibit cell division. The dose rate effect in that range is strongly conditioned by the extent of repair of sublethal damage which takes place during the radiation exposure. The biologic effect on tumor cells varies quite rapidly within this dose-rate spectrum of 1–100 rads/min. This low dose rate effect leads to greater cell kill effectiveness in systems having a longer cell cycle time when continuous, low dose rate irradiation is delivered.

Cell Kinetics

Factors of importance in any tumor system include the following: 1) cell cycle time; 2) growth fraction; 3) cell loss fraction; and 4) potential and observed volume-doubling time (25,51,74,130,157,158,249,250).

The average time interval between successive cell divisions is called the cell cycle time. Because the only event which can easily be distinguished is the actual process of mitosis itself, a number of ingenious techniques have been devised to arrive at the cell cycle time. The method of autoradiography lies at the heart of these techniques (117,118). When growing cells are fed radioactive labeled thymidine, the DNA synthesis phase can be easily determined. The percentage-labeled mitosis technique can then be utilized in conjunction with a complex computer program to arrive at a mean cell cycle for a tumor population, as the latter is made up of cells with a wide range of cell cycle times (51,74,157,212). From a number of experiments, it seems that the cell cycle time of malignant cells is less than that of their normal counterparts and can vary from 10 to 60 hr.

The growth fraction in experimental animals seems to vary from 25% to 80%, indicating that few solid tumor systems consist entirely of proliferating cells (51,52).

Of importance also is the cell loss fraction. The overall growth of a solid tumor seems to be the balance between cell proliferation and cell loss. The cell loss factor is an expression of the loss of growth potential by the tumor. Various animal experimental data reveal this factor to range between 0% and 90% (74,249).

Potential doubling times of human tumors have been calculated from labeling indices. Steel reported values ranging from 1.5 days for a lymphosarcoma to 43 days for breast carcinoma (250). However, the volume doubling times as reported by various authors range between 40 and 105 days, with a median doubling time of 65 days. Labeling indices and potential doubling times have been carried out in human gliomas. Johnson et al. (108) in 1960 reported a labeling index of 0.6% in a high-grade lesion. *In vitro* studies by Kury and Carter (125) revealed labeling indices of 3.0% and 3.6% in high-grade lesions versus 2.0% in low-grade astrocytomas. Hoshino et al. (100–102) described 12 patients with brain tumors. Labeling indices of 5.0–10.0% were found in glioblastomas, compared to 1.0% in astrocytomas. As shown in other tumor systems, the duration of the DNA synthetic phase remained constant within a range of 7–10 hr. Derived values of potential doubling times of 7 days with a cell loss factor of 80.0–85.0% were obtained. Similar values have been described from other studies, as described by Steel (248,249), with potential doubling times of 10 days in glioblastomas and 36 days in low-grade astrocytomas.

Data from Hoshino et al. (100–102) reveal that a glioma at the time of initial presentation may weigh 50–100 g and may contain approximately 10^{11} cells. For nongliomatous tumors in an adult human, the lethal amount of tumor is estimated to be 1 kg. However, because of the rather limited confines of the intracranial space and the usual amount of edema associated with a glioma, the lethal amount of tumor is more likely to be in the range of 100 g or more. It is believed that a long preclinical phase exists in all tumors prior to their diagnosis. Approximately 30 doubling times are needed to achieve a size of 1 g. From that point on, only six to seven more doublings are necessary before the patient succumbs to his tumor. Hence the importance of doubling times is increased in patients with gliomas.

Even though the above-mentioned concepts have a more theoretical than practical bent, they have shed a great deal of light on the radiation response of mammalian cells and possible ways to enhance this response. Brachytherapy has been an important tool in enhancing local control of tumor cells. The low dose rate irradiation is thought to be superior over the acute, protracted fractionations of teletherapy.

Brachytherapy

Radionuclides

Brachytherapy (*brachy* = short, *therapy* = treatment) is the therapeutic use of radioactive nuclides inserted close to a tumor. Brachytherapy came into being in 1901 when radium was inserted into a tumor by Danlos 3 years after the discovery of radium by Marie Sklodowska Curie (26). Various systems of dosimetry were developed over the next few years. Paterson and Parker (192) developed a system during the 1930s whereby a uniform dose ± 10% was achieved within the implanted area. At Presbyterian Hospital in New York Quimby (200) developed a system whereby the minimum dose on the surface on an implant instead was obtained. A varied number of radionuclides have been untilized in interstitial brachytherapy. The following are the most common: radium-226, cobalt-60, iridium-192, iodine-125, gold-198, cesium-137, and yttrium-90 (Table 8–2) (89,116,123,140,188).

We have been mainly interested in the use of iridium-192 and iodine-125 seeds. Iridium-192 seeds have a half-life of 74.2 days and gamma

Table 8–2 Radioisotopes Used in Brachytherapy

Isotope	Symbol	Gamma Energy (KeV)	Average Photon Energy (KeV)	Half-life
Radium-226	^{226}Ra	180–2,220	780	1,604 years
Cesium-137	^{137}Cs	660	660	30 years
Cobalt-60	^{60}Co	1,170–1,330	1,250	5.26 years
Tantalum-182	^{182}Ta	1,120–1,190	590	115 days
Iridium-192	^{192}Ir	300–610	350	74.2 days
Iodine-125	^{125}I	28–35	27	60.2 days
Radon	^{222}Rn	220–2,200	780	3.83 days
Gold-198	^{198}Au	410	410	2.7 days
Yttrium-90	^{90}Y	0	0	2.7 days

energies of 0.3–0.61 MeV. The theoretical advantages are as follows: They can be used for longer periods of time; they are ideally suited for a temporary, removable implant; and they are much more economical than similarly active iodine-125 seeds. Iodine-125 seeds, on the other hand, have a half-life of 60.2 days and a gamma energy of 28 KeV. The highly energetic seeds are quite expensive, a factor which has so far prevented us from using them in permanent implants. We have also dealt mainly with highly aggressive or recurrent tumors that require very intense, short-term irradiation. We believe that the iridium-192 seeds with their greater versatility are the better radionuclides in those situations.

Iridium seeds for implantation are obtained from Alpha Omega Services and consist of an extruded wire made up of a platinum and iridium matrix. This wire is surrounded by a platinum sheath with a wall thickness of 0.1 mm. The finished product has a diameter of 0.5 mm and a length of 3 mm.

Iridium has an atomic weight of 192.2, the result of naturally occurring iridium consisting of iridium-191 and iridium-193 in almost equal amounts. When natural iridium is sent to the reactor to collect neutrons, the radioactive products are iridium-192 and iridium-194. The seeds are therefore left at the reactor until the iridium-194 has gone through a sufficient number of its 18-hr half-lives to render it impotent.

Calibration of Sources and Dosimetry

On first calibration of these seeds, a two half-life curve is analyzed to determine the postreactor time necessary to negate the effect of iridium-194 contamination. It is generally agreed that the erroneous results of numerous iridium-192 calibration attempts may have stemmed from remnants of iridium-194 in the samples. Another possible source of calibration error may stem from the fact that some manufacturers of iridium-192 seeds encapsulate the wire case with 304 stainless steel. This material contains cobalt, manganese, phosphorus, and other trace elements. When these seeds are activated, not only do they produce iridium-192 and iridium-194 but a host of other nuclides including cobalt-60.

Iridium-192 has a complex decay scheme with gamma rays of 0.1–1.1 MeV arising from both β^- and V (E.C.) emissions. Lithium fluoride (TLD) was therefore selected as a medium for determining the clinical dose from these "iridium-192" seeds because of its energy independence over this range. An ion chamber calibrated by the U.S. National Bureau of Standards (NBS) for cobalt-60 is used to establish a calibration curve for the dose deposited in tissue as determined with TLD. The calibrated TLD is then used to determine the dose deposited in a phantom from a selected set of iridium-192 seeds. Because conversion from curies to milligrams radium equivalent (mg Ra eq) could not be agreed on (in the literature or otherwise), these seeds are assigned values of milligrams radium equivalent without regard to their activity in curies. Meisberger (158a) established that the dose deposited from iridium at increasing distances from the source can be modeled by a rather complex polynomial and is dependent on the combination of buildup and attenuation. His efforts were incorporated into the calculation of milligrams radium equivalent. The sources thus calibrated are then used to establish the calibration of a well type of ionization chamber, and an NBS-calibrated radium source is used to verify the constancy of that chamber.

Each batch of seeds returned to AOS from the reactor is polled by random selection and an analysis performed to determine the mean activity in milligrams radium equivalent, the standard deviation (SD), and the total spread of the sample. Typical results show that 1 SD varies about 5% from the mean, but that in an implant of more than 10 seeds the value of the total dose deposited varies by less than ± 3%. AOS verifies this accuracy by counting 10 individual seeds out of each batch shipped.

The dosimetry of an implant continues the tortuous trail in that the spatial position of each iridium-192 seed is determined from orthogonal x-rays. This, of course, requires corrections for magnification, which are accomplished with an ARS-1000 treatment planning computer. Having once established these positions as actual coordinates, the computer maps out two-dimensional grids and calculates the three-dimensional distance of each seed to each point on the grid. It then applies appropriate correction factors for distance and attenuation buildup to give the total dose to each point. These points then (up to 3,000) are further mapped to "connect the dots" that all give the same dose (87–89,130,140). These "isodose curves" are the basis for determining the length of time an implant must remain *in situ* to deliver a prescribed dose.

General Indications for Brachytherapy

Interstititial implantation at multiple sites has been utilized since the early 1920s. It has been shown to be well tolerated if excision of the tumor is to involve extensive dissection. Interstitial implantation permits a much higher dose to be delivered to the tumor site compared to that applied by external irradiation, while at the same time sparing the normal tissue from unnecessary ionizing radiation. The isodose curves show that with implantation the localization of the tumor dose is more precise, and its dose distribution can be easily patterned to an irregular tumor dose. A higher depth dose to the tumor bed can be delivered to the more hypoxic cells at the center of the tumor. It must also be remembered that for an interstitial implant a tumor dose means the minimum tumor dose because the dose is always greatly increased in the immediate vicinity of the radioactive seeds owing to the effects of the inverse square law.

Radionecrosis at the tumor site is not considered clinically significant because high local doses seem to be well tolerated. There are enough data in the literature, however, to suggest that extremely high doses of external beam radiation lead to radionecrosis if large volumes are treated. This limitation has been circumvented by using high-velocity nuclear particles employing the Bragg peak effect. However, the number of units capable of generating such particles is limited. A natural outgrowth of this dilemma has been the use of interstitial brachytherapy. Radioactive isotopes have been quite popular since the 1930s, but only recently has there been a resurgence of interest in implanting primary brain tumors. Computerized dosimetries can be calculated ahead of time in these patients and a tumor volume of interest predetermined. One could theoretically limit the radionecrotic effect to the tumor volume. By applying large enough doses (12,000–16,000 rads) to the center of the hypoxic tumor-bearing area, it is conceptionalized that the majority of those cells could be effectively destroyed. Because the centers of these tumors show poor vascularity and hypoxemic changes, a greater radioresistance is expected. A 50–100% increase in the radiation dose needs to be delivered to those cells. Mundinger and co-workers analyzed the radiotherapeutic difference between brachytherapy and permanent curietherapy (166,172). Less perifocal edema was detected with protracted long-term irradiation. A less oxygen-dependent effect with a reduced oxygen enhancement ratio (OER) is seen in those hypoxic cells. However, with brachycurietherapy (short-term irradiation), they theorized that a direct ionization effect with formation of short-lived intermediate products is the main reason for its effectiveness.

Interstitial brachytherapy has been combined with other modalities to good advantage. This includes implantation of the residual tumor volume after excisional surgery and combination of the implantation with external beam irradiation. The two main methods of interstitial brachytherapy consist of temporary or permanent implantation. For an implant to be "temporary" all the encapsulated radioactive sources are removed after the desired dose has been delivered. Permanent implants are those which are left implanted in the tissues permanently.

The advantages of a temporary implant include the possibility of better control of the distribution of the radioactive sources and of the total tumor dose delivered. This is to be contrasted to a permanent implant, where neither the dose nor the distribution can be changed after the initial insertion. The "afterloaded" technique is now utilized principally in temporary implants. A catheter is inserted into the tumor-bearing site at the time of surgery, and the radioactive material is then inserted ("afterloaded") after the patient returns to his or her room. One advantage here is the elimination of radiation exposure in the operating suite or the recovery room. Moreover, changes within the implanted site can be made at will because the operator is not working with radioactive materials; hence the position and accuracy of the implant is markedly enhanced.

Results of Brachytherapy

Early data from patients with brain implants were recorded by Talairach et al. (260) in 1961. They implanted isotopes into the tumor bed after surgical resection of the lesion. Klar et al. (116a) in 1959 had previously reported on the use of cobalt in the form of beads threaded on a string and left in place in the surgical bed. A prolonged postoperative survival was seen in their patients. However, this procedure utilized a loaded radioactive nuclide at the time of surgery and resulted in considerable exposure to all personnel. Cobalt-60 has a high-energy gamma radiation of 1.13–1.7 MeV. Its half-life is 5.3 years, and it therefore cannot be left in place as a permanent implant.

Sachs et al. (219,220) reported on the use of implanted gold radon seeds in patients with glioblastoma multiforme. They showed that a larger tumor dose could be delivered to the area of interest than that with external irradiation while at the same time sparing normal tissues. However, this free-hand technique was lacking in precision, as some of the seeds seem to migrate in brain tissue, accounting for areas of over- or underdosage.

Interstitial brachytherapy by stereotactic implantation of radioisotopes into brain tumors has been utilized since the early 1950s. Numerous head frames have been developed since the early description of the stereotactic apparatus of Horsley and Clarke used in animals in 1908. Spiegel et al. (247) described their technique in 1947. Since then the neurosurgical stereotactic literature abounds with advances and refinements of those devices. The commonest types in use today consist of the Leksell frame device (133–135), the target apparatus of Riechert (209), the Riechert-Mundinger modification (162,164,165,167,168,170), and the Talairach device (256–259).

Since the advent of computerized tomography during the early 1970s, the field of stereotactic neurosurgery has experienced a remarkable resurgence. Not only is the clinician able to accurately localize and delineate intracranial masses, but information regarding the nature of the contents of these lesions (whether solid or cystic) can be obtained and an exact volume determination prepared from the same data. The exact localization of one or multiple target points within these tumors can now be reproduced quite accurately in any plane. The accurate placement of radioisotopes within the tumor site is easily performed, allowing increased sparing of normal tissue. The stereotactic method allows the clinician the possibility of performing a stereotactic CT-guided biopsy for tissue diagnosis as well as the choice of aspiration and implantation of the lesion when appropriate. The field of stereotactic brain implantation continues to expand quite rapidly. However, this expansion has been aided by additional data collected during the 1950s.

Correll et al. (44) in 1961 reported on the use of iridium-192 seeds in a nylon ribbon with seed spacing of 1.0 cm in a patient with glioblastoma multiforme. A Patterson-Parker distribution was utilized with the ribbons spaced 1.0 cm apart. A tissue dose of 5,000–6,000 rads was delivered within 4–7 days. The authors also reported on the decrease in vascularity of a recurrent cerebellar hemangioblastoma with this technique. They were quite optimistic in regard to its potential in partially resected tumors.

Drake et al. (56) in 1963 used iridium-192 and cesium-137 in special applicators to deliver a minimum tumor dose of 5,000 rads within 2–5 days in nine patients with malignant gliomas. This special applicator was left in place in the cavity of the tumor at the time of surgery. Of the six patients they reported on, only one showed a prolonged useful life, a 17-year-old boy with a malignant astrocytoma. Pathologic analysis revealed recurrence of tumor in four of five patients, necrosis of residual tumor in all patients, and necrosis of surrounding normal tissue from radiation in three of the five. Degenerative changes were found in the white matter associated with evidence of reaction by astrocytes and histiocytes.

Doses of 10,000–58,000 roentgens at the surface and 2,500–7,200 roentgens at a depth of 2.5 cm were delivered. The white matter showed partial demyelinization with astrocytic gliosis. Fibrinoid necrosis of vessel walls with fibrin exudation into adjacent tissues was also discovered. This white matter necrosis was thought to be secondary to a delayed reaction caused by progressive ischemia related to alterations in the vasculature.

Chase et al. (38) in 1961 reported a 45-year-old man with a recurrent glioblastoma multiforme who had had an implant 10 days after resection. External radiotherapy had previously been delivered to the primary tumor to a tumor dose of 4,000 roentgens. Nylon ribbons, each containing eight iridium-192 seeds separated by 1 cm, were implanted at the time of craniotomy after resection of the tumor. A Patterson-Parker distribution of sources was utilized. A tumor dose of 6,000 rads was delivered. Obviously this was a preloaded application leading to a high radiation exposure of all medical personnel involved in the care of the patient. Partial return of neurologic function was described in their patient, although the patient expired 251 days after implantation. This was described in 1961 and helped stimulate further studies in the use of interstitial implantation of brain gliomas.

Rougie et al. (214) reported on 111 patients treated during 1978 and 1979. They adhered strictly to three guiding principles: 1) a surgical resection must be performed to debulk as much of the tumor burden as feasible; 2) a histologic diagnosis must be obtained either at the time of resection or by a stereotactic approach; and 3) all other prognostic factors (e.g., the grade of the lesion, age of the patient, and Karnofsky's status) must be taken into account (112). Eighty percent of their patients underwent stereotactic biopsies utilizing the apparatus developed by Talairach (257,260). The surgical indications comprised three subsets. The first group consisted of patients whose lesion could totally be excised as in the frontal lobe area. The second group consisted of patients clinically able to tolerate a biopsy only. Finally, the last group consisted of patients with lesions either localized too deeply or abutting against functional areas; those patients were subjected only to an interstitial stereotactic implantation. This procedure was performed for lesions less than or equal to 3.5 cm in diameter. If the diameter was greater than 3.5 cm, external beam irradiation alone was delivered. External beam irradiation was also delivered to the first two groups to a total tumor dose of 5,000 rads. Forty-six percent of their patients underwent a surgical resection; 26% underwent external beam irradiation only; and 20% underwent stereotactic interstitial irradiation. Overall the median survival rate was 34 months for patients with grade III astrocytoma who underwent surgery and external irradiation versus 15 months for patients with grade IV astrocytomas who underwent surgery plus external irradiation and/or interstitial implant plus chemotherapy (four cases).

Their experience is to be contrasted with that reported by Szikla et al. (253–255), who utilized the temporary interstitial implantation of iridium-192 wires. Their report includes also the experiences developed in Bordeaux, Grenoble, Rennes, and Marseille (11). Eleven patients with glioblastoma multiforme, whose lesions were greater than 5 cm in 70% of the cases, were analyzed. A second group of 28 patients with grade II–III gliomas with lesions measuring from less than 3 cm to 5 cm were also analyzed. Both groups tolerated the interstitial implant procedure quite well. The median survival rate in patients with grade IV lesions was 12.7 months. Of those with grade II–III gliomas, 70% showed stabilization of their disease for as long as 3 years after implantation. The immediate surgical morbidity was minimal and the late functional losses were low at the 3-year evaluation. Interstitial implantation was accompanied by successive biopsies which revealed evidence of involvement of the surrounding tissue beyond the area visualized on CT scans in some of their patients. Previously collected data seemed to indicate the appearance of radiation necrosis within the center of the lesion when doses of 6,000–7,000 rads were delivered. This late incidence of necrosis was seen at 1–2 years after implantation. Post-radiation edema was also noted, particularly in patients with lesser-grade lesions. A latent period of 6–

16 months is noted initially. This is then followed by cerebral edema lasting approximately 2–3 months, after which there is an atrophic retraction at the level of the lesion. These findings are negligible for lesions measuring less than 3 cm but become more important with lesions measuring over 5 cm. Finalized protocol, including the role of surgery and external beam irradiation in conjunction with interstitial implantation, are still being enunciated.

Mundinger and Riechert in 1962 (205) reported on the average survival of patients with a wide variety of tumors of the cerebral hemisphere treated by interstitial irradiation with various isotopes. They analyzed an initial series of 121 patients treated between 1954 and 1959. A 46.9% survival rate was found in this group compared to a 29.2% survival rate in patients undergoing surgery and external irradiation.

Serious disadvantages to the intraoperative technique of radionuclide implantation is the considerable radiation exposure to the medical staff within the operating room. For this reason, afterloaded applications were developed; moreover, in order to better localize the isotopes, interstitial stereotactic implantation was developed as described previously.

Scarabin et al. (229) described the advantages of stereotactic evaluation of 200 supratentorial brain tumors. Tissue diagnosis is easily obtained with such a technique. Localization of the lesion as well as its treatment, e.g., cyst evacuation and interstitial irradiation, can also be easily performed. Scarabin et al. described the case of a 12-year-old child with a right thalamic lesion whose cystic content was evacuated and biopsied. A diagnosis of pilocytic astrocytoma was made, followed by the insertion of four iridium-192 wires. A repeat CT scan at 6 months revealed regression of the lesion.

Kelly et al. (113,114) also reported on the stereotactic implantation of iridium-192. CT scan localization and stereotactic angiography were performed. A Todd-Wells stereotactic frame was utilized and serial biopsies taken. One patient was described in whom six iridium-192 wires were implanted into an oligodendroglioma. Personality changes and hemiparesis almost totally cleared at 2 months after implantation. This was associated with liquefaction of the tumor on CT scan.

Interstitial brachytherapy has been well described by Mundinger et al. (161–167,176). A recent review of their data (167) revealed a total of 983 patients who had undergone interstitial brachytherapy from 1952 through 1979. The majority of their patients received iridium-192 implants (488 patients); 267 patients with deep-seated midline tumors were stereotactically implanted with iridium-192 (173,174).

The initial series was difficult to evaluate because a multitude of brain tumors were analyzed as a group, and the grade of the astrocytomas was not clearly defined. However, in 66% of their patients, local neurologic destruction and mental disturbances were reported to have disappeared. Forty-eight patients with hemispheric tumors were analyzed. These authors believed that grade III–IV astrocytomas would require not only an iridium-192 implant but also external beam irradiation as a boost technique. In their hands, iodine-125 implants were used mainly for slow-growing tumors and pituitary adenomas.

Mundinger et al. favor interstitial implantation for the following reasons: 1) feasibility of the stereotactic implantation; 2) shortened hospitalization time; 3) shortened irradiation schedule; 4) good neurologic recovery; 5) good useful and productive function after the procedure; and 6) increased overall survival rate.

Stereotactic biopsy is also discussed in some of their articles (162,-163,167,171,176). The mortality rate has been 2.3%. A 95% positive correlation between paraffin-embedded material and smear preparations was obtained in 300 cases. Mundinger et al. have stereotactically implanted radioactive nuclides in over 1,200 patients since the 1950s. Survival rates were broken down by grade of glioma and are as follows: 19% 2-year survival rate with glioblastoma multiforme among 17 patients, and 47% 5-year survival rate among 34 patients with grade III astrocytoma.

An earlier evaluation of grade I and II gliomas in 108 patients undergoing iridium-192 implants was analyzed from 1965 to 1977. Three-year survival rates of 74% and 53% were found among patients with grade I and II astrocytomas, respectively. The corresponding 5-year survival rates were 63% and 32%. Deep midline tumors as well as hemispheral tumors were amenable to stereotactic implantation. A discussion of the dosages delivered include a tumor margin dose of 10,000–14,000 rads (100–140 GY) delivered with iridium-192 or iodine-125 seeds. In 65 patients with midline grade I and II gliomas, a 3-year survival rate of 63% and a 5-year survival rate of 46% were obtained. Forty percent of their patients with initial symptoms of seizure disorder remained free of attacks, and over 66% showed no neurologic deterioration.

Hosobuchi et al. (103) published a study of 10 patients undergoing stereotactic interstitial implantation with iridium-192 and gold-198. Seven of their 10 patients had tumor recurrence after previous therapy. A tumor dose of 4,000–12,000 rads was delivered to the tumor periphery. The Leksell stereotactic apparatus was utilized by their group. However, they performed a two-stage procedure by initially inserting a "dummy" copper seed into the center of the tumor. This was followed a few days later by insertion of the radionuclide seed. Seven of the 10 patients showed an initial response with tumor regression and neurologic improvement lasting 5–22 months.

This series was followed by a more recent analysis. Gutin et al. (83) reported on a total of 37 patients; 25 had recurrent primary gliomas refractory to previous therapy, and seven had evidence of solitary brain metastasis. Again, a Leksell stereotactic apparatus and a two-stage procedure were utilized. A total of 40 implants were performed, 16 of which were of the permanent type. Iridium-192, iodine-125, and gold-198 were the radionuclides used. A total dose of 4,000–12,000 rads was delivered to the periphery of the lesion. Of 35 evaluated patients, 17 responded for a period of time ranging from 4 to 37+ months. They concluded their study by stating that the final value of interstitial brachytherapy for brain tumor is still under evaluation.

Another interesting report by Mundinger and Hoefer (173) concerns small midline and deep-seated hemispheric gliomas traditionally not amenable to surgical intervention. They described a series of 98 patients with CT-delineated lesions stereotactically biopsied which received an iridium-192 permanent implant. The majority of these lesions were pilocytic grade I and II gliomas. A 90% improvement rate in neurologic and mental symptomatology was obtained. The mortality rate was less than 2% in their hands.

A more recent report on the use of the CT scan to allow for biopsy, aspiration, and assessment of operative results during surgery has been discussed by Lunsford et al. (143). They described the construction of a low-artifact frame as well as the development of computer software programs designed to develop data related to patient and stereotactic frame coordinates. Eleven patients with deep-seated midline intracranial lesions were described. Procedures ranging from brain tumor biopsies to cyst and abscess aspiration were performed without the development of any neurologic deficit. Instant data feedback was available with their integrated CT operative system. Not only were biopsies and aspirations feasible, but target confirmation as well as the immediate effect of the stereotactic surgical procedures were easily verified. A similar methodology has been utilized by our group.

Stereotactic Brachytherapy Technique

Localization of Target Points

Since the advent of computed tomography, brain lesions are being documented and detected with increasing regularity. It is now quite feasible to obtain the exact coordinates of such lesions (11,143). This enables the neurosurgeon to biopsy as well as evaluate such lesions. It has also aided in the exact placement of radioactive nuclide sources. A method for target points determination, based on Mundinger's technique, is presented here.

Patients are taken to the operating room where the Mundinger-Riechert base ring is inserted onto the patient's skull. The ring is secured by four screws to the skull, after which the patient is moved to the CT scanner suite. A GE 8800 head scanner is used in all of our stereotactic interstitial implantations. The base ring is secured in place at the head of the CT table where a special CT table adaptor apparatus has been installed. The ring is tightened into the table adaptor. Side lasers are used to line up the ring and the CT scanner. A reference point on the base ring is lined up with the same reference point of the CT scanner. The CT resident programs allow us to calculate stereotactic coordinates by obtaining a scout view CT scan in a frontal and sagittal plane. Multiple CT scans are obtained parallel to the stereotactic base ring. The reference slice lies at the reference plane of the stereotactic ring. A scan of 5 mm thickness is then obtained at zero location. This checks that the horizontal pins on the base ring located at 0° and 180° are really at grid zero. If the horizontal pins are seen to be superimposed on the grid, this confirms the center of the ring.

An abbreviated lateral scout view is then obtained to visualize the base ring only, confirming that the ring is perpendicular to the table top. A cursor is deposited at the zero point and another cursor at the center of the ring. The distance and the angulation are measured; the angulation should be 0°.

Scout scans are then performed because now the computer can accurately define all areas of the brain in the X, Y, and Z axes relative to the base ring. Below the top of the ring, the brain is poorly visualized because of artifacts created by the pins and the base ring. The scanning therefore is started at the level of the ring and every 5 mm cuts above it to the vertex.

Localization of the target point is then defined. The lowest and highest slices containing the tumor are determined. Depending on the thickness and length of the lesion, one or multiple target points can be obtained.

A grid is deposited over the lesion, and measurements are obtained with the use of depositing cursors. The X and Y coordinates and their numerical values are thus delineated. The Z coordinate is at the level of the slice being studied. Pictures of the slices with the above measurements are then gathered. The next step is to calculate the trephination point(s).

A reformatted sagittal image is now obtained at the level of a "center" slice. The target point is then located exactly on the sagittal image, and the cursor is moved to the estimated trephination point. All X, Y, and Z coordinates of the trephination point are then calculated and pictures again taken.

Target coordinates and trephination coordinates are then entered in the Mundinger/Birg software program of the TI-59 calculator, and the angles of entry are calculated. The values obtained are the depth of the needle of the biopsy forceps and the angular adjustment parameters. The target point is then duplicated on the test-phantom apparatus in the operating suite.

This phantom consists of a ring base with four ball-catch-secured legs inserting into the phantom ring. The phantom ring holds in place rulers in the X, Y, and Z coordinates. The target point is then located on the phantom ring, and the semicircular target arc is inserted into the phantom ring. The target arc describes a spherical shell by swinging around the X axis. The target arc angle is then set into place.

A segment arc is inserted through the center of the semicircular target arc and secured on the base ring. The segment arc angle is then also set in place. Finally, the electrode holder (all-round adjustable) vernier angles are adjusted to the previously obtained values (Figure 8–10). A guide cannula is then inserted into the guide and covering track of the electrode holder and advanced until it meets the target point.

In this fashion the target point is exactly localized prior to any manipulation on the patient. A small skin incision and burrhole are then made over the designated point on the patient's skull. All bleeding points are coagulated. The dura is entered and the whole apparatus dropped into place. An adjustable stop crank for the depth gauge is then placed in position and the stereotactic biopsy forceps is inserted through it into the guide tracks and through the dura toward the target site. The diameter of the biopsy forceps is 0.8 mm. The amount of the tissue sample

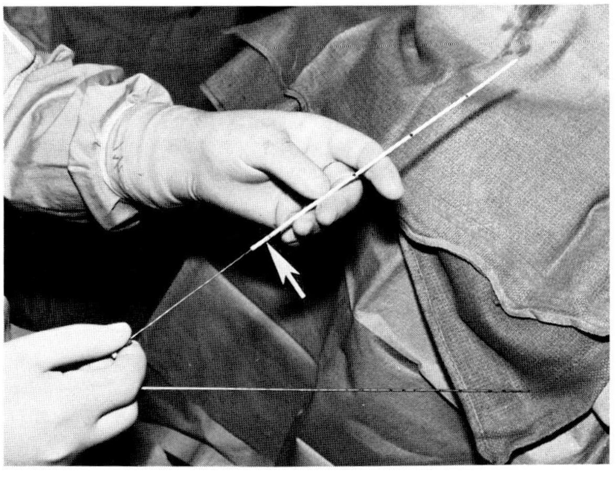

Figure 8–10 Standard CSF afterloading catheter with stylet in place and black markers visualized at 5-cm spacing.

consists of approximately 1 mm^3. Biopsies are carried out at successive levels 0.5–1.0 cm apart. Biopsies are taken above, into, and below the visualized lesions. The pathologist, who is present in the surgical suite, then instantly screens the obtained specimens. Permanent samples are also obtained at all levels.

A smear or squeeze preparation is made intraoperatively. An accurate diagnosis has been made by smear specimens in 85% of our cases (17/20 cases) on examination of the smear preparation. A definite diagnosis was made in 19 of our 20 patients (95%) when smeared and paraffin-mounted tissues were examined.

As soon as a diagnosis is obtained, the biopsy forceps is removed and an interstitial afterloaded catheter is left in place in the same biopsy tracks. A polyethylene catheter is pushed into this track with the help of a guiding cannula (Figures 8–11 and 8–12). This is fabricated from a silicone elastometer tubing rendered radiopaque by being impregnated with barium sulfate. Black markers made of graphite-impregnated silicone elastometer material are located at 5-cm intervals, acting in accurately localizing the depth of insertion of the catheter at the time of implantation. Multiple holes are located at the distal end of the catheter. This has allowed for drainage of cystic contents and bleeding sites. It also easily detects when the ventricular system has been entered, allowing for easy replacement of the catheter away from the ventricles (Figure 8–13).

A predetermined number of such catheters are left in place separated by a distance of 1.25–1.50 cm. The catheters are anchored to the patient's scalp and protected by a sterile clear "medicine cup" which allows for instantaneous visualization of the implanted site. They are then sutured to the scalp after the skin incision has been closed. The "dummy seeds" (consisting of inert alloy seeds mounted onto a plastic catheter) are then inserted inside the afterloaded catheter. Orthogonal films of the implanted site for dosimetry purposes are obtained and checked prior to sending the patient to the recovery room.

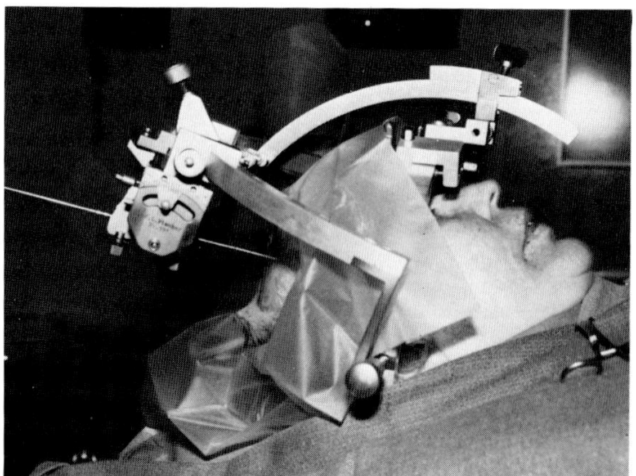

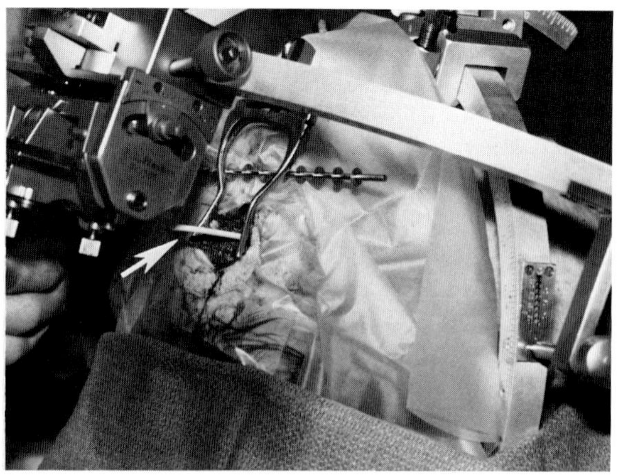

Figure 8–11 Mundinger frame in place. Biopsy forceps are being inserted into the intracranial contents while the patient is awake. Successive biopsies are obtained at 0.5-cm intervals.

Figure 8–12 In the operating suite an afterloaded catheter is being inserted (*arrow*) with the Mundinger frame in position. The magnification corkscrew is also in position.

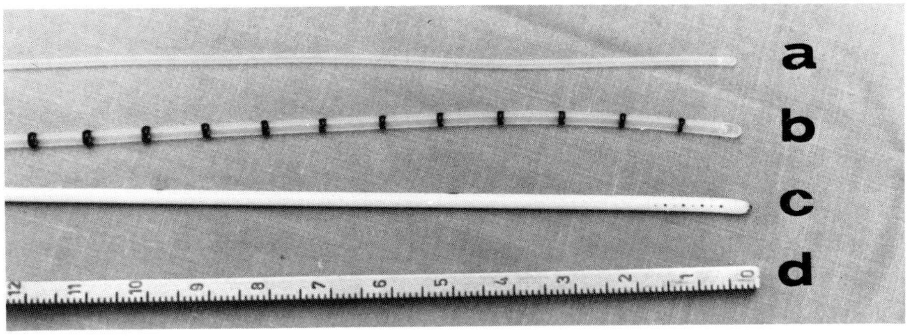

Figure 8–13 Afterloaded catheters. (*a*) Polyethelene hollow catheter with blunt end. (*b*) Modification of (*a*) with markers at 1-cm spacing. (*c*) CSF-ventricular catheter with the black markers at 5-cm spacing.

Dosimetry Calculations

As soon as a histologic diagnosis has been obtained, a therapeutic approach is formulated, taking into account the volume of tumor, the vital structures surrounding the area of interest, and the histologic grade of the tumor. From our extensive experience with interstitial implants at other organs (i.e., prostate, lung, breast, head and neck, and pancreas), a decision is reached as to the number of afterloaded catheters, length of iridium-192 ribbons, and the number and activity of iridium-192 seeds that will be required to deliver a minimum tumor dose of 5,000 rads to the periphery. Computer calculation of dose distribution is then performed after orthogonal films of the implanted site are obtained in the operating suite. We have employed iridium-192 exclusively as the radionuclide in all implanted patients. The reasons for selecting this isotope are multiple: 1) the greater technical availability of iridium-192 ribbons; 2) the lesser cost of iridium-192 seeds; 3) the use of permanent versus removable implants; 4) the greater technical flexibility of iridium-192 ribbons; 5) the longer half-life of iridium-192 (74.2 days versus 60.2 days for iodine-125); 6) the more energetic gamma rays from iridium-192 (0.3–0.61 MeV versus 0.028–0.035 MeV for iodine-125); 7) the half-layer in tissue of 6 cm for iridium-192 versus 2 cm for iodine-125.

The only advantages of iodine-125 seeds are the somewhat better protection of the hospital personnel and family members from radiation, as well as the theoretical advantage of continuous low-dose-rate irradiation obtained in permanent interstitial implantation.

The afterloaded catheter utilized has been a standard ventricular shunt catheter with side perforations allowing for egress of cerebrospinal fluid (CSF) tumor cyst, or blood leakage. These catheters have allowed for close scrutiny of the above fluids at the time of surgery. In one patient a biopsy led to a sudden surge of blood which stopped spontaneously after 2–3 min in a patient with a high-grade glioma. We have not seen any episodes of sepsis with the use of such catheters because the high-intensity radiation leads to local sterilization of the tissues. This particular fact had been determined previously at other implanted sites by the culture of such catheters before and after interstitial brachytherapy.

After the stereotactic biopsy and catheter insertion is completed, orthogonal x-ray films are obtained in the operation suite. The "dummy" ribbons are inserted into the afterloaded catheter. These ribbons consists of inactive radiopaque markers located 1 cm apart from one another. Radiographs taken at right angles, an anterior-posterior (AP) film, and a lateral film are developed before the patient leaves the operating room.

Magnification factors are easily obtained by placing a corkscrew magnification marker of a specified length within the AP and lateral images. The origin of the coordinate system is then selected by the dosimetrist, usually the end of one of the iridium-192 ribbons. The source coordinates are then determined and a computer calculation of dose distribution obtained (Figure 8–14).

Multiple dosimetries were calculated initially prior to determining the best possible implantation volumes in our patients (Figures 8–15 through 8–19). Because of the location and size of these tumors, multiple catheter insertion may not be feasible. The close proximity of vital structures (speech, motor, sensory, visual) as well as strategic vasculature does not always allow for a perfect homogeneous dose distribution.

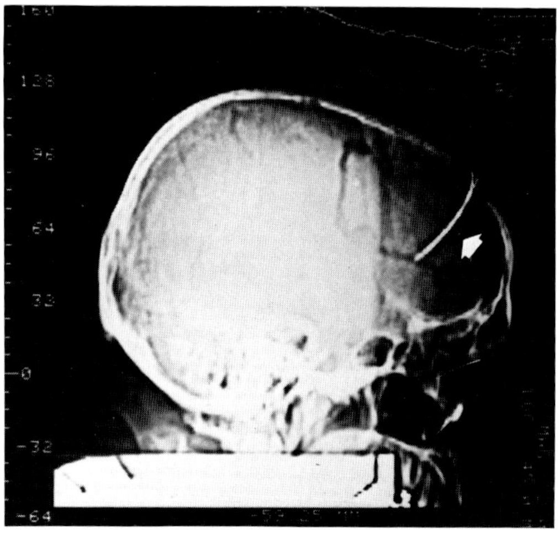

Figure 8–14 X-ray view of a single afterloaded catheter with "dummy" seeds in place.

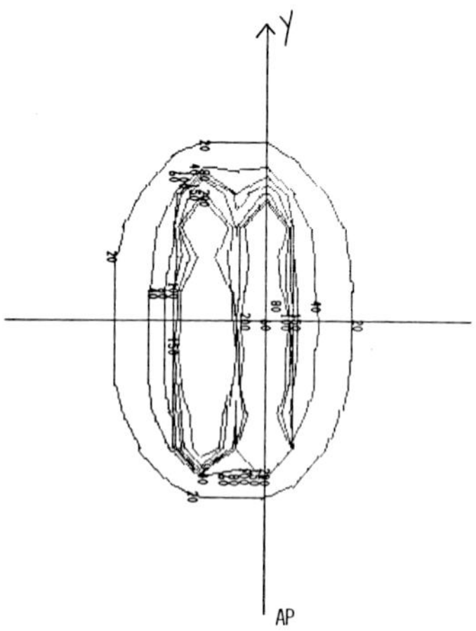

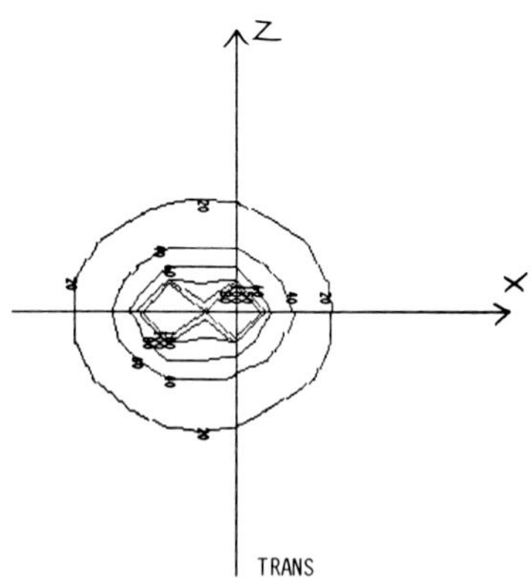

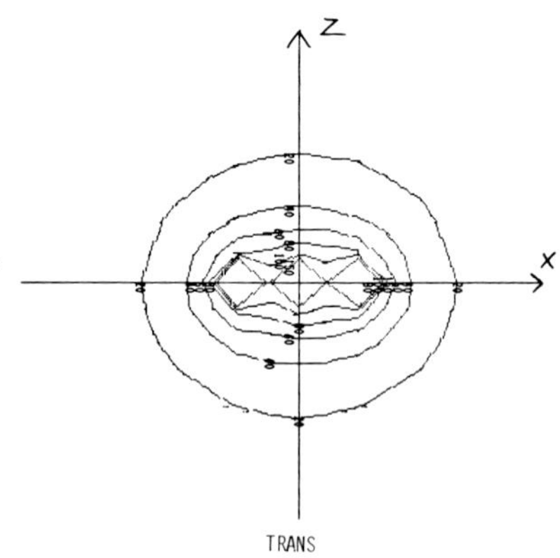

Figure 8–15 Anteroposterior (*AP*) dosimetry of a two-ribbon (catheter) implant. The dose rate varies between 200 rads/hr (at the center of the tumor) to 40 rads/hr at the periphery of the tumor. Each iridium-192 ribbon consists of 20 seeds laid end to end, with each seed's activity being 0.6 mg radium equivalent.

Figure 8–16 Transverse view of a two-ribbon (catheter) implant. Dosimetry reveals a dose rate varying between 150 rads/hr at the center of the tumor to 40 rads/hr at its periphery. Each ribbon contains 20 seeds, and each seed has an activity of 0.6 mg radium equivalent.

Figure 8–17 Transverse dosimetric view of a three-ribbon implant. The isodose curves are more elongated than in the two-ribbon implant.

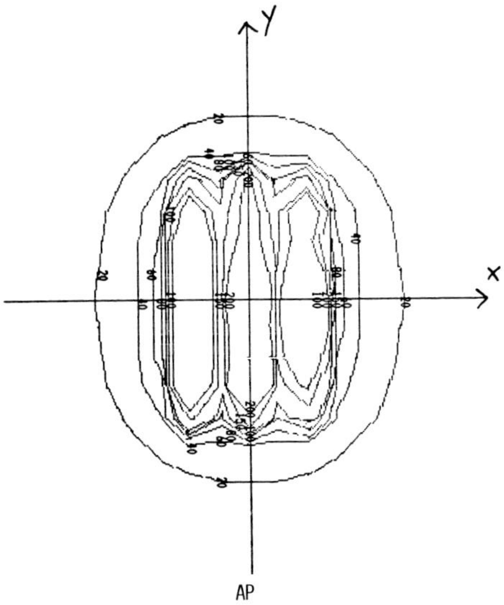

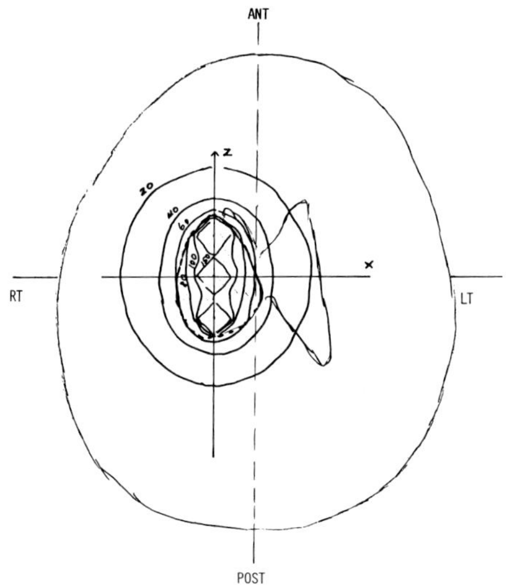

Figure 8–18 Anteroposterior (*AP*) dosimetry of a three-ribbon (catheter) implant. The dose rate varies from 100 rads/hr to 40 rads/hr at the tumor periphery.

Figure 8–19 Tumor volume (*broken lines*) localized by CT scan data. A three-ribbon implant with the dosimetry superimposed over the tumor volume is shown. The minimum tumor dose is 60 rads/hr. The center of the tumor will receive doses varying between 150 and 100 rads/hr.

However, the application of theoretical catheter insertions as determined by computer dosimetry has revealed that a dose rate of 50–60 rads/hr can be obtained at the periphery of the tumor region, with much higher doses up to 200 rads/hr found in the hypoxic center of these tumors (Figures 8–20 through 8–23).

Dose Rate

We have theorized that the high dose rate at the center could be advantageous because gliomas show evidence of focal as well as diffuse necrotic areas, particularly within the center of these tumors (111). Those areas consist of hypoxic cells which have been shown to be protected against the damage induced by x-irradiation. This has been shown elegantly in the split-dose experiments performed by Elkind and his colleagues (62,63). The increase in survival of those cells is affected by the repair of sublethal damage. This damage is reduced if a low level of hypoxia is present during the time the cells are exposed to radiation. Multiple experiments by Suit and his colleagues (251) have revealed the following: Chemically hypoxic cells are unable to repair sublethal damage to a great extent; however, cells which are just hypoxic enough to be protected and still able to repair sublethal damage constitute the core cells for tumor regrowth. This dependence of the cell survival curves on oxygen is best described by the oxygen enhancement ratio (OER). This is the ratio of the radiation dose required to affect certain biologic damage in the absence of oxygen/radiation dose required in a fully oxygenated state.

A possible benefit of interstitial implantation appears to be dependent on the OER, as this is reduced with dose rates of 30–60 rads/hr

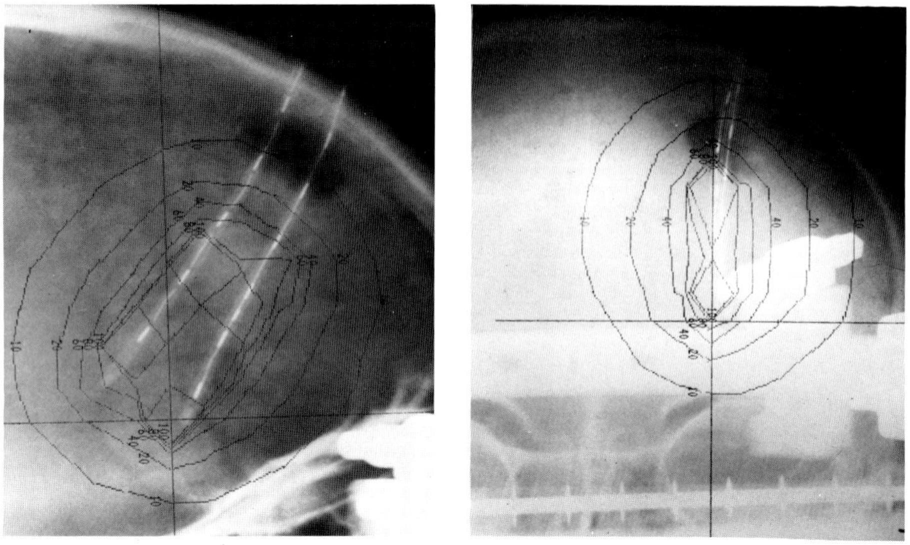

A B

Figure 8–20 Dosimetry of a two-catheter brain implant. **A:** Lateral view of a two-catheter implant with "dummy" seeds in place. The tips of the afterloaded CSF ventricular catheters are easily visualized. A maximum tumor dose rate of 100 rads/hr is obtained. The minimum tumor dose rate is 40 rads/hr. **B:** Anteroposterior view of a similar two-catheter implant showing the same dose rates.

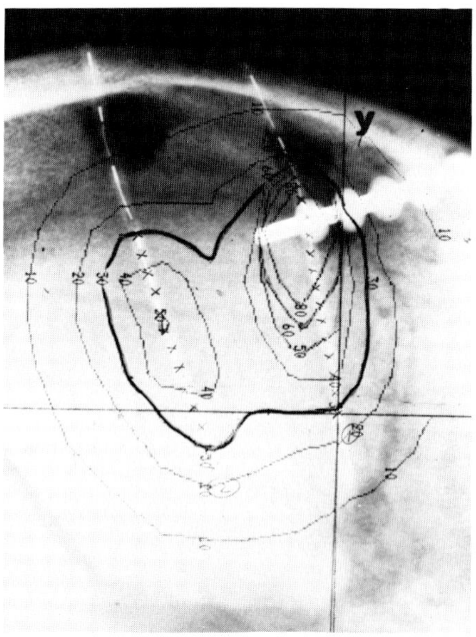

Figure 8–21 Dosimetry of two afterloaded catheters. "Dummy" seeds are within the afterloaded CSF ventricular catheters in this AP view. The dose rate ranges between 80 and 30 rads/hr. There is a cold spot between the two catheters because of the wide spacing between the radioactive iridium-192 ribbons.

as obtained in our brain implants (42). Finally, continuous irradiation might allow for relatively hypoxic cells to enter the more oxygenated compartment as tumor cell kill takes place in a continuous fashion.

As we aim to deliver doses of 3,000–10,000 rads either singly or in combination with previous external irradiation, these sources remain in place 50–120 hr. The patient remains on steroids during this period (152). Decadron is used initially in the operating suite and is then continued intravenously in a dose of 6–8 mg every 6–8 hr. The dose is sharply reduced over the next few days, and its administration is changed to the oral route as soon as the clinical situation permit. For patients with small lesions, we have had no difficulty sharply reducing these amounts

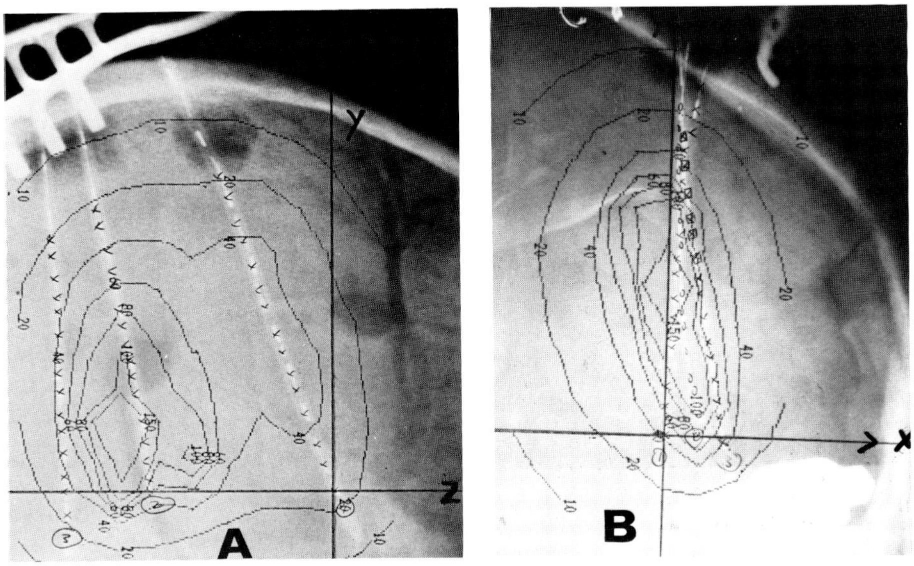

A B

Figure 8–22 Dosimetry of three afterloaded catheters. **A:** Lateral view showing a wide range of dose rates, which vary between 150 and 20 rads/hr. A cold spot developed between the more widely spaced iridium-192 ribbons. **B:** AP view shows the dose rate to vary between 150 and 40 rads/hr at the edge of the lesion. This view does not reveal the cold spot as well as was observed on the lateral projection.

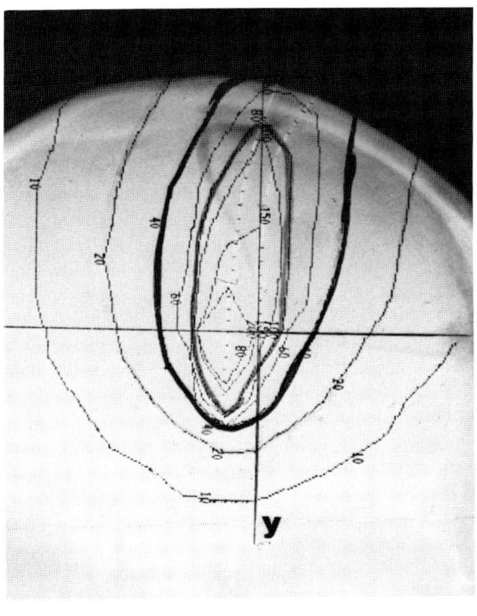

Figure 8–23 AP view of the dosimetry of two afterloaded catheters. A hot spot of 200 rads/hr is visualized. The minimum tumor dose rate was 40 rads/hr. An 80 rads/hr isodose curve comprises most of this tumor.

prior to discharge from the hospital. For larger lesions, however, a greater dose has been necessary at the time of discharge.

Other radiobiologic advantages of stereotactic brachytherapy include low-dose-rate irradiation and continuous irradiation at the implanted sites.

Lajtha and Oliver (127) derived survival curves for cells irradiated at dose rates varying between 10 rads/hr and greater than 200 rads/hr. Their findings reveal that as the dose rate is decreased the shape of the survival curves becomes flatter, with evidence of a greater surviving cell fraction.

The principal dose-rate effect in terms of cell killing seems to take place between 100 and 1 rad/min. Below 60 rads/hr (1 rad/min), little cell killing takes place because all sublethal damage is repaired during the exposure.

The effect of continuous low-dose irradiation could be expected to take on greater importance when a comparatively rapidly growing tumor (e.g., a glioma) is surrounded by normal tissues whose cell cycle is much slower, as found in nervous tissues.

The aim of our therapy in malignant gliomas is to reduce not only the proliferating cells but the nonproliferating cells as well, because these can always reenter the proliferative pool.

Interstitial local irradiation, by virtue of its low-dose-rate continuous irradiation and relative independence of the oxygen effect, could be quite beneficial since it affects both proliferating and nonproliferating pools. As the nonproliferating cells enter the proliferating pool, the local, continuous irradiation could effectively destroy them at the time of their division.

After the sources are removed, the catheters are then gently brought out through the implanted site at the patient's bedside. The skin is approximated with 2–0 silk sutures and covered with Bacitracin ointment. Opsite is then placed over the area to maintain sterility; the Opsite is changed daily.

We have not seen any incidence of local or central infection, nor have we seen any incidence of intracerebral or local bleeding at the time of removal of the sources. Postremoval CT scans were performed in our first series of 10 patients and showed no evidence of bleeding into the cerebral lesions. There was only minimal evidence for enlargement in the zone of edema (Figure 8–24).

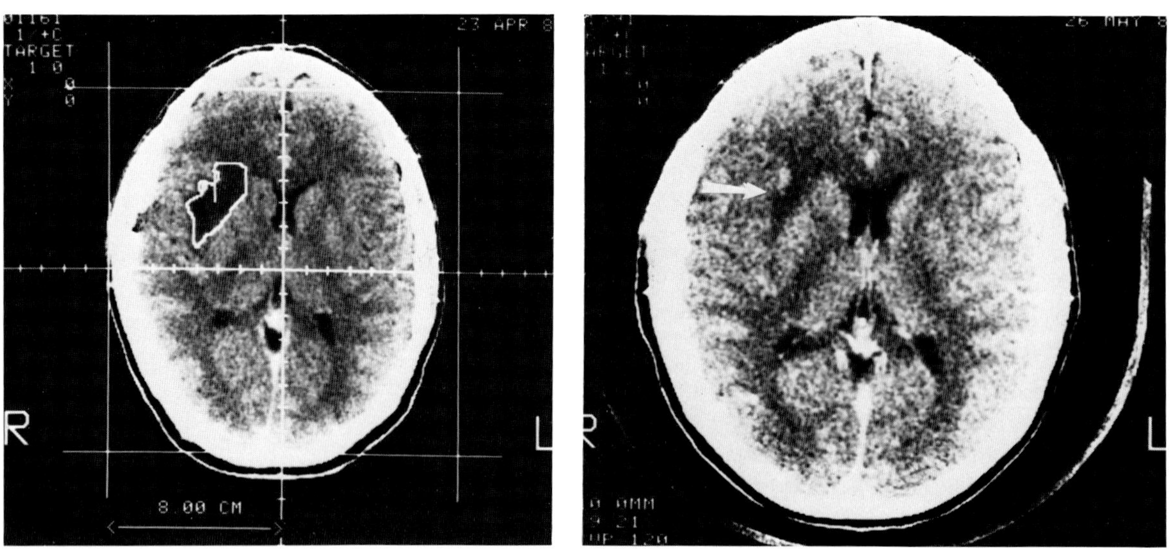

A **B**

Figure 8–24 Deep frontal lobe tumor associated with (**A**) peritumoral edema and (**B**) a small nucleus of increased staining (*arrow*) and compression of the frontal lobe.

Nursing Precautions

Maximum Permissible Dose Concept

The nursing precautions used in our stereotactic brain implants have been derived from acknowledged protocols used at other operative sites, e.g., lung, pancreas, head and neck, and gynecologic sites. A number of concepts need to be understood. The concept of maximum permissible dose lies at the core of the radiation protection protocols.

The human population is considered to be exposed to background radiation from natural causes as well as to manmade sources. The REM is the unit of dose equivalent used in radiation protection. It depends on the absorbed dose of ionizing radiation expressed in "rads" multiplied by a correction factor to allow for the fact that different types of radiation produce different biologic effects in humans.

The average annual dose to the population in millirems (1/1,000 REM) from natural background radiation is approximately 125 mREM/year to which approximately another 100 mREM/hr is added from medical uses, e.g., nuclear medicine, diagnostic radiography, and radiotherapy.

The maximum permissible dose has been developed in both the general population as well as the more specific subset of persons whose occupation exposes them to a higher level of radiation than the general public.

Maximum permissible dose (MPD) to the whole body (blood-forming organs, gonads) is described as 5 REM/year for the occupational subset and 500 mREM/year for the nonoccupational group. The respective figures are: for the extremities 75 REM/year and for the skin of the whole body 30 REM/year. These limits represent the upper levels of radiation exposure at which a negligible probability of either somatic or genetic damage is to be encountered. The use of afterloading techniques and lower energy sources (e.g., iridium-192 and iodine-125) has markedly diminished the radiation exposures in the occupational group.

Radiation Protection

The principal factors to be considered in decreasing the radiation exposure in those patients are: 1) distance from the radioactive sources; 2) the time spent near the patient; and 3) the shielding available. We have monitored our first series of 10 patients to delineate the various exposure values with iridium-192 sources at various sites from the implanted area. The amount of activity of our sources varied from 20 to 30 mCi of iridium-192. Each seed used varied in activity between 0.3 to 0.5 mg rad equivalent. We have used iridium-192 ribbons manufactured by the Alpha-Omega Company. Various computerized dosimetries were developed to determine the best dose rate available. We have found that seeds manufactured end to end in a linear fashion delivered the best volume distribution around the tumor-bearing region and its periphery.

An active length of 2–5 cm has been used. Two to four ribbons have been utilized in those patients. The total activity is derived from the number of seeds multiplied by their activity plus a factor for iridium-192.

Radiation Monitoring

The Geiger counter has been used to record the measurements of patient exposure in rates of millirads per hour. On the side of the implanted isotope, the following values were obtained:

At the surface of the implant	100–70 mR/hr	(70–100 mR/hr)
At 1 foot away from the patient	30–20 mR/hr	(20–30 mR/hr)
At 1 meter away from the patient	2–5 mR/hr	(2–5 mR/hr)
At the foot of the bed	1–2 mR/hr	(1–2 mR/hr)
At the door	0 mR/hr	
On the contralateral side of the implant	50–40 mR/hr	(40–50 mR/hr)

It is obvious from these figures that radiation exposure can be reduced considerably with greater distance from the patient. Indeed this exposure varies with the inverse square law. Because we are performing only afterloaded stereotactic interstitial implants at this time, no exposure occurs until after the patients return to their rooms, where they are loaded.

At the time of surgery the afterloaded catheters are inserted stereotactically into the tumor substance and anchored with 2–0 silk into the patient's scalp. We have found this simple technique to be quite effective in anchoring the catheters. A sterile plastic cup is placed over the catheters until they are loaded with the radioactive ribbons. The iridium-192 ribbons are inserted into the catheters and then secured in place by "stapling" the shaft of the catheters. The average length of time that these catheters remain in place varies from 50 to 100 hr. The dose rate usually varies from 50 to 60 rads/hr.

Dosimeters are worn by the nurses caring for the patient. Inasmuch as the first 24 hr are spent in the intensive care unit and the rest of the hospitalization in our oncology unit, the exposure of the hospital personnel is markedly reduced because of the different sets of medical personnel caring for the patients. The nursing staff wears the photographic film badge for 1 month, at which time it is processed to indicate the level of radiation exposure.

Specific precautions should be taken with the patient's family and visitors. We have continued to use precautions initially developed for patients having radium-226 intracavitary insertions because those are the most stringent ones developed. No pregnant visitors or medical personnel are allowed in the patient's room, nor are individuals under the age of 18 years allowed to visit. Because the half value layer of iridium-192 in lead is 1.5 mm, a lead shield at the head of the bed is quite effective in reducing the radiation exposure. Communication with both the medical staff caring for these patients and their family is of the utmost importance. Staff conferences have been held to discuss the issues involved in radiation protection and have helped to alleviate most radiation exposure fears in the majority of personnel. The patients and their family are also instructed in radiation safety precautions. Questions such as whether the patient will remain radioactive, if their excretions or sweat are radioactive, and if contamination of the family members will occur are discussed pre- and postoperatively. Because we have been performing two to four such implants per month, it is becoming more imperative to designate a nurse coordinator to answer the above issues in addition to the physicians involved in the care of these patients. Reinforcement of these issues is continuously required for both medical staff and family members.

Conclusion

Extensive data in the use of stereotactic interstitial implant have been published in the world literature (38,44,46,56,73,83,85,103,114,213,-214,219,220,227,229,232,253 –259). Mundinger's guidelines suggest that the more anaplastic gliomas (grade III–IV) respond best to a combination of interstitial irradiation (in the form of a temporary iridium-192 implant) and external beam irradiation (161,176). If these tumors are smaller than 3 cm in diameter, he favors the sole usage of interstitial brachytherapy. The lesser-grade gliomas (grade I–II) have responded best to a permanent interstitial implantation with iodine-125 or iridium-192. The grade II–III lesions also undergo external beam irradiation as dictated by the tumor volume (161,176) (Table 8–3).

Mundinger's conclusions were based on results from CT-directed stereotactic biopsies in areas of low-grade gliomas that received external radiation doses to 6,000–7,000 rads. Those biopsies revealed no sign of tumor regression (171,176).

For highly anaplastic tumors with rapid cell division, a rapidly accumulated tumor dose is preferred. This can easily be delivered with a temporary iridium-192 or iodine-125 implant. The aim has been to deliver a tumor surface dose of 9,000–12,000 rads. The dosimetry can be worked out ahead of the implantation procedure. If a course of postoperative radiation is to be delivered, the total dose remains the same for the combined procedures.

Complications were described by Mundinger and consist of the following: Cerebral hemorrhage occurred in 1.3% of their patients at the time of biopsy. Transient functional deficits, e.g., intensification of previous motor or sensory pareses, can be brought on by increasing edema. These changes are usually transitory (175,176).

We have had one case of intracerebral bleeding that occurred at the time of biopsy. The patient had been responsive and oriented prior to the biopsy, but a sudden deterioration in his mental status accompanied by tonic deviation of the eyes to the left side appeared suddenly. The rapid insertion of the fenestrated afterloaded catheter decompressed the

Table 8–3 Primary Lesions: Mundinger's Data

Hemispheric lesions
Fast-growing lesions
Iridium-192 implant–temporary plus Gamma-medical treatment
Low-grade lesions
Iridium-192 implant
Iodine-125 permanent implant
Midline tumors
Low-grade lesions
Iridium-192 permanent implant
Iodine-125 permanent implant

References 167, 172.

bleeding site fully. The patient regained consciousness with loss of the oculomotor changes instantaneously. Two of 26 patients suffered an episode of intra-operative bleeding. This resolved spontaneously without the need for surgical intersection. No mortality has incurred intraoperatively.

Mundinger's experience is to be contrasted to that of Szikla and his collegues (253,254) at the Hospital Saint-Anne in Paris. Astrocytomas of grade II–IV were implanted with iridium-192 sources only if the lesions were less than 5 cm in diameter, and additional external radiation was given if they were greater than 5 cm. A median survival rate of 12.7 months was obtained in 11 patients, all of whom expired from their disease.

In another 28 cases of grade II–III lesion, 80% showed complete remission over a 2-year period. Their data seem to favor the technique of interstitial implantation for the more active grade II–III lesions as compared to glioblastoma multiforme.

From these studies and others we have developed our own set of guidelines (Tables 8–4 through 8–6). We subdivide our patient population into two major groups: 1) patients with primary brain gliomas; and 2) those with metastatic brain tumors. We use a temporary, removable afterloaded iridium-192 stereotactic interstitial irradiation technique exclusively. This choice was based on criteria delineated previously. To reiterate, the criteria are as follows:

1. Availability of the radionuclide source
2. Need for strict radiation protection for our medical personnel
3. Improved cosmetic response if external beam irradiation is not utilized
4. Faster postoperative recovery period when afterloaded catheters alone are utilized
5. Flexibility in the tumor dose afforded by a temporary implant

The first group can be further subdivided into high-grade (III–IV) and low-grade (I–II) gliomas. A biopsy is mandatory in all those groups. Our policy has been to subject those patients to stereotactic biopsies. The diagnostic rate in our initial series of 20 patients was 17/20 diagnosed by the "smear" preparation and 19/20 by the paraffin-mounted sections. We have aimed for a total tumor dose of 8,000–12,000 rads. The more anaplastic lesions receive the higher doses. If external beam radiation

Table 8–4 Primary Lesions: Indications for Stereotactic Brachytherapy

Hemispheral lesions >3.5 cm
- Grade I–II lesions
  - Brachytherapy alone 6000–7500 rads at periphery
- Grade III–IV lesions
  - Brachytherapy 5500–6500 rads
  - External radiation therapy boost 2500–3500 rads

Hemispheral lesions <3.5 cm
- Grade I–II lesions
  - Brachytherapy alone 6000–7000 rads at periphery
- Grade III–IV lesions
  - Brachytherapy 5000–6000 rads
  - External radiation therapy boost 2000–3000 rads

Table 8–5 Treatment of Deep-seated Midline Lesions

Brachytherapy 4500–6000 rads to tumor periphery
1. If Grade I–II
   No additional external irradiation
2. If Grade III–IV
   Add external radiation therapy 2000–4000 rads

Table 8–6 Treatment of Metastatic Brain Lesions

If the lesion is:
1. Solitary and
2. Metastatic work-up is negative
   a. Brachytherapy 4500–5500 rads to tumor periphery
   b. Boost with external irradiation if the lesion recurs.

was previously delivered, the total tumor dose remains at the same level for the combined procedures. For the lesser-grade gliomas we have attempted to deliver a total tumor dose of 6,000–7,000 rads at the time of the stereotactic interstitial implant.

Debulking has not been used in our series unless the patient was previously subjected to a surgical resection prior to our evaluation for an interstitial implantation. Our assumptions that local irradiation could be as effective as whole brain irradiation have been based on data previously published by Hochbert et al. (92,95). Their study revealed that of 127 autopsied patients dead of untreated glioblastoma 96% showed evidence of nonmulticentricity. They also determined that, contrary to previously published data (221), 80% of 35 autopsied glioblastomas could be localized accurately by CT scans performed within the 2 months prior to the patient's demise. Finally, they also determined that recurrence of glioblastoma was detected either within the primary site or close to it in 90% of a group of 42 patients. Other series (28,184,185,228,231) supported the fact that local irradiation seems to be as effective as whole brain irradiation.

Of interest is a recent report by Fossati et al. (71) that the 2-year survival rate for patients receiving whole brain irradiation was 3.7% as compared to 27% for more local irradiation therapy. Because local recurrence is the major factor in causing death in these patients, theoretically a sound concept would consist of delivering a higher local dose to the tumor site. This would spare the normal brain tissue and has been found to be associated with a lesser incidence of brain necrosis and/or intellectual deterioration. Of great clinical interest also are the findings of enlarged ventricles and sulci associated with hypodense white matter as seen on CT scan (148,159,160,192). There is autopsy evidence of brain atrophy (27) and reduction in mental status (93,95) in patients undergoing external irradiation. Other studies have revealed similar findings. Norman et al. (182) reported ventricular enlargement without obstruction on CT evaluation of glioma patients pre- and posttherapy in 32% of the population undergoing irradiation and chemotherapy. A 24% incidence of similar findings was described by Marks and Gado (148). This same study showed a higher incidence of hydrocephalus and cerebral atrophy in patients receiving whole brain radiation than in those with more localized irradiation. Furthermore, not only is one now capable of delineating precisely those lesions by Ct scan, but the availability of three-dimensional computer reconstruction of brain lesions is now feasible. An excellent series by Batnizky et al. (9) describes the use of computer graphics for three-dimensional reconstruction of various brain lesions ranging from a suprasellar dysgerminoma to a brainstem glioma. They also describe the use of such a technique for stereotactic surgical and radiation treatment regimens. Rhodes et al. (209) and McKay et al. (144,145) reported similar data. Of particular interest to physicians interested in a stereotactic interstitial implantation is the fact that the tumor volume can be accurately quantitated and a dosimetry therefore obtained ahead of time. An accurate isodose can thus be developed that enables the clinician to decide on the number of ribbons or seeds needed for implantation. It should now be quite evident to the reader that the choice of the best therapeutic modalities for brain gliomas is still under vigorous discussion.

A multitude of rather sophisticated techniques are currently available to the team of physicians involved in the care of glioma patients.

Adjunctive modalities of treatment have been described with regularity and range from chemotherapy radiosensitizers (23,67,105,199), to high-LET radiation and hyperthermia, to laser therapy.

In Europe as well as in the United States there is a solid basis for the use of stereotactic interstitial implantation in brain tumors. However, a number of important questions related to the latter modality remain to be answered. The controversy regarding the use of temporary versus permanent implantation needs to be resolved. The choice of radioactive nuclides and total tumor dose needed requires further evaluation. Decisions regarding the extent of surgical resection and the postoperative use of external radiation remain to be fully answered. That our work is preliminary is quite obvious, although some statements can already be made.

The present stereotactic technique has been easily reproduced in our initial series of 26 patients. There is a minimal amount of morbidity associated with it and no mortality. It allows for the accurate placement of afterloaded interstitially implanted catheters.

Our own guidelines are presented in Tables 8–4 through 8–6. Mundinger's guidelines are introduced in Table 8–3. These guidelines remain somewhat fluid, however, and are subject to change as more experience is being gathered.

We have been quite encouraged by our early data (as reported in Chapter 7). We will continue to pursue not only temporary stereotactic brain implantation but also permanent implantation of radionuclides. Cooperative efforts with other groups working actively in this field are in progress. As a final word of caution, only centers showing a close interrelationship between the neurosurgical specialists, radiation oncologists, radiologists, and pathologists should attempt these procedures. A close cooperative effort between these specialists is paramount to the success of these techniques. Only as more and more centers enter these cooperative investigations will the previously asked questions be fully answered.

Acknowledgments

I want to acknowledge Sidney R. Stevens Ph.D. for his role in the evaluation of the source calibrations. I also extend my deepest gratitude for the supportive efforts of my partners Dr. Robert J. McKenna, Dr. S. Barry Sakulsky, and Dr. J. Douglas Smith. I want to extend my deepest thanks to Lucy Dario, Jeannette Taylor, and Kathy Scott for their dedicated efforts in the preparation of this manuscript.

References

1. Anderson AP: Postoperative irradiation of glioblastomas: results in a randomized series. Acta Radiol Oncol Radiat Phys Biol 17:475–484, 1978
2. Anderson AP: Scandinavian glioblastoma study group: combined modality therapy of operated astrocytomas grade III and IV: confirmation of the value of postoperative irradiation and lack of potentiation of bleomycin on survival time. Cancer 47:649, 1981
3. Aristizabal SA, Boone JLM, Laguna JF: Endocrine factors influencing radiation injury to central nervous tissue. Int J Radiat Oncol Biol Phys 5:349–353, 1979

4. Aristizabal SA, Caldwell WL: Time-dose volume relationships in the treatment of glioblastoma multiforme. Radiology 101:201–202, 1971
5. Arnold A, Bailey P, Harvey RA, et al: Changes in the central nervous system following irradiation with 23-MeV x-rays from the betatron. Radiology 62:37–46, 1954
6. Asquith JC, Foster JL, Willson RL: Metronidazole ("Flagyl"): A radiosensitizer of hypoxic cells. Br J Radiol 47:474–481, 1974
7. Bailey LP, Cushing M: A Classification of the Tumors of the Glioma Group on a Histogenic Basis with a Correlated Study of Prognosis. Lippincott, Philadelphia, 1926
8. Barendsen GW, Benstren TLJ, Vergresen AJ, et al: Effects of different ionizing radiation on human cells in tissue culture. II. Biological experiments. Radiat Res 13:841–849, 1960
9. Batnitzky S, Price HL, Lee KR, et al: Three-dimensional computer reconstructions of brain lesions from surface contours provided by computed tomography: a prospectus. Neurosurgery 11:73–84, 1982
10. Berg NO, Lindgren MK: Time-dose relationship and morphology of delayed radiation lesions of the brain in rabbits. Acta Radiol [Suppl 167] 1958
11. Betti O, et al: Combined interstitial and external irradiation of gliomas, a progress report. 6:329–338, 1979
12. Birg W, Mundinger F, Klar M: Computer assistance for stereotactic brain operations. Adv Neurosurg 4:287–291, 1977
13. Bleyer WA, Griffin TW: White matter necrosis, mineralized microangiopathy and intellectual abilities in survivors of childhood leukemia. In: Radiation Damage to the Nervous System: A Delayed Therapeutic Hazard, edited by HA Gilbert, AR Kagan. Raven Press, New York, 1980, pp 59–92
14. Bloom HJG, Peckham MJ, Richardson AE, et al: Glioblastoma multiforme: a controlled trial to assess the value of specific active immunotherapy in patients treated by radical surgery and radiotherapy. Br J Cancer 27:253–267, 1973
15. Boden G: Radiation myelitis of the cervical cord. Br J Radiol 21:464–469, 1948
16. Boden G: Radiation myelitis of brain stem. J Radiol 2:79, 1950
17. Boldrey EB: Initial surgical management of primary brain tumors. Semin Oncol 2:11–13, 1975
18. Boldrey E, Sheline G: Delayed transitory clinical manifestations after radiation treatments of intracranial tumors. Acta Radiol 5:5–10, 1967
19. Bouchard J: Radiation Therapy of Tumors and Diseases of the Nervous System. Lea & Febiger, Montreal, 1966
20. Bouchard J: Central nervous system. In: Textbook of Radiotherapy, ed 2, edited by GH Fletcher. Lea & Febiger, Philadelphia, 1973, pp 366–418
21. Bouchard J, Peirce C: Radiation therapy in the management of neoplasms of the central nervous system, with special note in regard to children: twenty years' experience, 1939–1958. Am J Roentgenol 84:610–628, 1960
22. Breuer AC, Blank NK, Schoene WC: Multifocal pontine lesions in cancer patients treated with chemotherapy and CNS radiotherapy. Cancer 41:2112–2120, 1978
23. Brisman R, Housepian EM, Chang C, et al: Adjuvant nitrosourea therapy for glioblastoma. Arch Neurol 33:745–750, 1976
24. Brismar J, Roberson GH, Davis KR: Radiation necrosis of the brain: neuroradiological considerations with computed tomography. Neuroradiology 12:109–113, 1976
25. Brown BW, Thompson JR, Barkley TB, et al: Theoretical considerations of dose rate factors influencing radiation strategy. Radiology 110:97, 1973
26. Brucer M: Brachytherapy. Am J Roentgenol 79:1080–1090, 1968
27. Burger PC, Mahaley MS, Dudka L, et al: The morphologic effects of radiation administered therapeutically for intracranial gliomas: a postmortem study of 25 cases. Cancer 44:1256–1272, 1979

28. Caldwell WL, Aristizabal SA: Treatment of glioblastoma multiforme: a review. Arch Radiol 14:503–512, 1975
29. Camins MB, Schleseeger EB: Treatment of tumors of the posterior part of the third ventricle and the pineal region: a long-term follow-up. Acta Neurochir (Wien) 40:131–143, 1978
30. Carella RJ, Pay N, Newall J, et al: Computerized (axial) tomography in the serial study of cerebral tumors treated by radiation, a preliminary report. Cancer 37:2719–2728, 1976
31. Cavanagh JB: The proliferation of astrocytes around a needle wound in the rat brain. J Anat 106:471–487, 1970
32. Caveness WF: Experimental observations: delayed necrosis in normal monkey brain. In: Radiation Damage to the Nervous System: A Delayed Therapeutic Hazard, edited by HA Gilbert, AR Kagan. Raven Press, New York, 1980, pp 1–38
33. Caveness WF: Pathology of radiation damage to the normal brain of the monkey. Natl Cancer Inst Monogr 46:57–76, 1977
34. Caveness WF, Carsten AL: Late effects of whole brain irradiation within the therapeutic range. In: Late Biological Effects of Ionizing Radiation, Vol 2. International Atomic Energy Agency, Vienna, 1978
35. Caveness WF, Carsten AL, Roizin L, et al: Pathogenesis of x-irradiation effects in the monkey cerebral cortex. Brain Res 7:1–119, 1968
36. Caveness WF, Tanaka A, Hess KH, et al: Delayed brain swelling and functional derangement after x-irradiation of the right visual cortex in the Macaca mulatta. Radiat Res 57:104–120, 1974
37. Chang CH, Seaman WB, Jacox HW: Clinical aspects of hyperbaric oxygen and radiotherapy. II. Clinical application. Br J Radiol 30:406, 1957
38. Chase NE, Atkins HL, Correll JW: Interstitial irradiation of brain tumors with iridium-192. Radiology 77:842–843, 1961
39. Cheek WR, Taveras JM: Thalamic tumors. J Neurosurg 24:505, 1966
40. Clemente CD, Holst EA: Pathological changes in neurons, neurologlia and blood-brain barrier induced by x-irradiation of heads of monkeys. Arch Neurol Psychiatry 71:66–79, 1954
41. Cohen L: Clinical radiation dosage. III. A biological factor in radon and isotope dosage. Br J Radiol 23:25, 1960
42. Cohen L: Theoretical iso-survival formulas for fractionated radiation therapy. Br J Radiol 41:552–528, 1968
43. Concannon JP, Kramer S, Berry R: The extent of intracranial gliomata at autopsy and its relationship to techniques used in radiation therapy of brain tumors. Am J Roentgenol 87:574–584, 1962
44. Correll JW, Chase NE, Atkins HL: New technique for interstitial irradiation of brain tumors. J Neurosurg 18:800–803, 1961
45. Cushing H: Intracranial Tumours: Notes upon a Series of 2,000 Verified Cases with Surgical Mortality Percentages Thereto. Charles C Thomas, Springfield, Illinois, 1932
46. D'Andrea F, de Divits E, Lignoretti CD, et al: Stereotaxic implantation of radioisotopes in brain tumors. Neurosurgery 3:86–92, 1972
47. Davis L: Neurological surgery, so to speak, out of roentgenology: Hickey Lecture, 1956. Am J Roentgenol 76:217–225, 1956
48. Davis L, Martin J, Padberg F, et al: A study of 182 patients with verified astrocytoma, astroblastoma and oligodendroglioma of the brain. J Neurosurg 7:299–312, 1950
49. Davis LL, Martin J, Golstein SL, et al: A study of 211 patients with verified glioblastoma multiforme. J Neurosurg 6:33–44, 1949
50. Denekamp J: The cellular proliferation kinetics of animal tumors. Cancer Res 30:393–400, 1970
51. Denekamp J, Fowler JF: Cell proliferation kinetics and radiation therapy. In: Cancer—A Comprehensive Treatise, edited by FE Becker. Plenum Press, New York, 1977, pp 101–137

52. De Reuck J, Van der Eeken H: The anatomy of the late radiation encephalopathy. Eur Neurol 13:481–494, 1975
53. Diengdoh JV, Booth AE: Post-irradiation necrosis of the temporal lobe presenting as a glioma: case report. J Neurosurg 44:732–734, 1976
54. DiLorenzo N, Nolletti A, Palma L: Late cerebral radionecrosis. Surg Neurol 10:281–290, 1978
55. Djordjevic B, Anderson LL, Kim SH: Oxygen enhancement ratios in Hela cells irradiated with californium and radium sources. Radiology 107:429, 1973
56. Drake CG, Pfalzner PM, Linell EA: Intracavitary irradiation of malignant brain tumors. J Neurosurg 20:428–434, 1963
57. Druckmann A: Schdatsucht als Folge der Rontgenbestrahling. Strahlentherapie 33:382, 1929
58. Dugger GS, Stratford JG, Bouchard J: Necrosis of the brain following roentgen irradiation. Am J Roentgenol 72:953–960, 1954
59. Duttera MJ, Bleyer WA, Pomenoy TC, et al: Irradiation, methotrexate toxicity, and the treatment of meningeal leukemia. Lancet 2:703–707, 1973
60. Earle KM, Rentschler EM, Snodgrass SR: Primary intracranial neoplasms: prognosis and classification of 513 verified cases. J Neuropathol Exp Neurol 16:321–331, 1957
61. Edland RW, Javid M, Ansfield RJ: Glioblastoma multiforme: an analysis of the results of postoperative radiotherapy alone versus radiotherapy and concomitant 5-fluorouracil (a prospective randomized study of 32 cases). Am J Roentgenol 3:337–342, 1971
62. Elkind MM, Han A, Volz KW: Radiation response of mammalian cells grown in culture. IV. Dose dependence of division delay and postirradiation growth of surviving and nonsurviving Chinese hamster cells. J Natl Cancer Inst 30:705, 1963
63. Elkind MM, Sutton H: Radiation response of mammalian cells growing in culture. I. Repair of x-ray damage in surviving Chinese hamsters cells. Radiat Res 13:556–593, 1960
64. Ellis F: Dose, time and fractionation: a clinical hypothesis. Clin Radiol 20:1–7, 1969
65. Elvidge AR, Penfield W, Cone W: The gliomas of the central nervous system. In: Tumors of the Nervous System, edited by EG Zabieskie AN Frantz, CC Hare. Williams & Wilkins, Baltimore, 1937, pp 107–181
66. EORTC Brain Tumor Group: Evaluation on survival rate of objective remission and duration of free interval in patients with malignant brain glioma. Eur J Cancer 14:851, 1978
67. EORTC Brain Tumor Group: Evaluation of CCNU, VM 26 and procarbazine in supratentorial brain gliomas: final evaluation of a randomized study. J Neurosurg 55:27, 1981
68. Eystee EF, Nielsen SL, Sheline GE, et al: Cerebral radionecrosis simulating a brain tumor. J Neurosurg 39:267–271, 1974
69. Fazekas JT: Treatment of grade I and II brain astrocytomas. The role of radiotherapy Int J Radiat Oncol Biol Phys Vol 2 #7 pp 661–666 1977
70. Foltz EL, Holyoke JB, Heyl HL: Brain necrosis following x-ray therapy. J Neurosurg 10:423–429, 1953
71. Fossati F, Tucker C, Tosi G: Effect of field size and unconventional dose fractionation in the radiotherapy of malignant cerebral gliomas. Presented at the International Symposium on Multidisciplinary Aspects of Brain Tumor Therapy, 1979, p 105
72. Frankel SA, German WJ: Glioblastoma multiforme, review of 219 cases with regard to natural history, pathology, diagnostic methods and treatment. J Neurosurg 15:489, 1958
73. Frazier CH: The effects of radium emanations upon brain tumors. Surg Gynecol Obstet 31:236–239, 1920
74. Frendel E, Malaise EP, Tubiana M: Cell proliferation kinetics in five human solid tumors. Cancer 22:611–620, 1968

75. Fu KK, Phillips TL, Kane LJ, et al: Tumor and normal tissue response to irradition in vivo: variation with decreasing dose rates. Radiology 114:709–716, 1975
76. Gehan EA, Walker MD: Prognostic factors for patients with brain tumors. Natl Cancer Inst Monogr 46:189–195, 1977
77. Gerstner L, Jellinger K, Heiss WD, et al: Morphological changes in anaplastic gliomas treated with radiation and chemotherapy. Acta Neurochir (Wien) 36:117–138, 1977
78. Gleason CA, Wise BL, Feinstein B: Stereotactic localization (with computerized tomographic scanning), biopsy, and radiofrequency treatment of deep brain lesions. Neurosurgery 2:217–222, 1978
79. Gozzano M, Reda GC: Necrosi cerebrale de raggi roentgen. Riv Neurol 19:145–165, 1949
80. Gray LH, Conger AD, Ebert M, et al: The concentration of oxygen dissolved in tissues at the time of irradiation as a factor in radiotherapy. Br J Radiol 26:638 1953
81. Green SB, Byar DP, Walter MD, et al: Comparisons of carmustine, procarbazine, and high-dose methylprednisolone as additions to surgery and radiotherapy for the treatment of malignant glioma. Cancer Clin Trials, in press
82. Gregersen MJ, Pallaricini C, Chien S: Studies on the chemical composition of the central nervous system in relation to the effects of x-irradiation and of disturbances in water and salt balance. Radiat Res 17:209, 1962
83. Gutin PH, Phillips TL, Hosobuchi Y, et al: Permanent and removable implants for the brachytherapy of brain tumors. Int J Radiat Oncol Biol Phys 7:1371–1381, 1981
84. Hall EJ: Radiation dose-rate: a factor of importance in radiobiology and radiotherapy. Br J Radiol 45:81–97, 1972
85. Hankinson J: Cerebral implantation of radio-active material. Ubt H Beyrik 5:94–104, 1965
86. Haymaker W: Effects of ionizing radiation on nervous tissue. In: The Structure and Function of the Nervous System, edited by GH Bourne. Academic Press, New York, 1969, pp 441–518
87. Henschler UK, Ceva P: Dimension averaging a simple method for dosimetry of interstitial implants. Radiat Biol Ther 9:287–298, 1968
88. Hilaris BS: Handbook of Interstitial Brachytherapy. Publishing Sciences Group Inc, Acton, Massachusetts, 1975
89. Hilaris BS, Kim HH, Tokita N: Low energy radionuclides for permanent interstitial implantation. Am J Roentgenol 126:171–178, 1978
90. Hindo WA, DeTrana FA, Lee MS, et al: Large dose increment irradiation in treatment of cerebral metastases. Cancer 26:138–141, 1970
91. Hitchcock E, Sato F: Treatment of malignant glioma. J Neurosurg 21:497, 1964
92. Deleted during production.
93. Hochberg FH, Linggood R, Wolfson L, et al: Quality and duration of survival in glioblastoma multiforme: combined surgical, radiation, and lomustine therapy. JAMA 241:1016–1018, 1979
94. Hochberg FH, Pruitt A: Assumptions in the radiotherapy of glioblastoma. Neurology 30:907–911, 1980
95. Hochberg F, Slotnick B: Neuropsychological impairments in astrocytoma survivors. Neurology 30:172–177, 1980
96. Hoffman WF, Levin VA, Wilson CB: Evaluation of malignant glioma patients during the post irradiation period. J Neurosurg 50:624–628, 1979
97. Holt G, Hilaris B, Balter S, et al: Experience with computerized implant dosimetry Am J Roentgenol 102:688–693, 1968
98. Horsley V, Clark RH: The structure and functions of the cerebellum examined by a new method. Brain 31:45–124, 1908
99. Deleted during production.

100. Hoshino T: The cell kinetics of gliomas: its prognostic value and therapeutic implications. Neurooncology 1:105–112, 1979
101. Hoshino T, Barker M, Wilson C, et al: Cell kinetics of human gliomas. J Neurosurg 37:15–26, 1972
102. Hoshino T, Wilson CB: Review of basic concepts of cell kinetics as applied to brain tumors. J Neurosurg 42:123, 1975
103. Hosobuchi Y, Phillips TL, Stupar TA, et al: Interstitial brachytherapy of primary brain tumors: preliminary report. J Neurosurg 53:613–617, 1980
104. Husain MM, Garcia JH: Cerebral radiation necrosis: vascular and glial features. Acta Neuropathol (Berl) 36:381–385, 1976
105. Irwin L, George F, Pitts F. et al: Hydroxyurea (HU) + radiation therapy (RT) in primary intracranial malignant glial tumors. Proc Am Assoc Cancer Res 16:243, 1975
106. Jelsma R, Bucy PC: Glioblastoma multiforme: its treatment and some factors affecting survival. Arch Neurol 20:161–171, 1969
107. Jelsma R, Bucy PC: The treatment of gliobastoma multiforme of the brain. J Neurosurg 27:388, 1967
108. Johnson MA, Haynaker WE, Rubini JR, et al: A radioautographic study of a human brain and glioblastoma multiforme after the in vivo uptake of tritiated thymidine. Cancer 13:636, 1960
109. Jones A: Transient radiation myelopathy (with reference to Lhermette's sign of electrical paresthesia). Br J Radiol 37:727–744, 1964
110. Kagan AR, Wollin M, Gilbet HA, et al: Comparison of the tolerance of the brain and spinal cord to injury by radiation. In: Radiation Damage to the Nervous System: A Delayed Therapeutic Hazard, edited by HA Gilbert, AR Kagan. Raven Press, New York, 1980, pp 183–190
111. Kal HB, Sissingh HA: Effectiveness of continuous low dose-rate gamma irradiation on rat skin. Br J Radiol 47:673–678, 1974
112. Karnofsky DA, Burchenal JH: The clinical evaluation of chemotherapeutic agents in cancer. In: Evaluation of Chemotherapeutic Agents, edited by CM McLeod. Columbia University Press, New York, 1949, pp 191–205
113. Kelly PJ, Alker GJ Jr: A sterotactic approach to deep-seated central nervous system neoplasms using the carbon dioxide laser. Surg Neurol 15:331–335, 1981
114. Kelly PJ, Olson MH, Wright AE: Stereotactic implantation of iridium-192 into CNS neoplasms. Surg Neurol 10:349–354, 1978
115. Kernohan JW, Sayre GP: Tumors of the central nervous system. In: Atlas of Tumor Pathology (Fascicle 35). Armed Forces Institute of Pathology, Washington, DC, 1952
116. Kim JH, Hiaris B: Iodine-125 source in interstitial tumor therapy: clinical and biologic considerations. Am J Roentgenol 123:163–169, 1975
116a. Klar E, Scheer KE: Die Kontaktherapie um malignen Hingeschwülsten mit Radiokobalt Co-Go IX Int Congr Radiologie, München, 148–149, 1959
117. Korr H, Schultze B, Maurer W: Autoradiographic investigations of glial proliferation in the brain of adult mice. I. The DNA synthesis phase of neuroglia and endothelial cells. J Comp Neurol 150:169–176, 1973
118. Korr H, Schultze B, Maurer W: Autoradiographic investigations of glial proliferation of neuroglia and endothelial cells. J Comp Neurol 160:477–490, 1975
119. Kramer S: Radiation Therapy in the Management of Milignant Gliomas. Seventh National Cancer Conference Proceedings. Lippincott, Philadelphia, 1973, pp 823–826
120. Kramer S: The hazards of therapeutic irradiation of the central nervous system. Clin Neurosurg 15:301–318, 1968
121. Kramer S, Kee KF: Complications of radiation therapy: the central nervous system. Semin Roentgenol 9:75–83, 1974
122. Kramer S, Southard ME, Mansfield CM: Radiation effect and tolerance of the central nervous system. Front Radiat Ther Oncol 6:332–345, 1972
123. Krishnaswamy V: Dose distribution around and iodine-125 seed source in tissue. Radiology 126:489–491, 1978

124. Kurland LT: The frequency of intracranial and intraspinal neoplasms in the resident population of Rochester, Minnesota. J Neurosurg 15:627–641, 1958
125. Kury G, Carter HW: Autoradiographic study of human nervous system tumors. Arch Pathol 80:38, 1965
126. Kusske JA, Williams JP, Garcia JH, et al: Radiation necrosis of the brain following radiotherapy of extracerebral neoplasms. Surg Neurol 6:15–20, 1976
127. Lajtha LG, Oliver R: Radiobiological considerations in radiotherapy. Br J Radiol 34:252–257, 1961
128. Lampert PW, Davis RL: Delayed effects of radiation on the human central nervous system: "early" and "late" delayed reactions. Neurology 14:912–917, 1964
129. Laramore GE, Griffin TW, Gerdes AJ, et al: Fast neutron and mixed (neutron/photon) beam teletherapy for grades II and IV astrocytomas. Cancer 42:96–103, 1978
130. Laughlin JS, Siler WM, Holodny EL, et al: A dose description system for interstitial radiation therapy. Am J Roentgenol 89:470–490, 1963
131. Lee F: Radiation of infratentorial and supratentorial brain stem tumors. J Neurosurg 43:65–68, 1975
132. Leibel SA, Sheline GE, Wara WM, et al: The role of radiation therapy in the treatment of astrocytomas. Cancer 31:1551–1557, 1975
133. Leksell L: A stereotaxic apparatus for intracerebral surgery. Acta Chir Scand 99:229–233, 1949
134. Leksell L: Stereotaxis and Radiosurgery: An Operative System. Charles C Thomas, Springfield, Illinois, 1971
135. Leksell L: The stereotaxic method and radiosurgery of the brain. Acta Chir Scand 102:316–319, 1951
136. Levy LF, Elvidge AR: Astrocytoma of the brain and spinal cord: A review of 176 cases, 1940–1949. J Neurosurg 13:413–443, 1956
137. Ley A, Ley A Jr, Guitard JM, et al: Surgical management of intracranial gliomas. J Neurosurg 19:365–374, 1962
138. Lindgren M: On tolerance of brain tissue and sensitivity of brain tumors to irradiation. Acta Radiol 170:1, 1958
139. Lindgren M: Roentgen treatment of gliomata. Acta Radiol 40:325–334, 1953
140. Ling CC, Anderson LL, Shipley WU: Dose in homogeneity in interstitial implants using iodine-251 seeds. Int J Radiat Oncol Biol Phys 5:419–425, 1979
141. Llena JF, Cespedes G, Hirano A, et al: Vascular alterations in delayed radiation necrosis of the brain: an electron microscopical study. Arch Pathol Lab Med 100:531–534, 1976
142. Lowenberg-Scharenberg K, Bassett RC: Amyloid degeneration of the human brain following x-ray therapy. J Neuropathol Exp Neurol 9:93–103, 1950
143. Lunsford DL, Rojenbaum AE, Perry J: Stereotactic surgery using the therapeutic CT scanner. Surg Neurol 18:116–122, 1982
144. MacKay AR, Gutin PH, Hosobuchi Y, et al: Computed tomography directed stereotaxy for biopsy and interstitial irradiation of brain tumors: technical note. Neurosurgery 11:38–42, 1982
145. MacKay A, Gutin PG, Hosobuchi Y, et al: CT stereotaxis and interstitial radiation for brain tumors. In: Interventional Radiological Techniques: Computed Tomography and Ultrasonography, edited by AA Moss, HI Goldberg. University of California Printing Department, San Francisco, 1981, pp 93–99
146. Mandybur TI, Gore I: Amyloid in late postirradiation necrosis of brain. Neurology 19:983–992, 1969
147. Marks JE, Baglan RJ, Pressad SC, et al: Cerebral radionecrosis: incidence and risk in relation to dose, time, fractionation and volume. Int J Radiat Oncol Biol Phys 7:243–252, 1981

148. Marks JE, Gado M: Serial CT of primary tumors following surgery, irradiation and chemotherapy. Radiology 125:119–125, 1977
149. Marra A, Guiffre R: Late cerebral radionecrosis. Eur Neurol 1:234–246, 1968
150. Marsa GW, Goffinet DR, Rubinstein LJ, et al: Megavoltage irradiation in the treatment of gliomas of the brain and spinal cord. Cancer 36:1681–1689, 1975
151. Marsa GW, Probert JC, Rubinstein LJ, et al: Radiation therapy in the treatment of childhood astrocytic gliomas. Cancer 32:646–655, 1973
152. Marshall LF, Langfitt TW: Needle biopsy, high-dose corticosteroids, and radiotherapy in the treatment of malignant glial tumors. Natl Cancer Inst Monogr 46:157–160, 1977
153. Martins AN, Johnston JS, Henry JM, et al: Delayed radiation necrosis of the brain. J Neurosurg 47:336–345, 1977
154. Matsumura H, Ono H, Mori K: Delayed radiation necrosis. J Electron Microsc 6:121–134, 1974
155. McDonald LW, Hayes TL: The role of capillaries in the pathogenesis of delayed radionecrosis of brain. Am J Pathol 50:745–764, 1967
156. McKissock W, Paine KWE: Primary tumors of the thalamus. Brain 81:41, 1952
157. Mendelsohn ML: The growth faction: a new concept applied to tumors. Science 132:1496, 1960
158. Mendelsohn ML: The kinetics of tumor cell proliferation. In: Cellular Radiation Biology. Williams & Wilkins, Baltimore, 1965, pp 498–513
158a. Meisberger LL, Keller RJ, Shale LR: The effective attenuation in water of the gamma rays, gold 198 Iridium 192, Cesium 137, Radium 226, Cobalt 60. Radiol 90:953–958, 1968
159. Mikhael MA: Dosimetric considerations in the diagnosis of radiation necrosis of the brain. In: Radiation Damage to the Nervous System: A Delayed Hazard, edited by HA Gilbert, HR Kagan. Raven Press, New York, 1980, pp 59–92
160. Mikhael MA: Radiation necrosis of the brain: correlation between computed tomography, pathology and dose distribution. J Comp Assist Tomogr 2:71–80, 1978
161. Mundinger F: Contributo alle indicazioni, all dosimetra ed alla tecnica di applicazione di radioisotopi per l'irradiazone interstiziale dei tumori cerebrali. Anat Chir 3:21–38, 1958
162. Mundinger F: Treatment of brain tumors with radioisotopes. Prog Neurol Surg 1:202–257, 1966
163. Mundinger F: Iridium-192—"GammaMed" a new irradiation for localized brachy-therapy of tumors. Excerpta Med Int Congr Ser 139, 1967
164. Mundinger F: Technik und Indikationen der interstitiellen Bestrahlung mit Radioisotopen bei Hirn- und Hypophysengeschwulsten. Kerntechnik Chemie, 11:333–345, 1969
165. Mundinger F: The treatment of brain tumors with interstitially applied radioactive isotopes. In: Radionuclide Applications in Neurology and Neurosurgery, edited by Yen Wang, P Paoletti. Charles C Thomas, Springfield, Illinois, 1970, pp 199–265
166. Mundinger F: Combined treatment of experimental DS-tumors and infiltrating cerebral glioma with interstitial curietherapy and radiosensitizing drugs. In: IV European Congress of Neurosurgery: Present Limits of Neurosurgery. Avicenum, Czechoslovak Medical Press, Prague, 1972, p 77
167. Mundinger F: Rationale and methods of interstitial iridium-192—brachycurietherapy and iridium-192 or iodine-125 protracted long term irradiation. In: Stereotactic Cerebral Irradiation, INSERM Symposium No. 12, edited by G Szikla. Elsevier/North-Holland Biomedical Press, Amsterdam, 1979, pp 101–116
168. Mundinger F: Stereotaktische Therapie nicht resezierbarer intracraniellar

Tumoren mit Ir-192 and Jod-125. In: Kombinierte chirurgische and radiologische Behandlung maligner Tumoren, edited by Wannenmacher, Schreiber, Gauwerky. Urban & Schwarzenberg, Munich, 1981

169. Mundinger F: Eine einfache Methode der lokalisierten Bestrahlung von Grobhirngesch wulsten mit radioaktivem Gold. Munch Med Wochenschr 98:23–25, 1956
170. Mundinger F, Birg W: CT-aided stereotaxy for functional neurosurgery and deep brain implants. Adv Neurosurg 10: 1981
171. Mundinger F, Birg W, Klar M: Computer-assisted stereotactic brain operations by means including computerized axial tomography. Appl Neurophysiol 41:169–182, 1978
172. Mundinger F, Busam B, Birg W, et al: Results of interstitial iridium-192 brachycurietherapy and iridium-192 protracted long term irradiation. In: Stereotactic Cerebral Irradiation, INSERM Symposium No. 12, edited by G. Szikla. Elsevier/North-Holland Biomedical Press, Amsterdam, 1979, pp 303–320
173. Mundinger F, Hoefer T: Protracted long-term irradiation of inoperable midbrain tumors by stereotactic curietherapy using iridium-192. Acta Neurochir (Wien) [Suppl] 21:93–100, 1974
174. Mundinger F, Metzel E: Interstitial radioisotope therapy of intractable diencephalic tumors by the stereotactic permanent implantation of iridium-192, including bioptic control. Confin Neurol 32:195–202, 1970
175. Mundinger F, Ostertag C: Postoperative stereotactic curie-therapy using iridium-192 Gamma Med® contact irradiation apparatus combined with radiosensitizers in treating multiforme glioblastomas. Acta Neurochir (Wien) 42:73–33, 1978
176. Mundinger F, Ostertag C, Birg W, et al: Stereotactic treatment of brain lesions, biopsy, interstitial radiotherapy (iridum-192 and iodine-125), and drainage procedures. Appl Neurophysiol 43:198–204, 1980
177. Nakagaki H, Brunhart G, Kemper TL, et al: Monkey brain damage from radiation in the therapeutic range. J Neurosurg 44:3, 1976
178. National Cancer Institute's Surveillance, Epidemiology and End Results (SEER) Program. CA 33:9–25, 1983
179. Netsky MG, August B, Fowler W: The longevity of patients with glioblastoma multiforme. J Neurosurg 7:261–269, 1950
180. Netsky MG, Shapiro J, Hoffman M, et al: The effect of single doses of roentgen radiation on experimentally induced gliomas: with a critical review of the effects of roentgen radiation on gliomas in man. Am J Roentgenol 76:351–366, 1956
181. Nias AHW, Howard A, Greene D, et al: The response of Chinese hamster cells to protracted irradiation from 252 cf and 60 Co. Br J Radiol 46:991, 1973
182. Norman D, Enzmann DR, Levin VA, et al: Computed tomography in the evaluation of malignant glioma before and after therapy. Radiology 121:85–98, 1976
183. O'Connor GT: Cancer—a general review. Primate Med 3:9–22, 1969
184. Onoyama Y, Abe M, Yabumoto E: Radiation therapy in the treatment of glioblastoma. Am J Roentgenol 126:481–492, 1976
185. Onoyama Y, Mitsuyuki A, Yabumoto E, et al: Radiation therapy in the treatment of glioblastoma. Am J Roentgenol 126:481–492, 1976
186. Orton CG, Ellis F: A simplification in the use of the NSD concept in practical radiotherapy. Br J Radiol 46:529–537, 1973
187. Ostertag CB, Mennel HD, Kiessling M: Stereotactic biopsy of brain tumors. Surg Neurol 14:275–283, 1980
188. Overton MC III: Radioactive chromic phosphate in cystic brain tumors. J Nucl Med 7:641–642, 1966
189. Overton MC III, Sheffel DD: Recurrent cystic formation in craniopharyngi-

oma treated with radioactive chromic phosphate: case report. J Neurosurg 20:707–710, 1963
190. Pancoast HK: Treatment of brain tumors by radiation. Am J Roentgenol 9:42–47, 1922
191. Paterson R, Parker HM: A dosage system for gamma ray therapy. Br J Radiol 7:592–612, 1934
192. Pay NT, Carella RJ, Lin JR, et al: The usefulness of computed tomography during and after radiation therapy in patients with brain tumors. Radiology 121:79–83, 1976
193. Peck FC Jr, McGovern ER: Radiation necrosis of the brain in acromegaly. J Neurosurg 25:536–542, 1966
194. Penman J, Smith MC: Intracranial Gliomata. Medical Research Council Special Report Series No. 284, MRC, London, 1954
195. Pennybacker J, Russell DS: Necrosis of the brain due to radiation therapy: clinical and pathological observations. J Neurol Neurosurg Psychiatry 11:183–198, 1948
196. Phillips TL, Fu KK: Quantification of combined radiation therapy and chemotherapy effects of critical normal tissues. Cancer 37:1186–1200, 1976
197. Poisson M, Haus JJ, Pouillart P, et al: Malignant gliomas treated after surgery by combination chemotherapy and delayed radiation therapy. Acta Neurochir (Wien) 51:27, 1979
198. Puck TT, Markus PI: Action of x-rays on mammalian cells. J Exp Med 103:653–666, 1956
199. Quagliana J, Eltringham J, Kushner J, et al: Radiation therapy and CCNU + procarbazine in patients with grade III and IV astrocytomas of the brain. Proc Am Assoc Cancer Res 17:21, 1976
200. Quimby EQ: Dosage table for linear radium sources. Radiology 43:572, 1944
201. Quinlan WS, Michaelson SM: The response of the dog to head irradiation. Aerospace Med 35:362–364, 1964
202. Ramsey RG, Brand WN: Radiotherapy of glioblastoma multiforme. J Neurosurg 39:197, 1973
203. Ransohoff J, Lieberman A, Walker MD: Multiple therapies in the management of malignant gliomas. Neurooncology 1:55–68, 1979
204. Reagan TJ, Bisel HF, Childs DS Jr, et al: Controlled study of CCNU and radiation therapy in malignant astrocytoma. J Neurosurg 44:186–190, 1976
205. Reichert T, Mundinger F: Indications, technique and results of the stereotactic operations upon the hypophysis using radioisotopes. J Neurol Ment Dis 13:1–9, 1966
206. Reinhold HS: The influence of radiation on blood vessels and circulation. Radiat Res 10:1–198, 1974
207. Reinhold HS, Busiman GH: Repair of radiation damage to capillary endothelium. Br J Radiol 48:727, 1975
208. Report No. 39: Basic Radiation Protection Criteria. National Council on Radiation Protection and Measurements, Washington, DC, 1971
209. Rhodes ML, Glenn WV, Azzawi UM: Stereotactic neurosurgery using 3D-image data from computer tomography. J Med Syst 6:103–117, 1982
210. Rider WD: Radiation damage to the brain: a new syndrome. J Can Assoc Radiol 14:67–69, 1963
211. Roth JG, Elvidge AR: Glioblastoma multiforme: a clinical survey. J Neurosurg 17:736, 1960
212. Rosenblum ML, Knebel KD, Vasques DA, et al: In vivo clonogenic tumor cell kinetics following BCNU brain tumor therapy. Cancer Res 36:3718, 1976
213. Ross JP: The treatment of cerebral tumours with radium. Br J Surg 18:618–635, 1931
214. Rougie A, Pigneux J, Richard R, et al: La prise en change diagnostique et therapeutiquedes gliomes malins. Neurochirurgie 27:315–320, 1981

215. Rubinstein LJ: Tumors of the Central Nervous System (Second Series, Fascicle 6). Armed Forces Institute of Pathology, Washington, DC, 1972
216. Rubinstein LJ, Herman MM, Long TF, et al: Disseminated necrotizing leukoencephalopathy: a complication of treated central nervous system leukemia and lymphoma. Cancer 35:291–305, 1975
217. Russell DS, Rubinstein LJ: Pathology of Tumors of the Nervous System, 4th ed. Williams & Wilkins, Baltimore, 1977
218. Rutten E, Kazen I, Sloaf JL, et al: Postoperative radiation therapy in the management of brain astrocytoma: retrospective study of 142 patients. Int J Radiat Oncol Biol Phys 7:191–195, 1981
219. Sachs E: The treatment of glioblastomas with radium. J Neurosurg 11:119–121, 1954
220. Sachs E, Rubinstein JE, Arneson AN: Results of roentgen treatment of a series of one hundred and nineteen gliomas. Arch Neurol Psychiatry 35:597–616, 1936
221. Salazar OM, Rubin P: The spread of glioblastoma multiforme as a determining factor in the radiation treated volume. Int J Radiol Oncol Biol Phys 1:627–637, 1976
222. Salazar OM, Rubin P, Felstein ML, et al: High dose radiation therapy in the treatment of malignant gliomas: final report. Int J Radiol Oncol Biol Phys 5:1733–1740, 1979
223. Salazar OM, Rubin P, McDonald JV: Patterns of failure in intracranial astrocytomas after irradiation: analysis of dose and field factors. Am J Roentgenol 126:279–292, 1976
224. Salazar OM, Rubin P, McDonald JV, et al: High dose radiation therapy in the treatment of glioblastoma multiforme: a preliminary report. Int J Radiol Oncol Biol Phys 1:717–727, 1976
225. Saleman M: Glioblastoma multiforme. Am J Med Sci 279:84–94, 1980
226. Saleman M: Survival in glioblastoma: historical perspective. Neurosurgery 7:435, 1980
227. Sargent P, Cade S: The treatment of gliomata and pituitary tumours with radium. Br J Surg 18:501–520, 1931
228. Scanlon PW, Taylor WF: Radiotherapy of intracranial astrocytomas: analysis of 417 cases treated from 1960 through 1969. Neurosurgery 5:301–308, 1979
229. Scarabin JM, Pecker J, Brucher JM, et al: Stereotaxic exploration in 200 supratentorial brain tumors. Neuroradiologie 16:591–593, 1978
230. Scholz W, Hsu YK: Late damage from roentgen irradiation of the human brain. Arch Neurol Psychiatry 40:928–936, 1938
231. Schryver de A, Greitz J, Forsby N, et al: Localized shared field radiotherapy of malignant glioblastoma multiforme. Int J Radiol Oncol Biol Phys 1:713, 1976
232. Sedan R, Peragut JC, Farnanier PH, et al: Place de biopsie en condition stereotaxique dans la tactique therapeutique des gliomes malins. Neurochirurgie 27:285–286, 1981
233. Seiler RW: Late results of multimodality therapy of high-grade supratentorial astrocytomas. Surg Neurol 15:88, 1981
234. Seiler RW, Greiner RH, Zimmerman A, et al: Radiotherapy combined with procarbazine, bleomycin, and CCNU in the treatment of high-grade supratentorial astrocytomas. J Neurosurg 48:861–865, 1978
235. Seiler RW, Zimmermann A, Bleher EA, et al: Preoperative radiotherapy and chemotherapy in hypervascular, high-grade supratentorial astrocytomas. Surg Neurol 12:131, 1978
236. Shapiro WR: Combined modality approach for brain tumors. In: Cancer: Achievements, Challenges and Prospects for the 1980s, Vol 2, edited by JR Burchenal, HF Oettgen. Grune & Stratton, New York, 1981, pp 379–389,
237. Shapiro WR: Management of primary malignant brain tumors. In: Weekly Update: Neurology and Neurosurgery, pp 1–8. Biomedia, Princeton, NJ, 1978

238. Shapiro WR, Young DF: Treatment of malignant glioma: a controlled study of chemotherapy and irradiation. Arch Neurol 33:494–500, 1976
239. Sheline GE: Conventional radiation therapy of gliomas. In: Recent Results in Cancer Research. Springer-Verlag, New York, 1974
240. Sheline GE: Radiation therapy of brain tumors. Cancer 39:873–881, 1977
241. Sheline GE: Radiation therapy of primary tumors. Semin Oncol 2:29–42, 1975
242. Sheline GE: The importance of distinguishing tumor grade in malignant gliomas: treatment and prognosis. Int J Radiat Oncol Biol Phys 1:781–786, 1976
243. Sheline GE, Boldrey E, Karlsbery P, et al: Therapeutic considerations in tumors affecting the central nervous system. Radiology 82:84–89, 1964
244. Sheline GE, Wara WM, Smith V: Therapeutic irradiation and brain injury. Int J Radiat Oncol Biol Phys 6:1215–1228, 1980
245. Silverberg E: Cancer statistics 1977. CA 27:26–41, 1977
246. Simpson WJ: Time and dose relationships in radiation biology as applied to radiotherapy. Presented at the NCI-AEC Conference, 1970
247. Spiegel EA, Wycis HT, Marks M, et al: Stereotaxic apparatus for operations on the human brain. Science 106:349–350, 1947
248. Stage WS, Stein JJ: Treatment of malignant astrocytomas. Am J Roentgenol 120:7, 1974
249. Steel GG: Cell loss as a factor in the growth rate of human tumors. Eur J Cancer 3:381–387, 1967
250. Steel GG: The Growth Kinetics of Tumors. Oxford University Press, London, 1977
251. Suit H, Urano M: Repair of sublethal radiation injury in hypoxic cells of a C_3H mouse mammary carcinoma. Radiat Res 37:423–434, 1969
252. Sweet DL, Hendler FJ, Hanlon K, et al: Treatment of grade III and IV astrocytomas with BCNU alone and in combination with VM 26 following surgery and radiation therapy. Cancer Treat Rep 63:1707, 1979
253. Szikla G (ed): Stereotactic Cerebral Irradiation: Proceedings of the INSERM Symposium on Stereotactic Irradiations. Elsevier/North-Holland Biomedical Press, Amsterdam, 1979
254. Szikla G, Betti O, Szenthe L, et al: L'experience actuelle des irradiation stereotaxiques dans le traitement des gliomes hemispheriques. Neurochirurgie 27:295–298, 1981
255. Szikla G, Peragut JC: Irradiation interstitielle des gliomes. Neurochirurgie (Suppl 2) 21:187–228, 1975
256. Talairach J, Aboulker J, Ruggiero G, et al: Essai d'un nouveau traitment des tumeurs cerebrales inoperables: mise en place d'or radio-actif par stereotaxie. Sem Hop Paris 31:1–6, 1955
257. Talairach J, Aboulker P, Ruggiero G, et al: Utilisation de la methode radiostereotaxique pour le traitement radioactif in situ des tumeurs cerebrales. Rev Neurol (Paris) 90:656–657, 1954
258. Talairach J, Bonis A, Szikla G, et al: Stereotaxic implantation of radioactive isotopes in functional pituitary surgery: technique and results. In: Radionuclide Applications in Neurology and Neurosurgery, edited by Y Wang, P Paoletti. Charles C Thomas, Springfield, Illinois, 1970, pp 367–299
259. Talairach J, Ruggiero G, Aboulker J, et al: A new method of treatment of inoperable brain tumours by stereotaxic implantation of radioactive gold—a preliminary report. Br J Radiol 2862–2874, 1955
260. Talairach J, Szikla G, Tournoux P, et al: Utilisation therapeutic des radioisotopes. Presented at the Second International Congress of Neurological Surgery, Washington, DC 1961
261. Taveras JM, Thompson NG, Pool JL: Should we treat glioblastoma multiforme? Am J Roentgenol 87:473–479, 1962
262. Todd IDH: Choice of volume in the x-ray treatment of supratentorial gliomas. Br J Radiol 36:645–649, 1963
263. Tonnis W: In: Kirschner-Nordmann Bd III, Gliome. 1961

264. Tonnis W, Walker W: Das glioblastoma multiforme. Acta Neurochir (Wien) [Suppl] 6:40–42, 1959
265. Tovi D, Schisano G, Liljequist B: Primary tumors of the region of the thalamus. J Neurosurg 18:735, 1961
266. Uihlein A, Colby MY, Layten DD, et al: Comparison of surgery plus radiation in the treatment of supratentorial gliomas. Acta Radiol [Ther] (Stockh) 5:67, 1966
267. Urtasun RC, Band PR, Chapman JD, et al: Radiation plus metronidazole for glioblastoma. N Engl J Med 296:757, 1977
268. Van der Kogel AJ, Barendsen GW: Late effects of spinal cord irradiation with 300 kv x-rays and 15 MeV neutrons. Br J Radiol 47:393–398, 1974
269. Wachowski TJ, Chenault H: Degenerative effects of large doses of roentgen rays on the human brain. Radiology 45:227–246, 1945
270. Walker MD: Brain and peripheral nervous system tumors. In: Cancer Medicine, edited by JF Holland, E Frei III. Lea & Febiger, Philadelphia, 1973, pp 1385–1407
271. Walker MD: Chemotherapy: adjuvant to surgery and radiation therapy. Semin Oncol 2:69–72, 1975
272. Walker MD: Chemotherapy of malignant glioma. In: Seventh National Cancer Conference Proceedings. Lippincott, Philadelphia, 1973, pp 817–821
273. Walker MD: Malignant brain tumors—a synopsis. CA 25:114–120, 1975
274. Walker MD, Alexander E Jr, Hunt WE, et al: Evaluation of BCNU and/or radiotherapy in the treatment of anaplastic gliomas: a cooperative clinical trial. J Neurosurg 49:333–363, 1978
275. Walker MD, Alexander E Jr, Hunt WE, et al: The evaluation of mithramycin in the treatment of anaplastic gliomas. J Neurosurg 44:655–667, 1976
276. Walker MD, Green SB, Byar DP, et al: Randomized comparisons of radiotherapy and nitrosoureas for the treatment of malignant glioma after surgery. N Engl J Med 303:1323–1329, 1980
277. Walker MD, Strike TA: An evaluation of methyl CCNU, BCNU and radiotherapy in the treatment of malignant glioma. Proc Am Assoc Cancer Res 17:163, 1976
278. Walker MD, Strike TA, Sheline GE: An analysis of dose-effect relationship in the radiotherapy of malignant gliomas. Int J Radiat Oncol Biol Phys 5:1725–1731, 1979
279. Wara WA, Phillips TL, Sheline GE, et al: Radiation tolerance of the spinal cord. Cancer 35:1558–1562, 1975
280. Weir B: The relative significance of factors affecting post-operative survival in astrocytoma grades 3 and 4. J Neurosurg 39:448, 1973
281. Weir B, Band P, Urtasum R, et al: Radiotherapy and CCNU in the treatment of high-grade supratentorial astrocytomas. J Neurosurg 45:129–134, 1976
282. Weir B, Elvidge AR: Oligodendrogliomas: an analysis of 63 cases. J Neurosurg 29:500–505, 1968
283. Whitmore GF, Gulyas S, Botond J: Radiation sensitivity throughout the cell cycle and its relationship to recovery. In: Cellular Radiation Biology. Williams & Wilkins, Baltimore, 1965, pp 423–431
284. Willson N, Duffy PE: Morphologic changes associated with combined BCNU and radiation therapy in glioblastoma multiforme. Neurology 24:465–471, 1974
285. Deleted during production.
286. Young DF, Posner JB, Chu F, et al: Rapid-course radiation therapy of cerebral metastases: results and complications. Cancer 34:1069–1076, 1974
287. Yung WK, Steward W, Marks JE, et al: Glioblastoma multiforme: treatment with radiation and triiodothyronine. Int J Radiat Oncol Biol Phys 1:645–650, 1976
288. Zeman W: Pathogenesis of radiolesions in the mature central nervous system. In: Proceedings of the Fifth International Congress of Neuropathology. Excerpta Medica Foundation, Amsterdam, 1966

289. Zulch KJ: Brain Tumors: Their Biology and Pathology. New York, Springer-Verlag 1965
290. Zulch KJ: Uber die Strahlensensibilitat der Hirngeschwulste und die sog. Strahlen-Spatnekros des Hirns. Dtsch Med Wochenschr 85:293–298, 1960

9

Interaction of Chemotherapy and Teletherapy

Peter S. Kennedy

Chemotherapy for brain tumors in adults has been largely the treatment of high-grade astrocytomas. Historically, the role of cytotoxic therapy was that of palliation for patients with recurrent tumors. A series of early uncontrolled studies (19) utilized patients with a variety of histologies who were generally heavily pretreated with surgery and irradiation, and who were debilitated in the bargain.

Recently, a more scientific approach has necessitated evaluation of the factors affecting response and survival which make results of chemotherapy given alone, or in combination with surgery and irradiation, more interpretable. Several prognostic variables affect survival duration in patients with malignant brain tumors. First, age varies inversely with survival (16). Other factors which have a negative impact on life span include prediagnostic symptom duration, the presence of personality change, an absence of seizures, the presence of a depressed level of consciousness at diagnosis, and low postoperative performance status. Studies by the Brain Tumor Study Group (BTSG, a multi-institutional cooperative research organization functioning under the auspices of the National Cancer Institute in the United States) have shown that patients with a Karnofsky status of ≤ 40 have an inferior survival when compared to patients with a performance status of ≥ 70 (p 0.0001) (22). Tumor grade is also an important determinant of survival. In general, treatment of slow-growing tumors produces a modest prolongation in survival when partial remission is achieved. Such remissions are not durable, however, in that cure is rarely produced. Conversely, survival advantages after treatment of rapidly growing tumors is even less impressive for patients with partial remission, but a plateau in survival curves after an initial steep decline suggests that some patients may be cured (23).

Individual brain tumors are characterized by cytologic and genetic heterogeneity. Multiple karyotypically defined subpopulations have been identified within a single tumor (15). The growth fraction at the periphery of a large lesion may approach 30%, whereas at the center values of 1% are common (6). Adequacy of blood supply, with subsequent variability of nutrient delivery, tissue Po_2 and tissue pH are important determinants of cell growth and drug delivery to the tumor. Calculated doubling times of 5 days for glioblastoma compare with an observed doubling time of 5 weeks, suggesting a cell loss factor of as much as 80% (7).

The blood-brain barrier (BBB) is of critical importance in the selection and success potential of chemotherapeutic agents. Aminoisobutyric acid (AIB) is an artificial amino acid which traverses a disrupted BBB and is taken up by adjacent cells. Blaisberg et al. (1) showed that AIB passes readily into the central portions of malignant gliomas but that the BBB is more consistently intact at the tumor periphery. Small molecules (<200 daltons) which are lipid-soluble (i.e., nonpolar) and nonprotein-bound serve as the best agents for delivery to tumor cells.

Measures of Tumor Response

Determinants of tumor response to treatment are variable but important to consider when evaluating efficacy of treatment. Clinical regression of tumor-related signs and symptoms (e.g., paresis, behavior abnormalities, seizure activity, headache) may be the result of tumor regression or a reduction in edema. Serial measurements by isotopic or computed axial tomography (CAT) brain scans are widely used but remain, at best, indirect measurements of tumor response. The resolution limits of these diagnostic tools and their inability to distinguish viable tumor from scar tissue and/or nonviable tumor represent limitations in their reliability in measuring response to therapy. Other parameters frequently measured when evaluating drug efficacy include median remission duration (time to progression), overall survival, disease-free survival, and rarely postrelapse survival.

Evaluative Studies of Chemotherapy

The first prospective controlled evaluation of drug efficacy in the treatment of malignant brain tumors was the BTSG evaluation of mithramycin. Patients were randomized to receive mithramycin (25 mg/kg/day q 21 days) or conventional supportive therapy starting 21 days after surgery. Median survival among 96 evaluable patients was 21 weeks for mithramycin-treated patients and 26 weeks for controls (21). The drug was considered ineffective, but a new era of brain tumor research had begun. During this time, low-molecular-weight, lipid-soluble compounds, including the nitrosoureas and procarbazine, were introduced.

In 1978 the BTSG published a prospective randomized trial of 303 patients who received "best conventional therapy," chemotherapy with BCNU $80/m^2/day \times 3$ every 6–8 weeks, identical chemotherapy plus radiotherapy consisting of 5,000–6,000 rads to whole brain, or radiotherapy alone. Patients were evaluated as to appropriate entry by neuropathology, steroid treatment, and therapeutic approach (222 patients), or as having received 5,000 rads of radiotherapy, two or more courses of chemotherapy, with a minimum survival of 8 weeks. In the last group, median survival was 17 weeks for conventionally treated patients, 25 weeks for chemotherapy-treated patients, 37.5 weeks for patients receiving radiation alone, and 40.5 weeks for patients receiving chemotherapy and radiation. There was no statistical difference in survival among patients receiving radiation or chemotherapy. All were superior to supportive treatment alone. All treatment groups were comparable with respect to age, sex, tumor location, histopathology, signs, symptoms, or steroid use (20).

A study utilizing combination chemotherapy was carried out by Seiler et al. in 1978 (14). Twenty patients with grade III–IV astrocytomas received 6,000–6,800 rads after gross total tumor resection. Chemotherapy consisted of CCNU, procarbazine, and bleomycin followed by maintenance with CCNU. The combination was used because previous studies by Brisman et al. (2), Reagan et al. (10), and others had failed to show an advantage for patients receiving CCNU when compared to radiation therapy alone. Seiler's study also showed a median survival of 56 weeks for combined-modality-treated patients compared to 51 weeks for 32 retrospective historical controls.

Following leads that suggested activity for the epipodophyllotoxin in VM^{26} against glioblastoma (9,17), Sweet et al. (18) randomized 21 patients to receive either BCNU alone or BCNU plus VM^{26} after surgery and radiation therapy; there was no difference in survival for the two groups (median 14 months versus 22 months, $p \geq 0.05$).

Furthermore, serial CAT scans could not document tumor regression in any patients receiving chemotherapy, and two patients died of BCNU-related pulmonary fibrosis. In a later study, the EORTC evaluated VM^{26} plus CCNU and found a 39-week median survival compared to a 30-week survival in controls receiving surgery and radiation (5,500–6,000 rads) only. A previous EORTC study had shown similar survival for adjuvant CCNU alone (4).

A further BTSG trial compared McCCNU, radiotherapy, BCNU plus radiotherapy, and McCCNU plus radiotherapy (22). A group of 358 patients comprised the "valid study group." Although no statistically significant advantage was found for combined-treatment patients, there was a greater number of "long-term" survivors in both combined-method groups. This confirmed findings of their previous study (20) and suggested that chemotherapy was advantageous to a small group of radiation-treated patients.

An interesting study "developed from animal data and human glioma cell kinetic studies" utilized 5-fluorouracil (5-Fu) given 2 weeks after BCNU. Although disease progression was said to be "temporarily arrested" in 83% of patients, this combination has not found its way into adjuvant trials (8). An earlier study utilizing concurrent radiation therapy and 5-FU given to the point of gastrointestinal and marrow toxicity showed no improvement in survival (3).

Salcmann reviewed 17 papers evaluating survival data on 1,561 patients with glioblastoma (12). When grouped by treatment, 349 patients receiving surgery alone had a median survival of 16 weeks. Surgery plus irradiation (568 patients) produced a median survival of 37 weeks. The addition of chemotherapy in 146 patients was associated with a 40-week survival. Although there are dangers in this kind of comparative trial, it has been advocated in other tumor systems (T. Moon, unpublished data) and supports the general impression that little survival advantage is gained by adding adjuvant chemotherapy to postoperative radiation.

The most recent BTSG trial has compared BCNU, high-dose methylprednisolone, procarbazine, and BCNU plus methylprednisolone (5). Once again, patients were comparable with regard to important prognostic factors as measured by multiple regression analysis. Unadjusted survival analysis showed inferior survival for patients receiving high-dose methylprednisolone compared to patients receiving BCNU or procarbazine ($p < 0.05$). When adjusted for eight variables found to have prognostic significance for survival (age, histopathology, performance status, ABO group, pretreatment white blood cell and platelet counts, duration of symptoms, and level of consciousness), methylprednisolone treatment was no longer statistically significantly inferior to the other treatment forms ($p > 0.20$). Although this finding does not conclusively suggest that high-dose steroid treatment is harmful, it indicates that standard-dose steroids often given in uncontrolled fashion in other clinical trails do not improve survival. Patients receiving BCNU plus steroids had an intermediate survival, but this is difficult to interpret in light of the predictably increased serious infection rate in these patients. When compared to previously studied patient groups receiving radiation alone, BCNU or procarbazine therapy was comparable, had only a slight impact on median survival, but again increases the number (25%) of long-term survivors at 2 years.

Quality of Survival

Equally important to improved survival among some patients receiving combined-modality therapy is the quality of survival in adjuvant-treated patients. Although the nitrosourea compounds are relatively simple to administer, there is little evidence that performance status is ever improved by their use (7). Additionally, reports of severe, irreversible pulmonary fibrosis, hepatocellular damage, and renal insufficiency are disturbing. Cases of acute leukemia among patients receiving nitrosoureas are few, but the finding is ominous and a potentially high price to pay for extended survival (11). Finally, it has been shown that patients surviving 3 years have an increased incidence of brain damage measured both clinically and pathologically (13). Overall, the advantage gained by adjuvant chemotherapy has been modest, and new approaches to chemotherapy and irradiation are necessary.

References

1. Blaisberg RG, Gazendam J, Patlak CS, et al: Changes in blood brain transfer parameters induced by hyperosmolar intracarotid infusion and by metastatic tumor growth. In: The Cerebral Microvasculature, edited by HM Eisenberg, RL Suddith. Plenum, New York, 1980, pp 307–319
2. Brisman R, Housepian EM, Chang C, et al: Adjuvant nitrosourea therapy for glioblastoma. Arch Neurol 33:745–750, 1976
3. Edland RW, Manucher J, Ansfield F: Glioblastoma multiforme—an analysis

of the results of postoperative radiotherapy alone versus radiotherapy and concomitant 5-fluorouracil. Am J Roentgenol 3:337–342, 1971

4. Evaluation of CCNU, VM[26] plus CCNU and procarbazine in supratentorial brain gliomas. J Neurosurg 55:27–31, 1981
5. Green SD, Dyar DP, Walker MD: Comparisons of carmustine, procarbazine, and high dose methylprednisolone as additions to surgery and radiotherapy for the treatment of malignant glioma. Cancer Treat Rep 67:121–132, 1983
6. Hoshino T, Wilson, CB: *J Neurosurg* 42:123, 1975
7. Jones A: Cerebral astrocytoma: trends in radiation therapy and chemotherapy—a review. J R Soc Med 71:661–674, 1978
8. Levin VA: Chemotherapy of Recurrent Brain Tumors in Nitrosoureas—Current Status and New Developments, edited by AW Prestayko, ST Crooke, LH Baker, et al. Academic Press, New York, pp 259–268, 1981
9. Muggin FM, Selaway OS, Hansen HH: Clinical studies with a new podophyllotoxin derivative epipodophyllotoxin, 4:demethyl-9-(4.6-0-2-thenylidine-β-D-glucopyranoside) (NSC-122819). Cancer Chem Rep 55:575–581, 1971
10. Reagan TJ, Risel HF, Childs DS Jr, et al: Controlled study of CCNU and radiation therapy in malignant astrocytoma. J Neurosurg 44:186–190, 1976
11. Robustellidilla Curia G, Paoletti P, Bernado G, et al: Clinical toxicity of combined modality treatment with nitrosourea derivatives for central nervous system tumors. Neurosurgery 11:408–411, 1982
12. Salcman M: Survival in glioblastoma—historical prospective. Neurosurgery 7:435–439, 1980
13. Schiffer D, Giordana MT, Paoletti P, et al: Pathology of human malignant gliomas after radiation and chemotherapy. Acta Neuroclin 53:205–216, 1980
14. Seiler RW, Greiner RH, Zimmerman A: Radiotherapy combined with procarbazine, bleomycin, and CCNU in the treatment of high-grade supratentorial astrocytomas. J Neurosurg 48:861–865, 1978
15. Shapiro JR, Jung W-KA, Shapiro WR: Isolation, karyotype and clonal growth of heterogenous subpopulations of human malignant gliomas. Cancer Res 41:2349–2359, 1981
16. Shapiro WR: Treatment of neuroechodermal brain tumors. Ann Neurol 12:231–237, 1982
17. Sklansky BD, Mann-Kaplan RS, Reynolds AF Jr, et al: 4:Demethyl-epipodophyllotoxin-B-D -thenylidine-glucoside (PTG) in treatment of malignant intracranial neoplasms. Cancer 33:460–467, 1974
18. Sweet DL, Handler FJ, Hanlon K, et al: Treatment of grade III and IV astrocytomas with BCNU alone and in combination with VM[26] following surgery and radiation therapy. Cancer Treat Rep 63:1707–1711, 1979
19. Walker MD: Brain tumors. In: Cancer Medicine, edited by JF Holland, E Frei. Lea & Febiger, Philadelphia, 1973, pp 1385–1407
20. Walker MD, Alexander E, Hunt WE: Evaluation of BCNU and/or radiotherapy in the treatment of anaplastic gliomas. J Neurosurg 49:333–343, 1978
21. Walker MD, Alexander E, Hunt WE: Evaluation of mithramycin in treatment of anaplastic gliomas. J Neurosurg 44:655–657, 1976
22. Walker MD, Green SB, Byar DP, et al: Randomized comparisons of radiotherapy and nitrosoureas for treatment of malignant glioma after surgery. N Engl J Med 303:1323–1329, 19xx
23. Wilson CB, Boldrey EB, Enot KJ: Cancer Chemother Rep 54:273–281, 1980

10

CT-Assisted Interactive Stereotactic Systems

Roger A. Slater
Michael L. Rhodes
William V. Glenn Jr

Several stereotactic systems using computed tomography (CT) data for precise placement of neurosurgical instruments have been introduced during the last 5 years. Using digital CT image data that are transformed to a patient-frame coordinate system, surgery can be simulated, planned, and executed with submillimeter precision. This chapter introduces two stereotactic systems that improve the speed, image resolution, accuracy, and patient comfort of past methods. Both frames and their computer programs were developed by a team of neurosurgeons and computer scientists for surgical procedures conducted entirely in the CT suite. The first part of this chapter describes the ongoing clinical development of the first all-plastic frame now used in over 30 procedures. Methods utilized in this early integrated system are discussed, special biopsy tools are described, an analysis of the histologic lesions identified is made, and the preliminary results of therapy utilizing this approach are presented.

Since 6 June 1980 we have used such an integrated system of technologies to biopsy intracerebral tumors via a burrhole and, where appropriate, to place isotopes (iridium-192) within the neoplastic lesions. Results at this time demonstrate that adequate tissue can be obtained for diagnosis via a burrhole without general anesthesia, formal craniotomy, or open biopsy. At this time results *do not* demonstrate conclusively a superior outcome as compared with the classic approach of craniotomy, biopsy, and external-beam irradiation. However, the system offers a practical alternative approach to the classic management of intracerebral gliomas. The implications of brachytherapy versus teletherapy and combinations of these modalities are discussed. Morbidity and mortality statistics are also reviewed.

The chapter's second half describes geometric resolution of a new system, its test procedures, and phantom results. The latter system is designed for higher-resolution CT scanners and their faster computer systems, and incorporates several frame modifications suggested by our past experience. At this writing, patient data are not yet available for the new or second generation system.

The First Frame and Clinical Results

The stereotactic systems described in this chapter are an integration of several technologies: computer-aided diagnostic medicine, computed tomography, interactive computer graphics, pathology, medical instrumentation, and treatment planning, including the use of brachytherapy, teletherapy, or subtotal resection of a lesion where indicated. Although this system approach has applications beyond biopsy and treatment of intracerebral neoplasms, our experience is limited to this area at the time of this writing.

The first system was developed at Memorial Hospital Medical Center of Long Beach during the late 1970s and has been used clinically since June 1980, at which time the first biopsy was obtained (Figure 10–1). Our first use of the device for biopsy and interstitial irradiation was begun on 15 July 1981. The second system described here (Figure 10–2) was developed during 1981 and 1982 by coresearchers at Multi-Planar Diagnostic Imaging, Inc., Torrance, California.

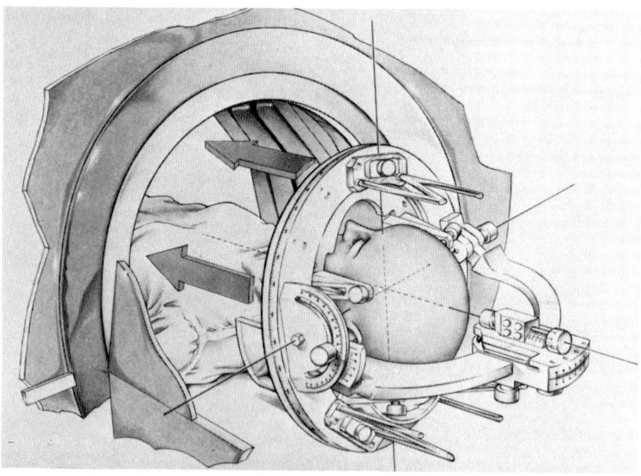

FIGURE 10–1 Memorial Hospital frame, 1980.

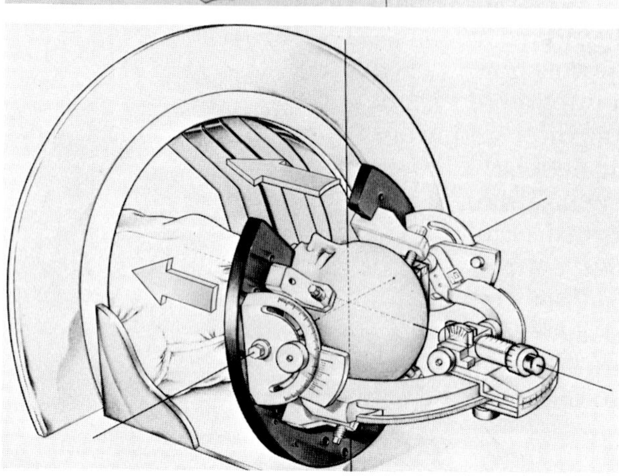

Figure 10–2 Multiplanar stereotactic (MPS) frame, 1982.

Background

A stereotactic system for neurosurgery requires three components: 1) an image-generation device—historically, plane-film x-ray systems (6–8,10), but more recently computed tomography (CT) scanners (1,3,16); 2) a mechanical frame; and 3) a procedure to transform image-system coordinates to frame positions. In the past, image-to-frame registration has been a manual triangulation approach (6–8,10). Now, more automated solutions have taken the form of computer programs (1,3,16). Together with these programs, new frames have been introduced that represent the key component of any stereotactic system. The frame provides a fixation mechanism to hold the skull firmly in place during the procedure, a known geometry to locate image-system pictures in the frame's coordinate system, and a platform for precise placement of surgical instruments.

Stereotactic frames have undergone several changes since the early work in England by Horsley and Clarke (6,7). Their frame was solid brass and designed primarily for neurostructure and neurofunction experimentation with cats. Wide acceptance for human neurosurgery procedures was aided by Professor Lars Leksell of the Karolinska Institute in Stockholm in his pioneering work (10) only three decades past. The dramatic introduction of the CT scanner revolutionized neuroradiology and neurosurgery during the early 1970s. CT's wide acceptance during the mid-1970s inspired innovations for frames that were originally designed for plane-film x-ray surgical procedures. Notably, Mundinger et al. (12–14) have made extensive use of CT image information to treat cerebral gliomas with long- and short-term irradiation. Brown (3) and later Kelly and Alker (9) attached geometry to a Trent Wells (Trent Wells, Inc., South Gate, California 90280) frame for CT scanning. CT images then were used to select a target and instrument trajectory for surgery. In both cases additional apparatus was manufactured to transport the patient out of the CT scanning suite to the operating room for the actual procedure.

The frames described here are designed for CT scanner suite operations to speed the procedure and to ensure extreme accuracy. Simple tumor biopsy, ablation, or radioactive-seed placement should be complete within 1 hr, and in some cases less than one-half hour. Verification and postoperative scans can be taken easily and provide precise, timely localization of intracranial bleeding should any occur during the operation. An additional benefit, largely untapped in most neurosurgical procedures, is the numerical and image display power of the scanner's computer system. Three-dimensional presentations of neuroanatomy, isodose radiation therapy contours or surfaces, and quantitative anatomic measurements are now the exception but soon could become routine diagnostic aids.

CT Scanner, Computer, and Software

Surgical procedures reported here have used an EMI-5005 second-generation CT scanner. The interactive software on this early system allows registration of CT information from the slice coordinates to the stereotactic frame coordinates. Biopsy tools, afterloading catheters, radioactive sources, stimulating electrodes, or lesion electrodes can be directed to the target site through an aperture in the frame's probe-holding assembly. This assembly is mounted on a carriage that can be positioned along the frame's arch (Figure 10–3).

The frame is an 8-pound gas-sterilizable Delrin device mounted on an aluminum base ring. Use of these materials reduces artifact in the images generated by the CT scanner. A plastic base ring positioned over the aluminum base supports an arch that can swing through an angle of 135°. There is a carriage that slides along the arch through 0°–165°. This carriage includes a probe holder or bushing with a central aperture. The central aperture in the bushing and the appropriate "sleeves" provide the guided trajectory for inserting the biopsy needle into the brain. The probe holder may pivot through ±25° in the arch plane. A reference zero point is marked on the probe holder for setting the probe length. The probe holder can be advanced in 0.1-mm increments. These frame components and the coordinate system of the frame are illustrated in Figure 10–4.

To establish a reference system between the CT image and the frame spatial system, three N-shaped locators are used. These are illustrated in Figure 10–5 and can be seen in position around the frame base in Figure 10–1. The N-shaped locators are constructed of a high-density material, and hence the cross section of each locator produces three dots on the CT scan. These locators are mounted on the plastic base ring.

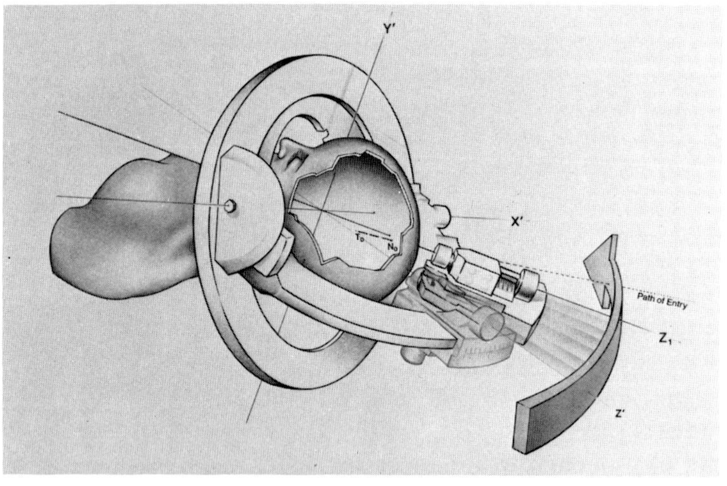

Figure 10–3 Memorial frame showing probe repositioned along the arch.

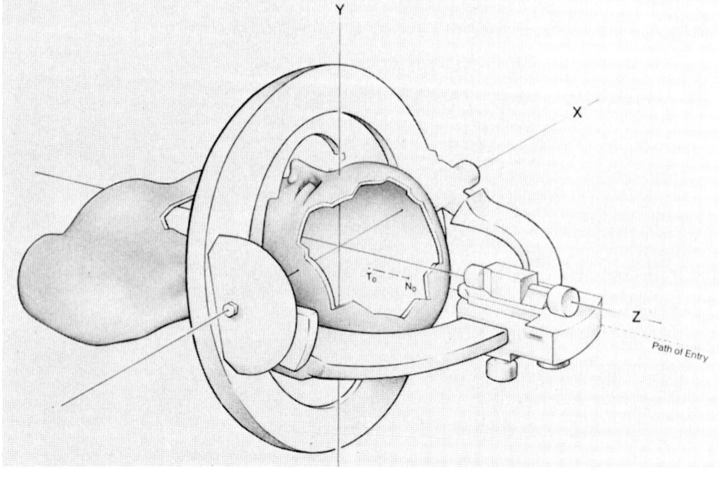

Figure 10–4 Coordinate system for the Memorial frame.

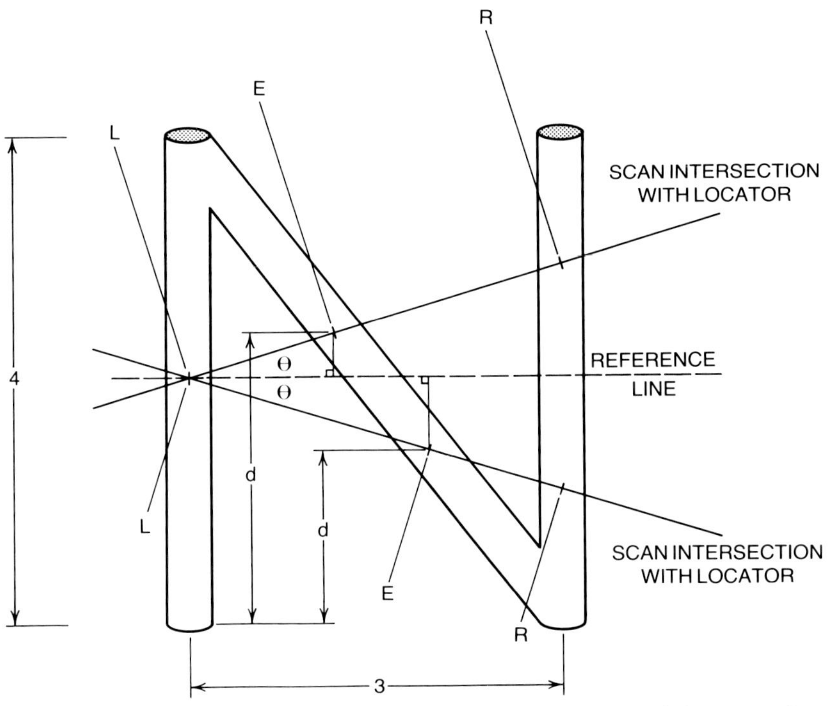

Figure 10–5 N-shaped locator assembly for the Memorial frame and MPS frame.

After the patient is scanned the N-shaped locators are removed. A typical CT image is shown in Figure 10–6. The locating information left by the nine dots of the three locators is used to determine the position of every point in each CT picture in terms of the three-dimensional coordinate system of the frame. This information is then used by the computer to calculate four angular settings and the probe length needed to reach the target. Trajectories for this target are determined using either an entrance point selected from CT picture data or a frame location designated by the surgeon. The procedure is a five-step process that has taken from 3 hr early in our development down to less than ninety minutes more recently. The sequence is described below.

Step 1. Mount the head frame to the end of the scanner's bed. Once attached, position the patient's skull within the frame and secure the patient to the frame using four fixation pins. Use the CT scanner to localize the target tumor within the appropriate horizontal section. (The patient has had a 5-min shampoo with pHisoHex the night before surgery. The points of fixation of the frame to the skull are shaved immediately prior to mounting the head frame.)

Step 2. The surgeon selects the optimum site for biopsy on the CRT display and uses a cross hair to designate the exact location desired to biopsy the tumor. This is the target point.

Step 3. Similar to step 2. The surgeon selects another location on a higher CT slice. This second point is selected to lie along the desired trajectory.

Step 4. As a reference to the surgeon, the computer indicates on the image display console where the trajectory intersects each scan slice. At the same time, the program prints out the frame settings needed to reach the designated target in the desired direction.

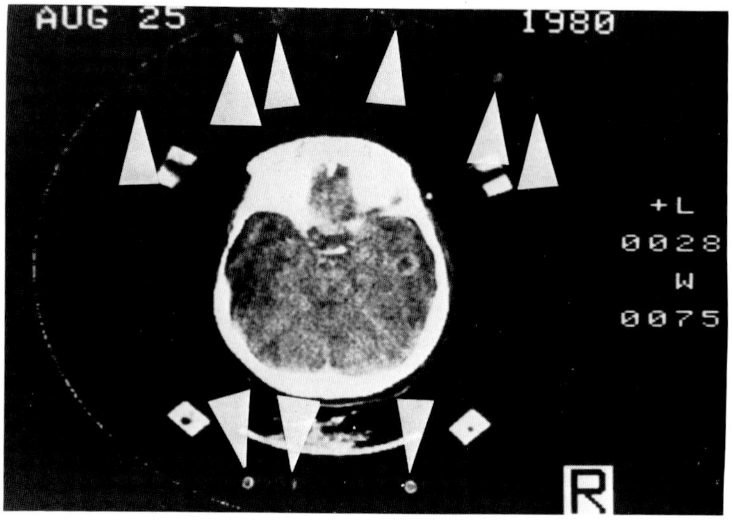

Figure 10–6 Second-generation scanner, EMI 5005, CT picture scanned through the frame's three locator assemblies (see the nine triangular arrows).

Step 5. The frame is reset to the parameters printed by the computer. The surgeon then prepares to perforate the patient's skull and to perform the insertion of the biopsy tool.

If the surgeon desires a fixed entrance point, steps 3 and 4 are replaced by steps 3′ and 4′ as follows:

Step 3′. The surgeon manipulates the frame and sets the length of the probe so the probe just touches the preferred entrance point.

Step 4′. These angular settings and the probe length are entered into the computer. The program is used first to calculate the position of this entrance point. Then the frame settings needed for the probe to reach the target through the entrance point are computed and printed. In order to access multiple targets the surgeon simply performs the above procedure repeatedly. The complete flow chart of the program for these procedures is given in Figure 10–7.

Biopsy Tool

The biopsy tool utilized is a modified Lee biopsy needle consisting of three parts: 1) an outer cannula; 2) an inner cannula; and 3) a biopsy cannula with an open side port 3.0 mm from the tip of the cannula.

Tissue is gently aspirated into the port of the biopsy cannula by attaching a 5.0-cc syringe to the luer lock on the proximal end of the biopsy cannula. A quick withdrawal of the biopsy cannula shears the tissue on a sharp edge of the inner cannula. A frozen section report is obtained within 30 min. Specimens are also taken for permanent section.

After biopsy, afterloading catheters are positioned into the tumor margins at appropriate points based on the geometric configuration of the lesion as demonstrated on the CRT terminal and on the estimated volume of tumor as calculated from the CT data. The afterloading catheters are loaded with a "dummy source" until permanent-section report is available (24 hr). The dummy sources are then removed and the radioactive isotopes introduced into the lumen of the afterloading catheter in the patient's room. A postoperative scan is taken to confirm the biopsy site and the catheter placement and to check for evidence of bleeding.

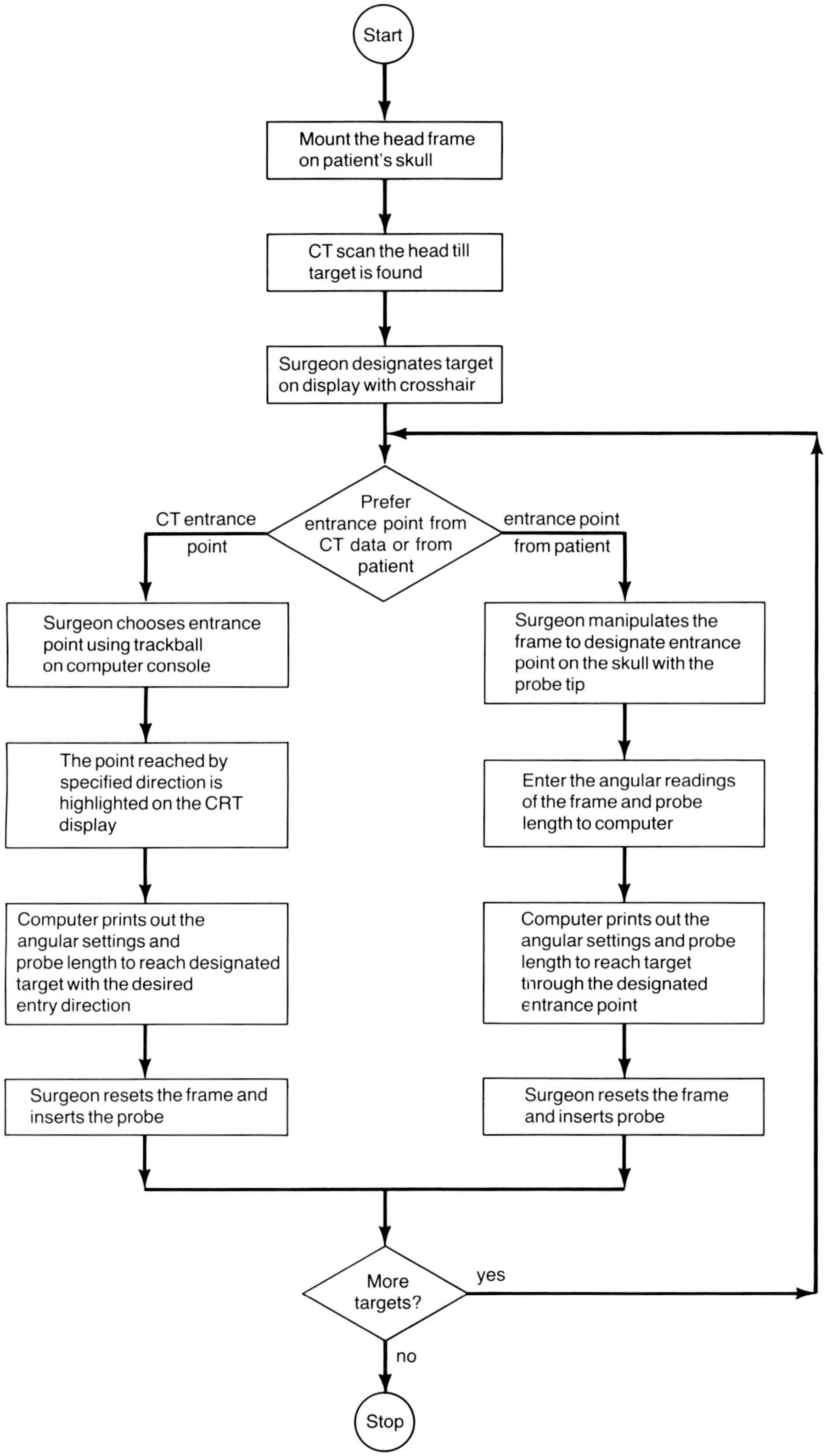

Figure 10–7 Flow chart outlining the stereotactic procedure.

Clinical Results

Our initial efforts were directed to intracranial gliomas. Patients were selected who had tumors that were usually solitary and nonhomogeneous. Gliomas rarely metastasize outside the central nervous system—they grow by direct extension—and so are ideal biopsy targets to determine subsequent treatment. Most tumors targeted in our study were positioned where external-beam radiation could not be delivered in sufficient dose to destroy the tumor without affecting normal tissue. Because of their position, total excision of these lesions is possible only rarely.

Survival Data

The national brain tumor study group demonstrated survival curves for patients with malignant gliomas (Figure 10–8). These survival curves varied as follows: 1) best conventional care but no radiotherapy or chemotherapy; 2) BCNU; 3) radiotherapy; 4) BCNU and radiotherapy.

Our limited series includes 13 biopsies without irradiation performed between 6 January 1980 and 15 July 1981. Since 15 July 1981, 20 stereotactic biopsies with interstitial irradiation and supplementary external-beam irradiation have been performed. No procedures have been performed since December 1982 because the therapeutic CT unit is being developed and the current EMI-5005 unit is being replaced with a Siemens scanner.

Complications

The significant complications, in order of their occurrence, are illustrated by the following case studies.

Case FH-57

A 57-year-old right-handed Caucasian female was admitted with history of headache, instability of gait, and removal of a left kidney for carcinoma in 1979. Neurologic symptoms began in the spring of 1980. When first seen the patient had evidence of multiple intracerebral deposits.

After biopsy on 7/11/80, the patient was awake and responsive, with no evidence of hematoma in the cerebellar biopsy site and a moderate amount of blood in the supratentorial biopsy site (5.0-mm biopsy tool).

The day after the procedure she was dull, arousable, and responsive to simple commands. Histologic diagnosis was confirmed as metastatic renal cell carcinoma. The second postoperative day, the patient deteriorated. After discussion with the family, no further therapeutic measures were instituted, and she expired.

Autopsy was performed. The autopsy surgeon's diagnosis was:

1. Status postnephrectomy for renal cell carcinoma, 1979
2. Metastatic renal cell carcinoma of the right kidney; adrenal gland, bilaterally; lung, bilaterally; pancreas; and brain
3. Generalized atherosclerosis, moderate
4. Myocardial hypertrophy, left ventricle

Lesson For *biopsy,* do not use an "open-bite" tool with a cup size of greater than 3.0 mm.

Case RLU-31

A 31-year-old right-handed white male was admitted for histologic diagnosis of a dominant hemisphere intracerebral tumor. CT-assisted biopsy was performed on 3 November 1980. Frozen-section diagnosis was malignant intracranial glioma.

The immediate postoperative scan demonstrated significant blood at the biopsy site. Under observation by the author (R.A.S.), the pupil on the left side (biopsy side) began to dilate in the recovery room. Immediate craniotomy was performed. The operative findings were as follows:

The brain was swollen, and there was evidence of subpial hemorrhage. Upon incision of the cortex, at a depth of approximately 4.0 cm there was a malignant glioma with a significant hematoma (40–50 cc). There were many vessels indicating neovascularization. After evacuation of the hematoma and subtotal resection of the glioma, meticulous attention was paid to hemostasis and the scalp was closed after removal of the bone flap. The dura was not completely closed.

On 20 November 1980 the craniotomy was reexplored, radioactive iodine was inserted into the margins of the tumor, and the bone flap was replaced. The patient was discharged on 26 November 1980, ambulatory, 23 days after biopsy. He returned to his father's ranch, improved for a few months, then expired.

Lesson An immediate postoperative CT scan can alert one to potential difficulty within the first few hours after biopsy.

Case GD-49

A 49-year-old gravida III, para II, had a known diagnosis of nondominant hemisphere oligodendroglioma after surgery in Washington state in 1979. The tumor was considered unresectable. Maximum-dose teletherapy was delivered postoperatively. The patient was admitted to the hospital ambulatory, alert, oriented, and with mild left hemiparesis.

On 25 August 1981 CT-assisted stereotactic brain biopsy was performed. Iridium-192 was utilized after biopsy: minimal tumor dose 2,525 rads; maximum tumor dose 4,040 rads. The catheter was removed 31 August 1981.

The patient did well postoperatively and was discharged ambulatory. She developed an indolent ulceration of the scalp at the site of biopsy through a prior burrhole.

Lesson In previously operated patients, do not make the entry point through a prior burrhole where scalp irradiation has previously occurred.

Case AK-57

A 57-year-old white male was admitted to the hospital with symptoms and signs of an intracerebral mass. CT scan demonstrated a corpus callosum glioma. Biopsy was performed 26 May 1982 from both the right and the left sides. Three afterloading catheters were inserted through each aperture. The catheters were loaded 27 May 1982 and removed 30 May 1982, having delivered a minimum of 4,690 rads and a maximum of 6,030 rads to the tumor. On 1 June 1982 the patient became more lethargic, and his neck was stiff. Lumbar puncture demonstrated 811 white blood cells, predominantly polymorphonuclear cells, and a glucose level of 27 mg%; gram stain showed rare gram-negative rods. The patient was treated with Moxalactam 12 g/day, gentamicin, 5 mg/kg, and nafcillin pending cultures. The patient improved under appropriate antibiotic regimen.

The patient was transferred from hospital to Long Beach V.A.H. and expired 26 September 1982. Autopsy was performed with the following findings: There was exudate over both frontal lobes, evidence of a basal meningitis, and evidence of exudative meningitis over the spinal meninges. There was no evidence of brain abscess on brain cutting.

Lesson With multiple entry sites and multiple use of afterloading catheters, meticulous attention must be paid to technique when removing the dummy sources and introducing the active isotope.

Summary of Clinical Trials

The method described differs in certain respects from similar systems and similar devices in use at other medical centers.

1. The entire procedure is performed in the CT suite.
2. The frame was manufactured by Howland Industries to integrate with a custom software program.
3. Our experience with CT-assisted stereotactic placement of radioactive isotopes is limited to a single source (iridium-192).
4. We have not used a smear technique for biopsy analysis, which has proved satisfactory in other centers (15).
5. We have not routinely performed angiography on all patients preoperatively.
6. An immediate postbiopsy CT scan is performed *before* removal of the head frame.
7. The entire procedure is performed under neuroleptanalgesia with local infiltration of the scalp (Marcaine).
8. Multiple afterloading catheters are utilized in appropriate lesions. Dose rates vary from 40 to 80 rads/hr. Sources remain in place up to, but not exceeding, 100 hr before the sources and afterloading catheters are removed.
9. Dosimetry calculations are performed by a physicist prior to initiation of external beam irradiation should this prove desirable.

The Second-Generation Frame

The Frame and Surgical Procedure

The all-plastic frame (Figure 10–2) and the software needed to plan stereotactic surgery are integrated with flexible imaging capabilities (4,5). As in its predecessor, this frame is made of gas-sterilizable Delrin, which is sufficiently hard to resist deflection under operating conditions yet easily machined to ±0.001-inch tolerance. The result is a head-mounted device that is attached to the CT scanner's patient table and causes no image artifacts.

The stereotactic operation begins by taking a series of parallel CT images (usually 12–16 slices) of the patient's skull with the frame attached. Although stereotactic software described here does not require parallel axial slices, sagittal and coronal reconstructions are important benefits realized when parallel scans are taken. Scans are taken to include the trajectory's target and skull entrance points for the surgical probe. Like any set of CT images, the CT scanner system provides a variety of image presentation options to review the anatomy, but once stereotactic planning is chosen CT scans are frame-registered (see following section) and additional, more powerful review capabilities are possible.

Figure 10–9 shows axial slices in a collage format used to select probe target and entrance point. The composite display is the result of choosing an image window on the axial slice containing the stereotactic

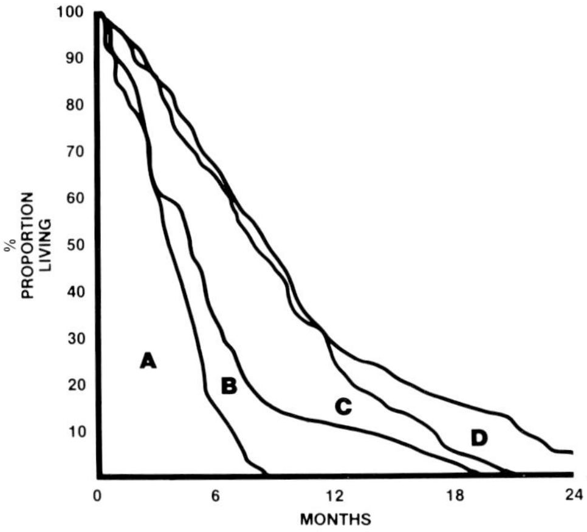

Figure 10–8 Survival curve for malignant gliomas. See for reference Journal of Neurosurgery, 49:333–343, 1978.

target. Window size is adjusted to include the likely point of probe entrance. Target and entrance location also can be chosen from an image display format that shows axial, sagittal, and coronal views simultaneously, as in Figure 10–10. Once the target and reference points are chosen, instructions are delivered by the computer to adjust the frame for precise probe placement (Figure 10–11). Adjustments are made corresponding to the five degrees of freedom the frame allows: a pitch of the arch, a carriage position along the arch, a probe-holder pitch, a probe-holder tilt, and probe length.

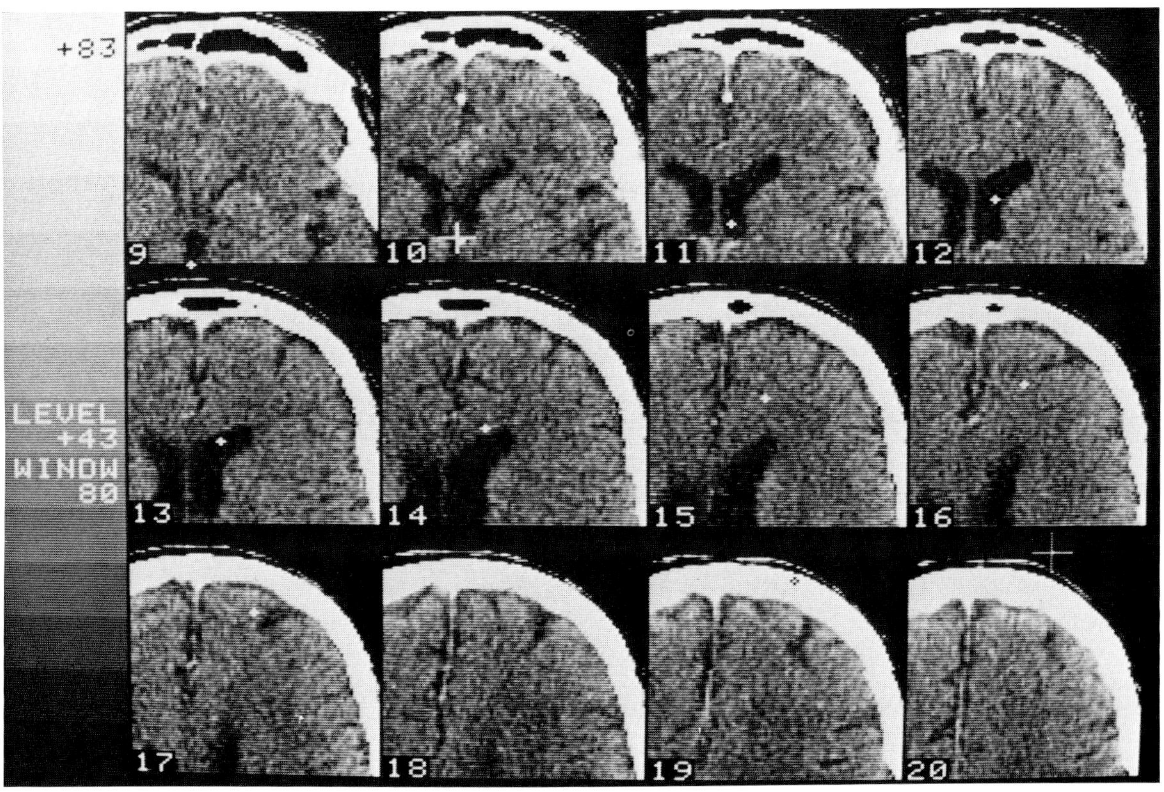

Figure 10–9 A collage of axial slices used to select the target and determine the stereotactic probe trajectory.

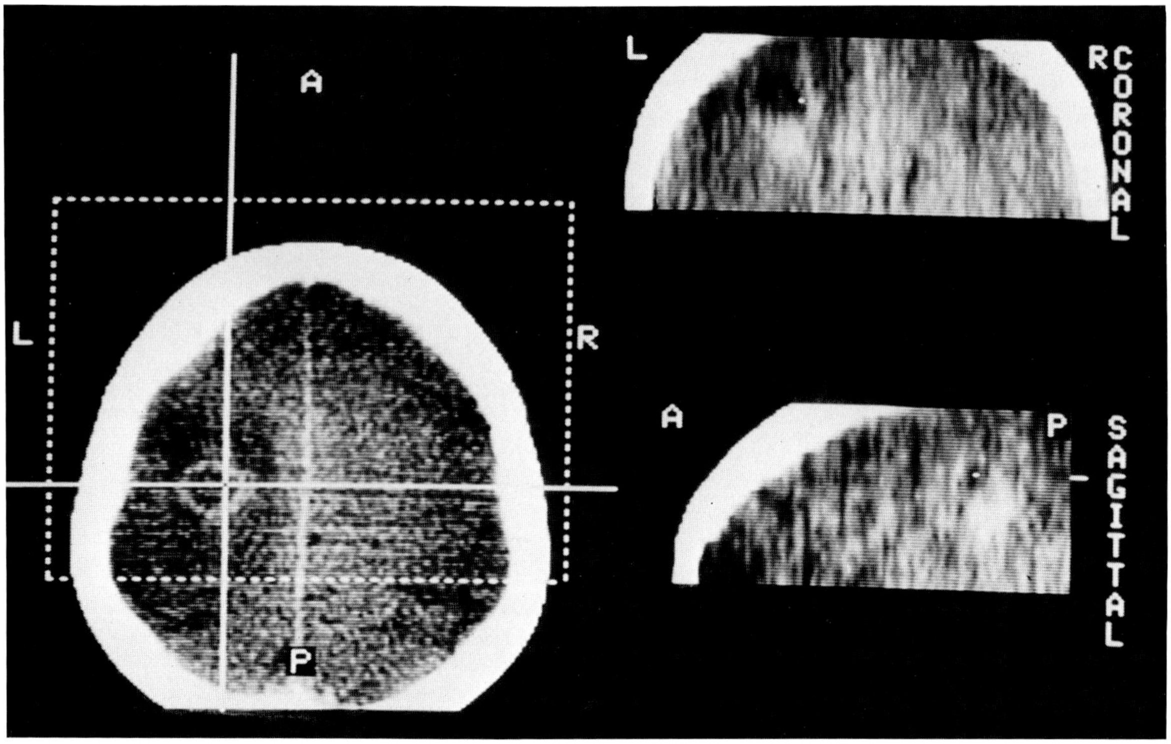

Figure 10–10 An alternative simultaneous display of axial, sagittal, and coronal CT images for selecting the target and stereotactic trajectory.

An important feature of this approach is illustrated in Figure 10–10. Prior to surgery several probe trajectories can be assessed by their representation in a CT image format that illustrates anatomy from three orthogonal points of view simultaneously: axial, sagittal (lateral), and coronal (frontal).

An especially useful simulation is that which shows anatomy touched by the probe as it is advanced along the chosen trajectory (Figure 10–12A-D). The intersecting axial, sagittal, and coronal image is presented automatically as the neurosurgeon moves a virtual probe down the selected trajectory. The simulated probe tip triggers the intersecting image from each of the three views. If the trajectory proves undesirable during

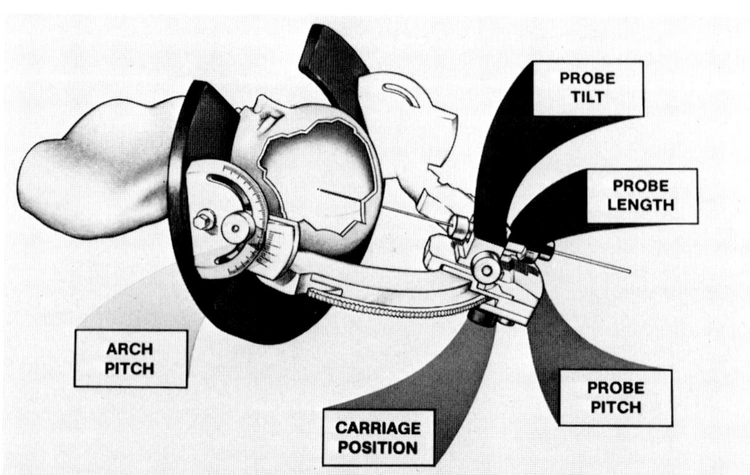

Figure 10–11 The MPS frame's adjustments.

this analysis, a new trajectory can be chosen. Figures 10–13A through 10–13C illustrate a similar presentation where oblique images that contain the entire trajectory are generated.

Improvements to Frame Design

Figure 10–1 illustrates the forerunner of this frame, shown in Figure 10–2. The most obvious difference between the two appears in the base geometry. Other software changes have been made to speed the overall procedure and to deliver a clear presentation of anatomy to the neurosurgeon. For example, image-to-frame registration now requires 20 sec *regardless* of the number of CT slices taken. The earlier system required 10 seconds of computer processing to register each CT slice to the frame coordinate system. Another software enhancement allows target point and trajectory to be selected by sagittal or coronal images in addition to axial views. Other more apparent changes are seen in the frame itself.

The new frame has a horseshoe-shaped base that reduces the claustrophobic effect such intimidating devices have on patients. The earlier frame formed a complete circle at its base. The new design eliminates base ring rotations that on occasion became difficult to reach and has been made more substantial than the earlier circular base to compensate for its open end.

The overall appearance is less cluttered than the earlier device. Large N-shaped locator assemblies on the earlier frame have become less than one-fourth in relative size and are permanently mounted, clear from normal surgical access. The locator assemblies are plastic blocks with an N shape drilled within. This approach permits the N-shaped cavity to be filled with oil for use on nuclear magnetic resonance (NMR) scanners.

Head mounting pins have been repositioned and better directed to support the skull firmly. Reliable fixation is more likely than in the past.

The arch now has two protractors, one at each end of its attachment to the base. The earlier frame had but one, which at times was positioned facing the floor and was difficult to read after a base ring rotation. In addition, locking pins are used on both ends of the arch to better secure the arch once adjusted.

All degrees of motion on the frame are color-coded to avoid confusion during a busy operation. All scales have been made in a similar, easy-to-read orientation.

Several quick-change probe bushings have been made for the frame to allow a variety of surgical instruments to be used easily. All the above improvements are incorporated in further enhancements to the interactive display program.

Image-to-Frame Registration

Common CT scans are rendered on digital displays without regard to patient-scanner orientation; no image orientation information is given other than that provided by the patient's anatomy. However, with the frame attached firmly to the skull, orientation of CT scans can be determined precisely using the frame as reference.

The frame's coordinate origin, illustrated in Figure 10–14, is located at the intersection of the arch axis and the base center. All image data measures are converted to the frame system as a prerequisite to frame

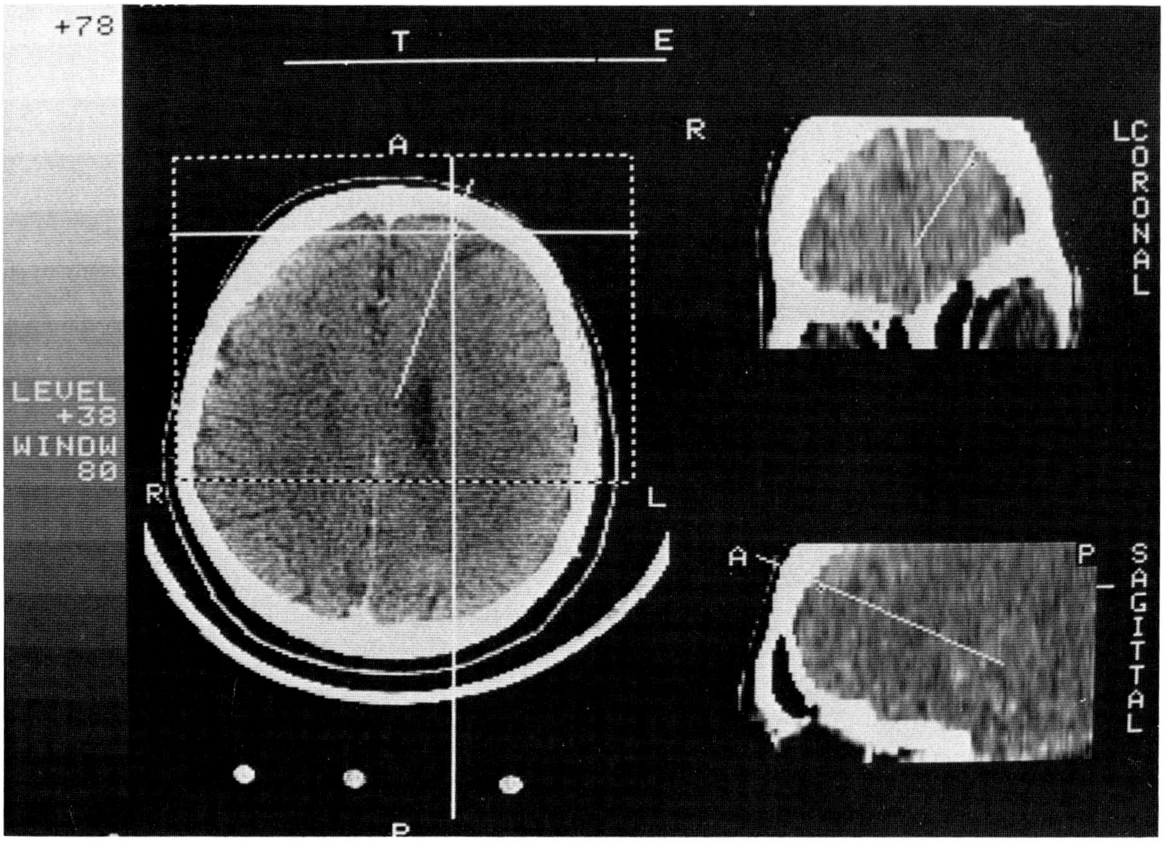

A

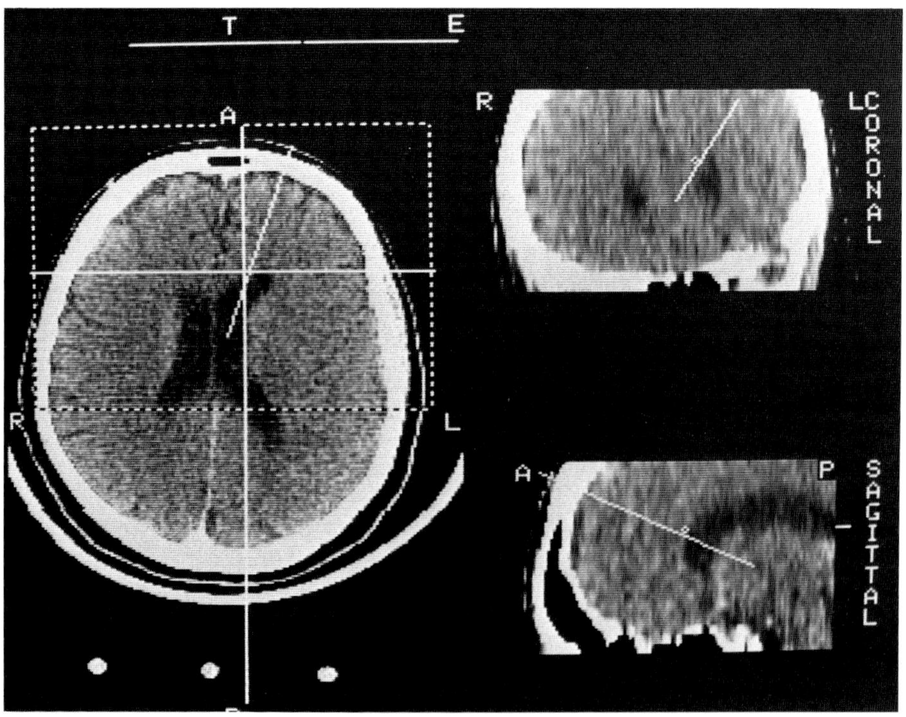

B

Figure 10–12 **A:** Simulated probe tip triggers display of intersecting axial, sagittal, and coronal pictures. **B:** Simulated probe tip advanced along proposed trajectory 25.1 mm from target.

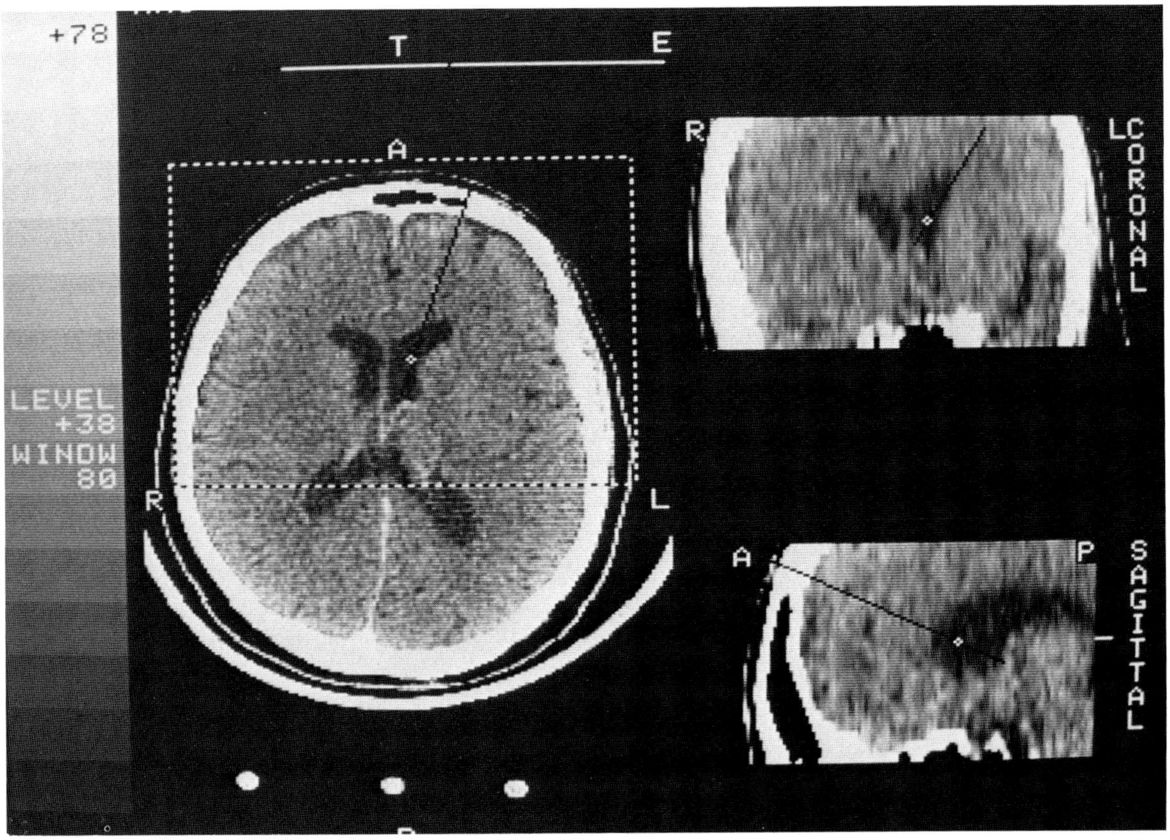

C

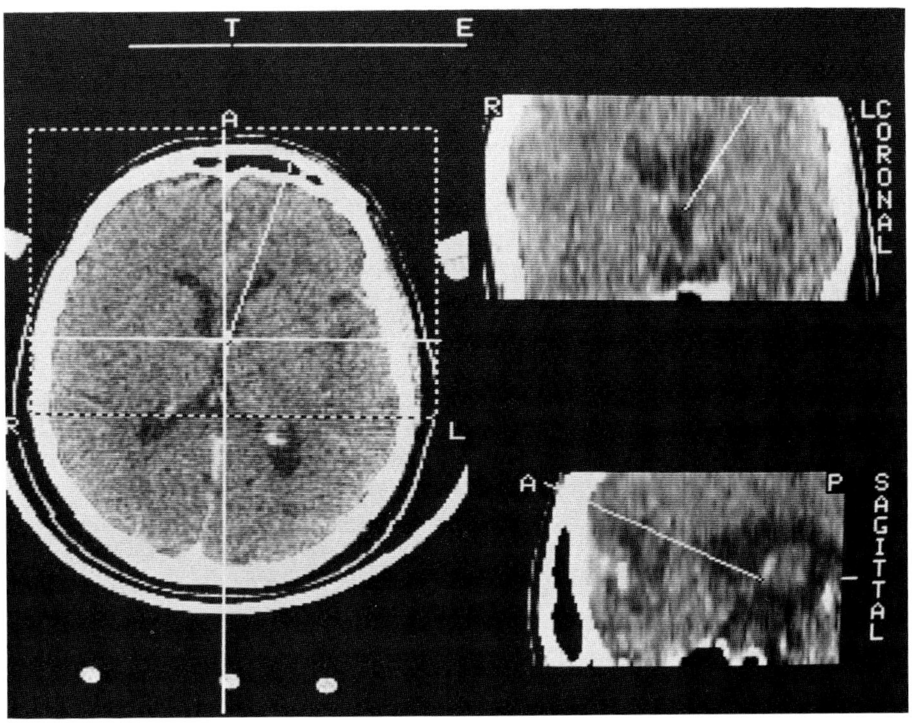

D

Figure 10–12 (cont.) **C:** Simulated probe tip 15.1 mm from target. **D:** Simulated probe tip at target; intersecting sagittal and coronal images also illustrated.

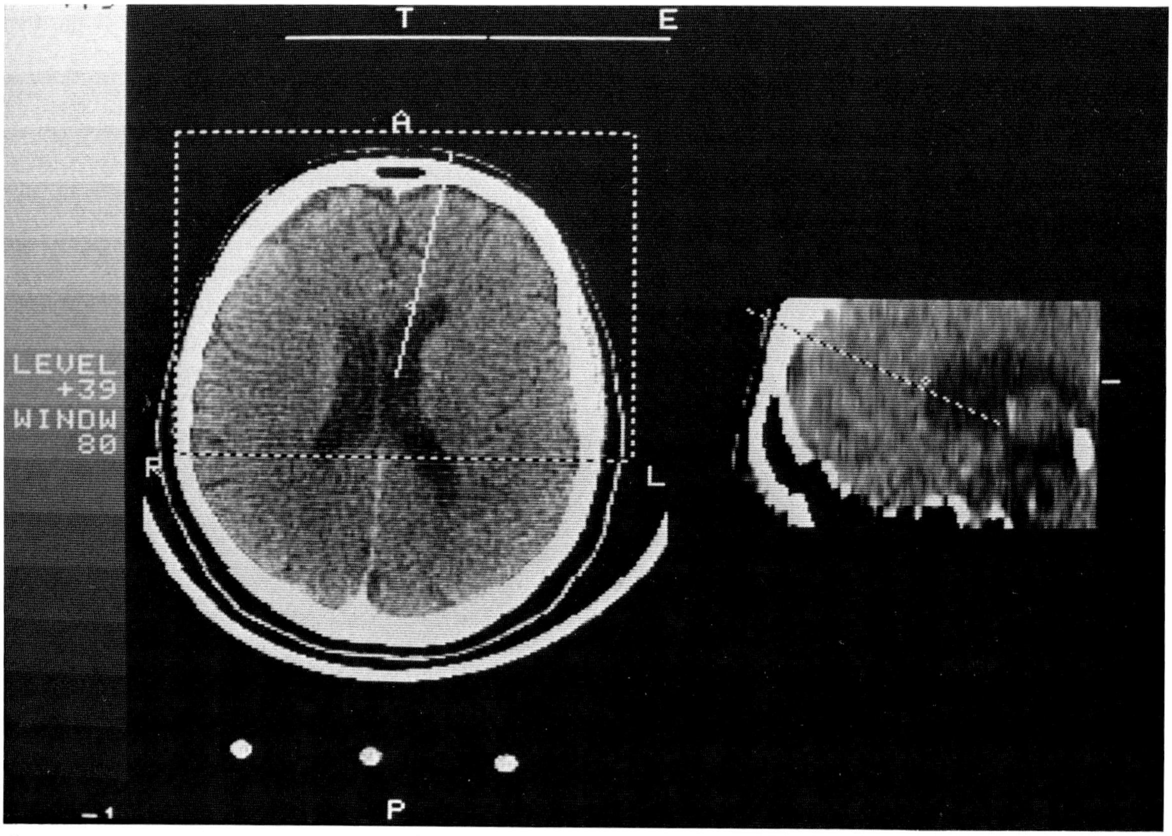

A

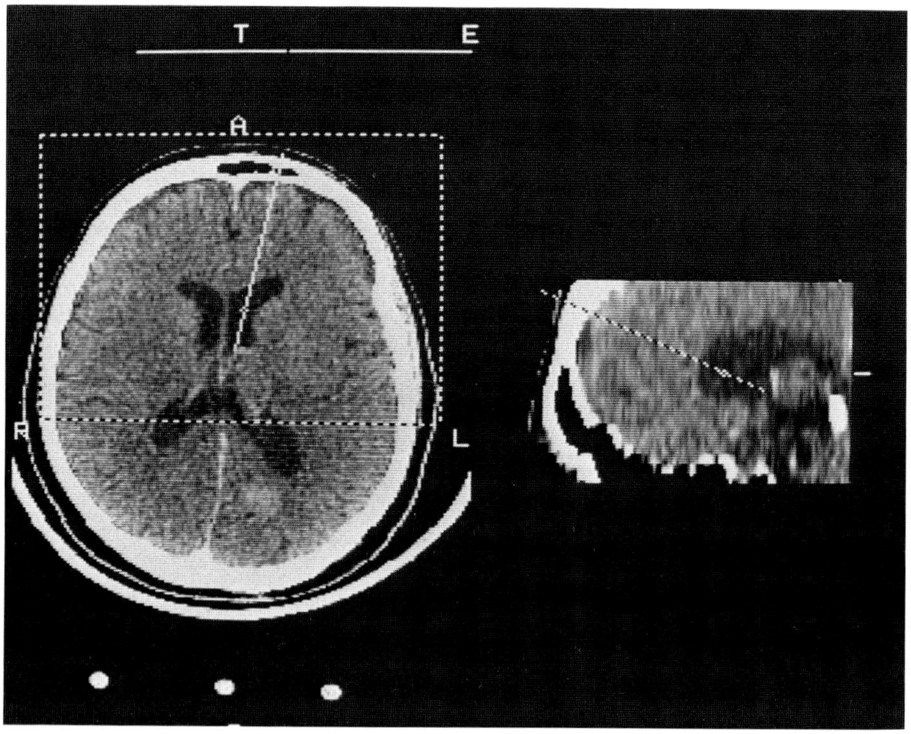

B

Figure 10–13 **A:** Oblique view of anatomy. The trajectory is contained entirely within this view. **B:** The axial image is triggered for presentation by the simulated probe tip.

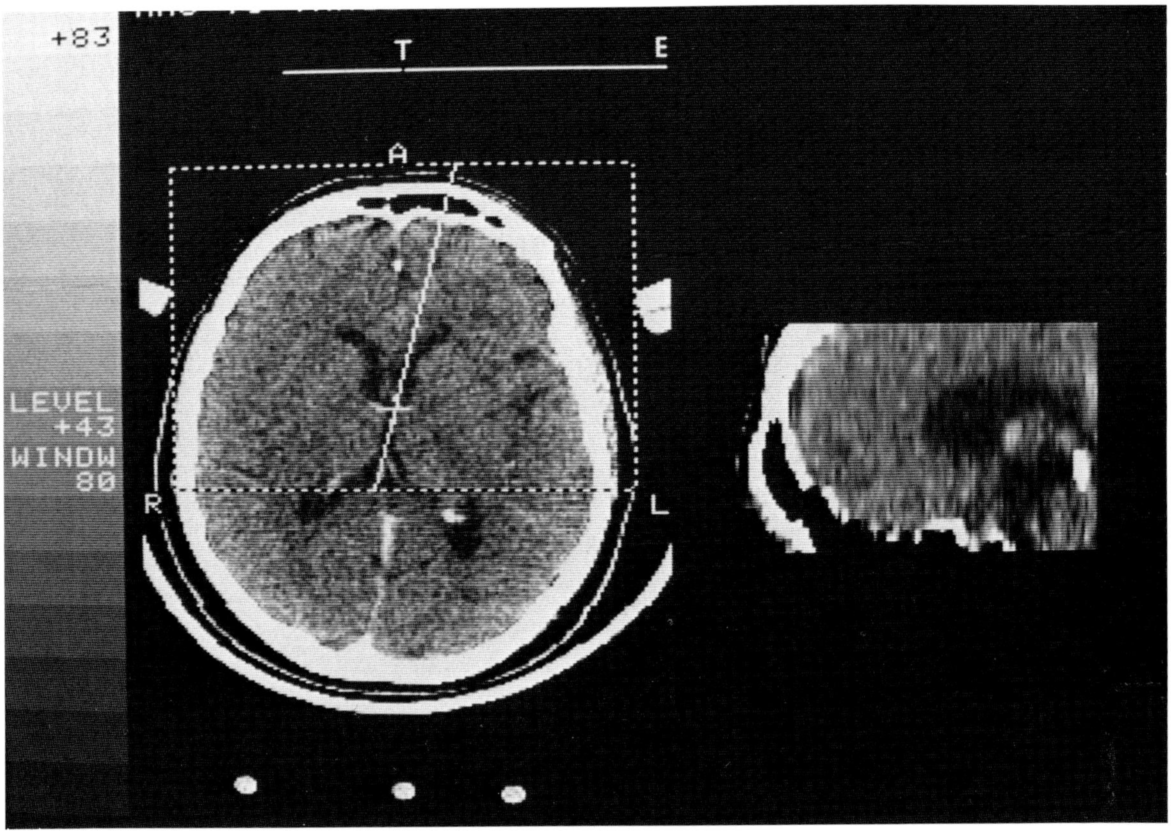

C

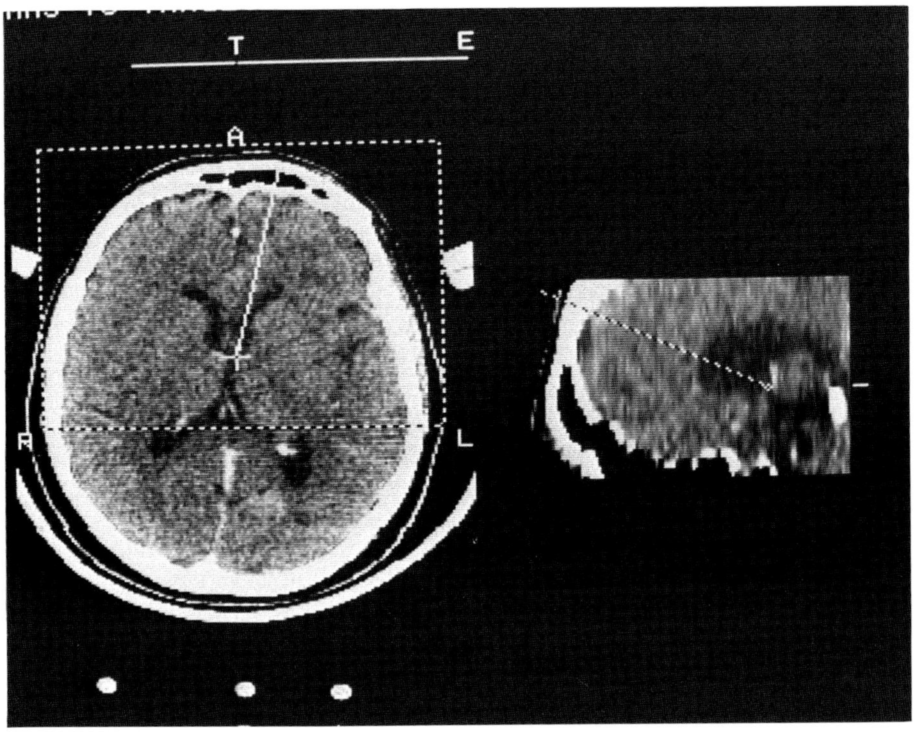

D

Figure 10–13 (cont.) **C:** For clarity the trajectory line can be removed. **D:** The oblique image is not changed as the simulated probe is advanced.

adjustment. Also shown in Figure 10–14 are hypothetical target (*T*) and entrance (*N*) points for a probe. Using N-shaped locator assemblies, permanently attached to the frame, three reference points are provided to describe completely the plane of each CT scan. These three frame system coordinate points are found automatically for any one scan used in the operation. This approach is quite different from that used in the past (16). The method here relates a single reference scan to the frame coordinate system; subsequent scans are then registered using the reference scan's orientation but offset in one dimension—along the direction of patient table incrementation between CT slices (Z coordinates).

Using the frame as reference, we extract third-dimension coordinates by planting Z-axis variant geometry to be detected in a reference scan. Locator assemblies stand on an X-Y plane at a calibrated position from the frame origin. A CT image is scanned by the stereotactic program to locate the diagonal and upright cross sections of each of the three N-shaped locators. Because frame system X and Y coordinates for the uprights are known and the relative distance between uprights and the locator diagonal indicates height from the frame base, Z-axis coordinates for the diagonal cross section result.

Figure 10–15 shows the geometric details that allow spatial coordinates to be extracted from each locator. As shown, the assembly forms a triangle that is intersected randomly by any CT scan. Pattern-scanning software (a subroutine that searches or scans the CT images) determines the size and location of points L, E, and R, corresponding to the center of the left upright, the diagonal ellipse, and the right upright for each assembly. Because CT image planes can have an oblique intersection with locator assemblies (as shown), orientation software used here further generalizes a similar method reported by Brown (3). The pattern scanning is entirely automatic once initiated. Users "page" through CT images to find a suitable reference scan—one that clearly shows the cross sections of the three locator assemblies. Then, after the left upright of the first locator is identified, all images are frame system registered without further interaction. This work uses the only such automatic registration system known for stereotaxis (16).

As shown in Figure 10–11, five frame adjustments are needed to orient the frame for probe trajectory and length. Geometric principles for finding these adjustments are given here using frame-registered CT images. The first task finds the arch pitch (*A*) and probe tilt (*PHI*) simultaneously, as they are interdependent rotations. Once these two rotations are found, carriage position, probe pitch, and length are more simply determined. Figure 10–15A illustrates the orthometric projection of the arch in a nominal position. Note that the arch itself is offset to allow the probe-holding assembly to position the probe through P_0 along the Z coordinate axis. Also shown is a target point (*T*) and an entrance point (*N*). Two rotations are required, one about the X axis and a second about a parallel axis through P_1. Figure 10–15B illustrates both rotations.

Both *A* and *PHI* rotations are found using an iterative process that begins by approximation but proceeds quickly to resolution. The first approximation is

$$PHI = 0 \text{ and } A = A_0$$

where A_0 is that rotation that begins P_1 to intersect the trajectory line $N - T$.

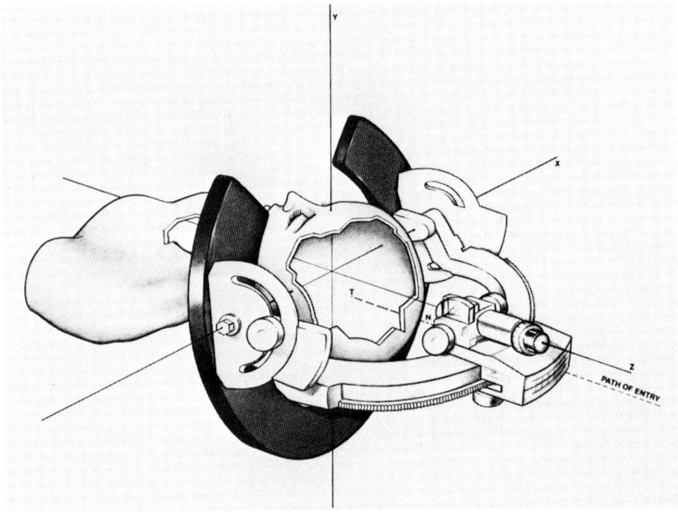

Figure 10–14 The coordinate origin for the MPS frame.

Equation 8, below, provides A_0, where $I = I_x, I_y, I_z$ is the intersection of the trajectory with the hemisphere having radius equal to the distance between P_1 and the origin (see Eqs. 1–7). In terms of the frame, the P_1 hemisphere is that surface described by rotating the arch about the X axis and simultaneously sweeping the carriage along the arch.

$$I_x = T_x + \cos X * k \qquad [1]$$

$$I_y = T_y + \cos Y * k \qquad [2]$$

$$I_z = T_z + \cos Z * k \qquad [3]$$

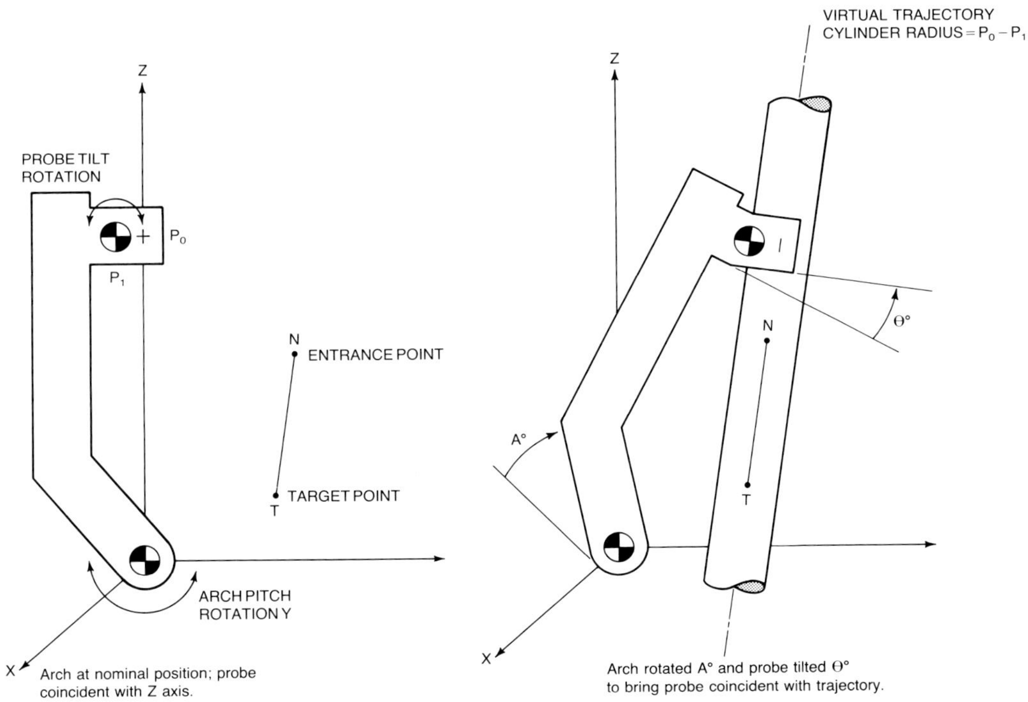

A **B**

Figure 10–15 **A:** Orthometric projection of arch in nominal position. **B:** Orthometric projection of arch positioned to align the probe holder with the trajectory.

In Eqs. 1–7, k is the variable of the parametric line equation of the trajectory whose value places I_x, I_y, I_z, on the P_1 hemisphere. cosX, cosY, and cosZ are constants for this equation and are determined directly from the line equation for entrance (N_x, N_y, N_z) and target point (T_x, T_y, T_z).

$$\cos X = (N_x - T_x) / \| N - T \| \quad [4]$$

$$\cos Y = (N_y - T_x) / \| N - T \| \quad [5]$$

$$\cos Z = (N_z - T_z) / \| N - T \| \quad [6]$$

$$I_x^2 + I_y^2 + I_z^2 = \| P_1 \|^2 \quad [7]$$

Substituting Eqs. 1–3 for I_x, I_y, and I_z in Eq. 7 reduces the expression to a quadratic in terms of T. Equations 1–3 then deliver the coordinates of the intersection point I_x, I_y, I_z. A_0 then can be found using Eq. 8, which is simply a transform expression for rotations about the X axis. There, the constant R is the distance between P_0 and the origin when the frame is at a nominal setting, as in Figure 10–15A.

$$A_0 = (-20 I_y + R * SQRT(1 - I_x^2 / R^2) * I_z) / (I_y^2 + I_z^2) \quad [8]$$

Once A_0 is determined, a counterrotation of A_0 is iteratively tested for intersection with the cylinder equation about the trajectory. As incremental adjustments to A_0 are tried, the distance between P_1 and the cylinder diminishes (P_1 approaches the cylinder surface). Iteration terminates at solution (A) when the P_1-to-cylinder distance is zero; P_1 is resting on the cylinder (call this coordinate position Q). Moreover, because the cylinder has radius $P_1 - P_0 = 20$ mm, a rotation parallel to the axis about Q (PHI) is known to exist to bring P_0 coincident with the trajectory.

After a reverse arch rotation (A), only the transformed X and Z coordinates of Q ($Q = Q_x, Q_y, Q_z$) are needed to position the carriage.

$$CP = \arctan (Q_z / Q_x) \quad [9]$$

The probe's pitch (PCH) and the probe's tilt (PHI) result from a transformation of the origin to Q. Using the line equation for the trajectory in this new coordinate system, we know that after the PCH and PHI rotations the trajectory is parallel to the new Z axis at Y = 20. Using the rotation matrix expression in Eq. 10 for any point along the trajectory (e.g., T_x, T_y, T_z), in the new coordinate system the resultant X coordinate is zero. This delivers probe pitch PCH in Eq. 11.

$$\begin{bmatrix} \cos(PCH) & 0 & -\sin(PCH) \\ \sin(PHI)\sin(PCH) & \cos(PHI) & \sin(PHI)\cos(PCH) \\ \cos(PHI)\sin(PCH) & -\sin(PHI) & \cos(PHI)\cos(PCH) \end{bmatrix} = \begin{bmatrix} T_x \\ T_y \\ T_z \end{bmatrix} \quad [10]$$

$$PCH = \arctan(T_x / T_z) \quad [11]$$

Knowing that the trajectory is on the Y = 20 line after both rotations in Eq. 10, Y coordinates for both the entrance point (N) and the target (T) points are equal; see Eqs. 12–14.

$$\sin(PHI)\sin(PCH) T_x + \cos(PHI) T_y + \sin(PHI)\cos(PCH) T_z = 20 \quad [12]$$

$$\sin(PHI)\sin(PCH) N_x + \cos(PHI) N_y + \sin(PHI)\cos(PCH) N_z = 20 \quad [13]$$

$$PHI = \arctan[-N_y - T_y) / (\sin(PCH) * (N_x - T_x) + \cos(PCH) * N_z - T_z)] \quad [14]$$

Because A is found, the position of the carriage along the arch (CP) follows. The location of Q positions both the carriage (CP) and the arch (A). CP can be found by transforming the coordinate system by an X-axis rotation of A degrees. In this new system, CP is that angle on the transformed Z-X plane formed by the origin-to-P_1 vector and the Z axis.

Frame settings are complete when the probe length (PL) is added to A, PHI, CP, and PCH. In Eq. 15 P_0' is that position of P_0 after rotations A, PHI, CP, and PCH. The incremental constant (C) is determined directly from the frame or its manufacturing drawings.

$$PL = \| P_0' - T \| + C \qquad [15]$$

Discussion

The preceding geometric resolution is executed by the computer entirely free from manual intervention. Stereotactic methods by Brown (3) and Kelly and Alker (9) require manual determination of actual frame settings. Although computer programs are used to register CT scans to their stereotactic frames, the settings of the frame are not delivered to these researchers by computer. The settings are determined by using a jig to simulate the actual target and entrance-point positions. During the surgical procedure, one of the surgery team members adjusts the frame containing the simulated target to determine its setting for the patient. These settings then are transferred to the patient-mounted frame.

The stereotactic system described in the first part of this chapter and that described in the second part are the only systems that have incorporated image-presentation software to carefully preview proposed trajectories simultaneously from an axial, sagittal, and coronal image point of view. No other stereotactic system is known to the authors that includes this surgery simulation capability.

Four generations of CT scanners have been developed during the last 10 years. In that time a typical CT-guided stereotactic surgical operation has been reduced from 3–5 hr to 90 min. This new frame and its software will further reduce the time needed for surgery. The entire procedure has taken less than 35 min for trials that contacted targets embedded randomly in watermelons. Prior to these trials, over 700 computer-generated random trajectories have shown accurate frame adjustment to never more than 1.5 mm distance from desired target.

Two objections to performing brain biopsies in a CT scanner suite are frequently raised by neurosurgeons. The objections are 1. the lack of sterility and 2. the distance from numerous life-supporting aids commonly available to the operating room. This distance is also often judged too remote from the CT scanner suite. The method described here minimizes both objections. First, by routine, precise probe placement, drill holes in the skull can be extremely small. Holes for simple biopsy or ablation can be as small as 3.0 mm in diameter. The risk of infection under these circumstances is remote with routine precautions. Second, we do not endorse use of the CT suite for all neurosurgical procedures. This does not invalidate our position that many procedures are appropriate for the CT suite, and such procedures will become more commonplace in the near future.

The second frame and its software have been designed for operation on GE 8800 and 9800 CT/T scanner systems. No additional hardware is needed. All image review features outlined here exploit standard CT system capabilities. Sagittal, coronal, axial, and oblique images are reviewed at the physician's console interactively; image data are adjusted in terms of CT number level and window, all under user control. All three planar views—sagittal, coronal, and axial—are displayed simultaneously to illustrate the three-dimensional context of anatomic structures.

Film documentation of selected trajectories at the intersected anatomy is provided using the scanner system's camera during the procedure. Postbiopsy CT scans can be documented in a similar way.

We are in the process of developing a therapeutic CT scanner suite immediately adjacent to the operating room in our radiology department. Such suites are also under construction in other centers (11).

Our protocol has been modified to exclude those lesions from the above-described biopsy methods if:

1. The lesion is calculated to be greater than 4.0 cm in any dimension
2. The lesion is accessible surgically without the likelihood of major damage to vital cerebral structures
3. There is evidence of major displacement of intracerebral structures that could be reduced by "debulking"
4. The intensity of therapeutic efforts is balanced and considered in relationship to the patient's age, neurologic deficit, and general health status

In such cases, the patient may undergo craniotomy, resection of the majority of visible tumor utilizing adjunctive techniques to better define tumor margins, and then placement of radiation sources directly into the tumor margins.

Utilizing the system described, with the addition of computer reference brain atlases, plans are under way to more accurately place deep-brain-stimulating electrodes in periventricular gray and periaquaductal gray to stimulate endogenous enkephalin and beta-endorphin release. Cerebrospinal fluid analysis of these endogenous opiates will be performed before, during, and after stimulation. Correlation, or the lack of it, with clinical response and endogenous opiate measurement will be evaluated.

Further uses, again with the addition of computer reference brain atlases, will allow improvement in target localization in the treatment of movement disorders, e.g., Parkinson's disease. Stimulation and ablation of appropriate sites should thus be enhanced.

Recent work in the use of microwave-generated hyperthermia will be pursued utilizing this tool as a device to introduce, within appropriate neoplasms, microwave antennae and thermisters to heat and monitor lesions within the range of 42°–40°C.

An entirely new application of CT-assisted stereotaxis is showing promise in orthopedic surgery. Efforts are now under way to develop a similar stereotactic frame and procedure to replace, percutaneously, damaged cruciate ligaments with biosynthetic ligament tissue.

Acknowledgments

Early enthusiasm in 1978 by Russell Brown, MD, at the Memorial Hospital Medical Center (MHMC), Long Beach, California, prompted our interest in stereotactic systems. Clinical evaluation by colleagues Robert W. Porter, MD, PhD, A. M. Nisa Syed, MD, and Ajmel Puthawala, MD, was instrumental in the development of both stereotactic systems. The authors are indebted to Robert S. Howland, Terril Grago, Donald J. Gabel (Howland Industries), Yik San Kwoh, PhD, T. K. Truong, PhD, and Irving S. Reed, PhD, who have worked with us on this and other projects over the last 5 years. Special thanks go to Yu-Ming Azzawi for her programming work on both systems and another version operational on Technicare CT scanners. Suggestions and encouragement by Nicholas Zervas, MD, and Robert Martuza, MD at the Massachusetts General Hospital, Roy A. E. Bakay, MD, at the Emory University Clinic, Stanley Goodman, M.D., at Torrance Memorial Hospital, Torrance, California, and Barry D. Pressman, M.D. at Cedars Sinai Memorial Center, Los Angeles, are sincerely appreciated.

References

1. Barcia-Salorio JL, Barbera J, Broseta J, et al: Tomography in stereotaxis: a new stereoencephalotome designed for this purpose. Acta Neurochir (Wien) [Suppl] 24:77–83, 1977
2. Brain Tumor Study Group: J Neurosurg 49:333–343, 1978
3. Brown RA: A computerized tomography-computer graphics approach to stereotactic localization. J Neurosurg 50:715–720, 1979
4. Glenn WV, Johnston RJ, Morton PE, et al: Image generation and display techniques for CT scan data: thin transverse and reconstructed coronal and sagittal planes. Invest Radiol 10:403–416, 1975
5. Glenn WV, Rhodes ML, Altschuler EM, et al: Multiplanar display computerized body tomography applications in the lumbar spine. Spine 4:282–352, 1979
6. Horsley VA, Clarke RH: On the intrinsic fibres of the cerebellum, its nuclei and its efferent tracts. Brain 28:13–29, 1905
7. Horsley VA, Clarke RH: The structure and functions of the cerebellum examined by a new method. Brain 31:45–124, 1908
8. Ingram WR, Ranson SW, Hannett FI, et al: Results of stimulation of the tegmentum with the Horsley-Clarke stereotaxic apparatus. Arch Neurol Psychiatry 28:513–541, 1932
9. Kelly PJ, Alker GJ Jr: A method for stereotactic laser microsurgery in the treatment of deep-seated CNS neoplasms. Appl Neurophysiol 43:210–215, 1980
10. Leksell L: The stereotactic method and radiosurgery of the brain. Acta Chir Scand 102:316–319, 1951
11. Lunsford LD, Rosenbaum AE, Perry J: Stereotactic surgery using the therapeutic CT scanner. Surg Neurol 18, 1982
12. Mundinger F: Rationale and methods of interstitial iridium-192 brachycurietherapy and iridium-192 or iodine-125 protracted long-term irradiation. In: Stereotactic Cerebral Irradiation, INSERM Symposium No. 12, edited by G Szikla. Elsevier/North Holland, Amsterdam, 1979
13. Mundinger F: The treatment of brain tumors with interstitially applied radioisotopes. In: Radionuclide Applications in Neurology and Neurosurgery, edited by Y Wang, F Paoletti. Charles C Thomas, Springfield, Illinois, 1970, pp 199–265
14. Mundinger F, Birg W, Ostertag CB: Treatment of small cerebral gliomas with CT-aided stereotaxic curietherapy. Neuroradiology 16:564, 1978
15. Oostertag CB, Mennel HD, Kiessling M: Stereotactic biopsy of brain tumors. Surg Neurol 14:275–283, 1980
16. Rhodes ML, Glenn WV, Azzawi YM, et al: Stereotactic neurosurgery using 3-D image data from computed tomography. J Med Syst 6:105–119, 1982

11

Method of Computer Assisted Stereotactic Implantation of Iridium-192 into CNS Neoplasms

Patrick J. Kelly

A lethal dose of radiation can be administered to any intracranial neoplasm by the stereotactic implantation of interstitial radioactive sources while minimal irradiation is delivered to surrounding brain tissue—if certain criteria are met. First, appropriate patients must be selected for the procedure. Secondly, careful acquisition of stereotactic tumor volumetric information by stereotactic computerized tomographic (CT) scanning and serial stereotactic biopsies is required. Finally, preoperative computer simulation of source placement improves the ultimate distribution of stereotactically implanted radionuclides to most efficiently treat the intracranial tumor volume. In this chapter we discuss these points and detail the method of stereotactic implantation of iridium-192 sources utilized at our institution.

Patient Selection

Tumor Size

The implantation of multiple radioactive sources interstitially results in trauma to brain and tumor tissue as well as edema. Postirradiation edema may also result in increased intracranial pressure (14). A patient having a tumor of significant mass may undergo cerebral herniation after implantation of several radioactive sources. Therefore it is recommended that intracranial tumors treated by this method be smaller than 5 cm in volume (14,15).

Histologic Aspects

The maximum therapeutic effect of interstitial irradiation requires several weeks (13). Therefore a slowly growing neoplasm has a greater chance of remaining within therapeutic isodose contours generated by the radioactive sources than one that is growing faster. A rapidly growing tumor may extend beyond the lethal radioactive dose lines before the maximal radiation effect has been achieved (8,13). Thus a patient with a tumor of a lower grade of malignancy does better with this form of treatment than those having more malignant varieties (15).

Tumor Geometric Considerations

An isodose contour produced by a finite number of radionuclide sources has a greater chance of fitting a neoplasm if the three-dimensional shape of the tumor is not complex. The radiation isodose contours produced by a series of interstitially placed sources have the general shape of a cylinder or sphere. Contours of a more complex shape require a greater number of sources. However, the risk of surgery increases in proportion to the number of sources inserted. Therefore in order to safely deliver a lethal dose of radiation to an irregularly shaped neoplasm, one has two choices: 1) underirradiate parts of a tumor that do not fit within the therapeutic isodose lines resulting from the interstitial radionuclides and supplement with external irradiation later; or 2) deliver a lethal dose of irradiation to surrounding brain tissue in order to therapeutically irradiate an irregular portion of a neoplasm.

Data Base Acquisition

CT Scanning

CT scanning provides precise three-dimensional data. CT data are obtained on a GE 8800 CT scanner under stereotactic conditions utilizing a CT compatible stereotactic head holder and localizing system as shown in Figure 11–1. The localizing system, described previously, creates a series of nine reference artifacts on each CT slice (2,4). The CT data

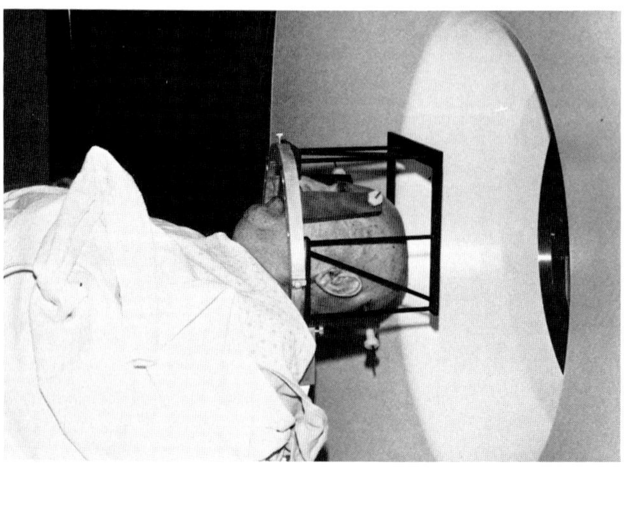

Figure 11–1 CT compatible stereotactic head holder is fixed by four carbon fiber pins inserted through the outer table of the skull into the diploë. A localizing system is attached to the head holder.

tape is put into the operating room computer system (Data General Eclipse S140; 128K RAM, 192 MBYTE disc). CT slices are displayed on a Ramtek raster scan display screen. The reference artifacts are digitized automatically by an intensity detection program. Outlines of the tumor are digitized on each CT slice using cursor and trackball (Figure 11–2). An interpolation program creates intermediate slices, and a volume algorithm is used to create a three-dimensional volume in stereotactic space (Figure 11–3).

CT data may also be utilized by an alternate method. Sagittal and coronal reconstructions of CT data are projected onto respective anteroposterior (AP) and lateral stereotactic radiographs or drawings of radiographs (7,8). The tumor volume is thus represented as a series of contours.

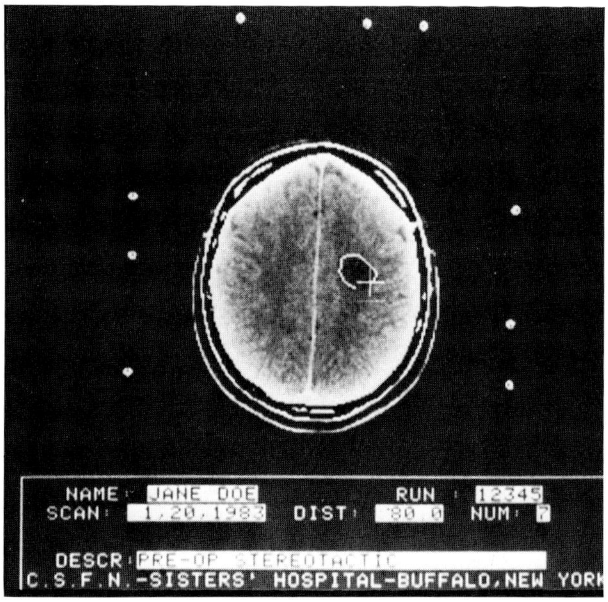

Figure 11–2 The localizing system creates a series of nine artifacts around each CT slice. The nine reference marks are digitized automatically by an intensity detection program. The surgeon outlines the boundary of the tumor on each CT slice utilizing cursor and trackball.

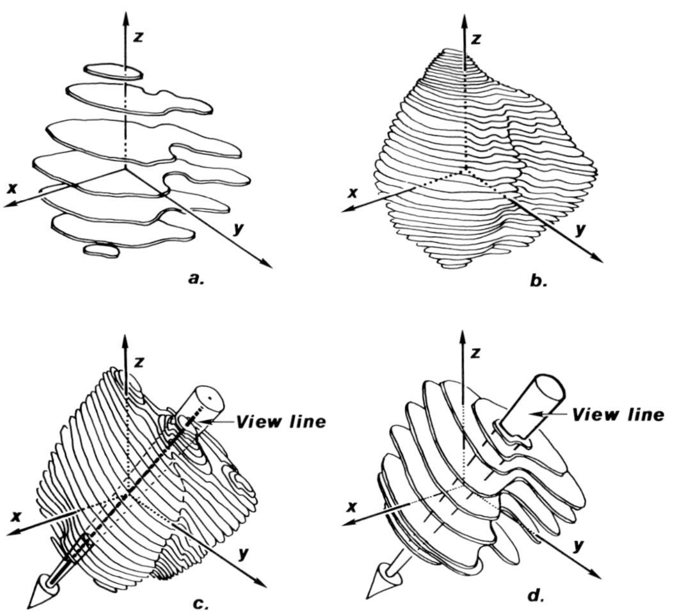

Figure 11–3 **a:** Tumor outlines are suspended in a computer matrix representing the stereotactic coordinate system. **b:** An interpolation program creates intermediate slices at 1-mm intervals. Each slice is given the thickness of 1 mm, and a volume and space are created. **c:** The tumor slices are then reformatted perpendicular to the surgical view line. **d:** The slices at any distance along the view line may be displayed on a computer monitor.

Stereotactic Biopsy

It is doubtful that CT scanning adequately defines the histologic limits of all intracranial neoplasms (1). Therefore one must verify the CT data base histologically by stereotactic serial biopsy (1,12). This CT-based procedure is done separately from and prior to the implantation procedure. Serial biopsies are obtained at 5-mm intervals along a trajectory which passes through the neoplasm. The position of each biopsy is confirmed by AP and lateral teleradiographs. After histologic examination the position and histology of each biopsy is inscribed on AP and lateral stereotactic radiographs or CT slices. These are compared to the boundaries of the tumor defined by CT scanning.

In our system the three-dimensional tumor volume derived from stereotactic CT scanning is retained in a three-dimensional computer storage matrix. The tumor volume may then be expanded or contracted within the computer matrix depending on the results of the stereotactic biopsy procedure.

Source Location Determination

The angle at which the radioactive sources are stereotactically inserted depends on the orientation of the long axis of the tumor and the location of important blood vessels and cerebral structures which must be avoided during the implantation procedure. The insertion angle or "surgical viewline" is actually two angles expressed in degrees from horizontal and vertical planes which relate to respective collar and arc angles on an arc-quadrant stereotactic frame. The three-dimensional tumor volumetric data are reformatted in the computer matrix along this surgical viewline and displayed as a series of contours on the Ramtek raster display terminal.

A computer simulation program allows the placement of simulated sources within these slices and allows the surgeon to view the isodose contours produced by the sources against serial tumor outlines. The isodose contours as a function of the total dose are represented by gray levels (Figure 11–4). Isodose contours which fit one tumor outline are viewed against the outline of the tumor at deeper or more superficial levels. If the isodose contour on deeper or more superficial slices does not fit the radiation isodose contour, sources may be subtracted or others added.

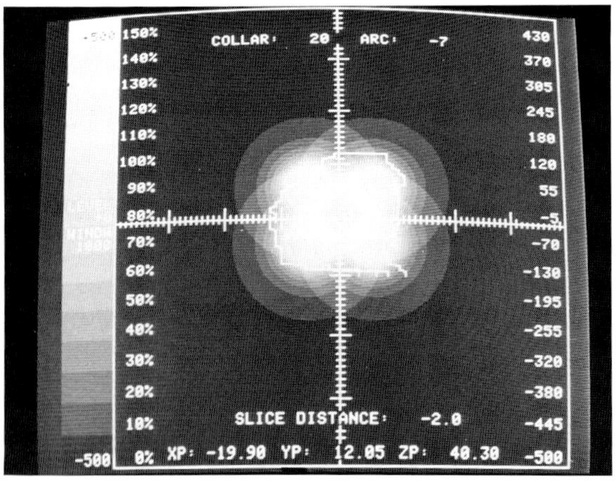

Figure 11–4 The tumor outline is displayed on a graphics monitor. Simulated radioactive sources are added by the surgeon, and the aggregate isodose produced by these sources is displayed in gray levels which relate to a percentage of the total radiation dosage.

Ultimately a satisfactory isodose configuration is determined. The computer outputs X, Y, and Z mechanical adjustments on the stereotactic frame to place the deepest end of each source into the focal point of the stereotactic frame. The computer also outputs the length of each source (Figure 11–5).

Implantation Instrumentation

Our system utilizes a double catheter afterloading technique. The afterloader or carrier consists of a hollow Teflon button to which is fixed a silicone catheter. The internal length of the catheter is related to the distance from the outer table of the skull to the target point given by the computer system. An inner catheter containing a precut length of iridium-192 fits inside the hollow Teflon button into the outer catheter.

A custom stereotactic frame has been developed which utilizes the arc-quadrant principle. The patient's head, fixed in the CT compatible stereotactic head holder, is moved with 3° of freedom within a fixed stereotactic sphere defined by the arc and the quadrant. The X, Y, and Z movements of the patient's head are controlled by servomotors operated by foot pedals. A digital readout in X, Y, and Z gives the position of the head at all times in stereotactic space. This custom stereotactic frame allows rapid access to multiple intracranial target points (Figure 11–6).

DATE: 3, 9,83 TIME: 12:24:24

ARC ANGLE: 5.
COLLAR ANGLE: 45.

WIRE #:	X:	Y:	BEGIN:	END:	DISTANCE:	DELT-X:	DELT-Y:	DELT-Z:
1	-4.64	4.14	-15.	10.	25.	-3.832	5.493	9.684
		XPOSITION:	3.83	YPOSITION:	-5.49	ZPOSITION:	-9.68	
2	5.14	3.64	-10.	12.	22.	-6.199	-4.076	11.341
		XPOSITION:	6.20	YPOSITION:	4.08	ZPOSITION:	-11.34	
3	-4.14	-4.39	-10.	10.	20.	-9.892	4.994	3.686
		XPOSITION:	9.89	YPOSITION:	-4.99	ZPOSITION:	-3.69	
4	5.89	-4.89	-15.	12.	27.	-12.274	-4.825	5.358
		XPOSITION:	12.27	YPOSITION:	4.83	ZPOSITION:	-5.36	
5	1.63	.38	-16.	12.	28.	-8.287	-.578	8.819
		XPOSITION:	8.29	YPOSITION:	.58	ZPOSITION:	-8.82	

Figure 11–5 Computer output of the mechanical settings on the stereotactic frame for the deepest end and the length of each source (distance).

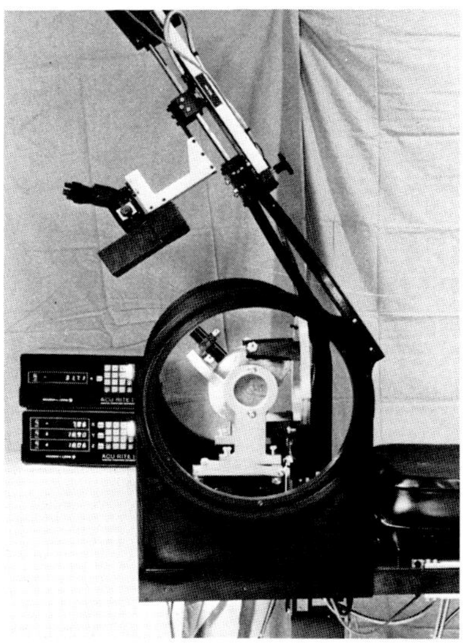

Figure 11–6 Custom stereotactic frame from a lateral view. This is based on the arc-quadrant principle. A CT-compatible head holder holds the skull. The target positions in x, y, and z are displayed on an optical digital readout system shown at the left. Also shown is a double-gimbled 400-mm arc used in stereotactic laser crainotomies.

Implantation Procedure

Implantation of radioactive sources is performed under local anesthesia. First, all of the Teflon button/outer catheter carrier devices are implanted. The X, Y, and Z mechanical adjustments on a custom stereotactic frame given by the computer program are performed which place the intracranial target point for the carrier at the focal point of the stereotactic arc-quadrant. A stab wound is made in the scalp under local infiltration anesthesia and a ⅛-inch drill hole is made in the skull. The dura is opened with unipolar electric cautery. An insertional tool with stylet is inserted through the Teflon button into the outer catheter (Figure 11–7). The carrier is then directed by a guide tube on the stereotactic frame to place the deepest portion of the stylet at the focal point of the stereotactic arc-quadrant. This is confirmed by AP and lateral teleradiographs (Figure 11–8).

After insertion of all of the carrier devices, an inner catheter containing a precut length of iridium-192 is placed. The length of the wires is determined by the computer simulation program. AP and lateral stereotactic teleradiographs are then obtained, as shown in Figure 11–9.

The wounds are then closed. The final AP and lateral stereotactic radiographs are used to perform a computer calculation of the dose rate at successive isodose lines considering the specific activity of the sources used. The sources remain in place until a 6,000-rad dose has been delivered to the peripheral margin of the tumor. These are superimposed on computer-generated sagittal and coronal reconstructions of the tumor volume. The carriers containing the sources are then removed under local anesthesia. External radiation therapy may be given to increase the radiation field outside the margins of a tumor which has a complex geometric shape or an aggressive histologic character.

Discussion

The technique described utilizes a variation of a double-catheter afterloading procedure described previously (7,8). This has several advantages over permanent implantation procedures utilized at some institutions (9–12). In an afterloading technique, a high-specific-activity removable source is used so that the radiation dosage is delivered within a shorter period of time. The surgeon and radiotherapist have better control of the radiation dosage, as sources may be retrieved at any time. Permanently implanted sources may shift in position as the tumor undergoes necrosis.

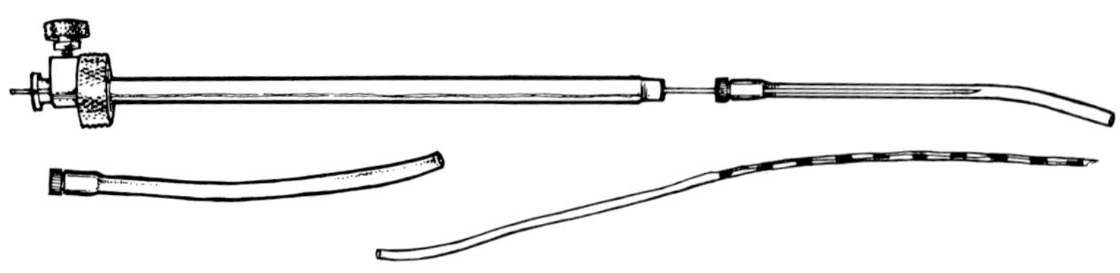

Figure 11–7 The double catheter afterloading system demonstrating a hollow Teflon button connected to a silicone outer catheter. This is implanted by means of an insertional tool and stylet. The stylet extends through the hollow Teflon button into the silicone catheter. An inner catheter containing a precut length of iridium wire is shown.

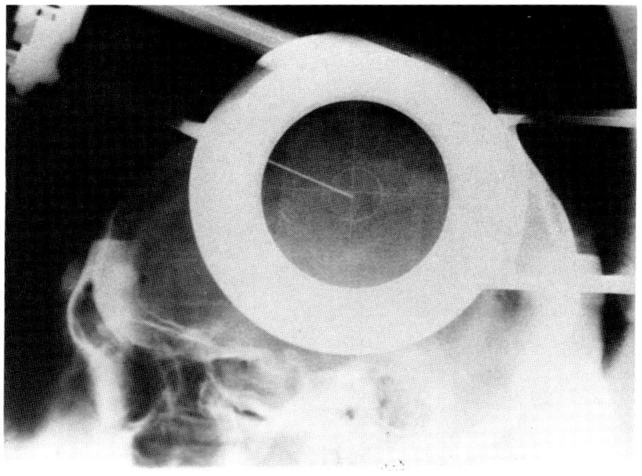

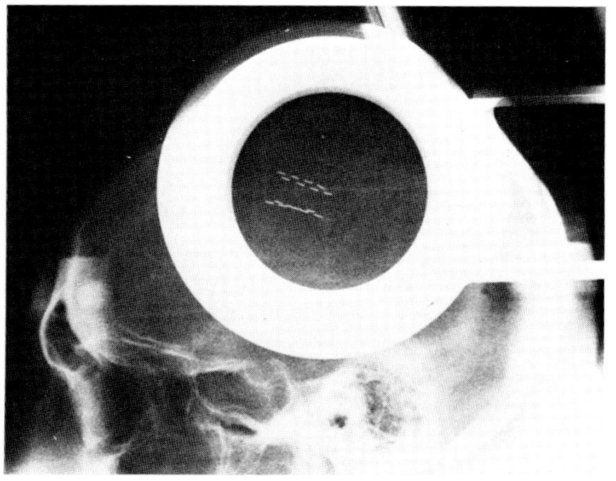

Figure 11–8 Stereotactic teleradiograph demonstrating the position of the insertional stylet after placement of a Teflon button outer catheter carrier.

Figure 11–9 Lateral stereotactic teleradiograph performed after insertion of inner catheters with iridium-192 sources.

In the past, the technique of cerebral interstitial irradiation has been limited by the method of determining source locations within the tumor volume. Tumor outlines were usually inscribed on two-dimensional x-ray pictures or drawings or, most recently, on CT scans. Geometric arrangements of proposed source placement were then superimposed. This could not adequately represent the three-dimensional nature of a tumor, especially when the geometry of the neoplasm was complex or when the sources were placed in a plane not perpendicular to that of the radiographs or CT slices.

Our method was derived from a similar program for stereotactic laser vaporization of central nervous system neoplasms (3–6). Here a tumor volume is created in a three-dimensional computer matrix corresponding to the stereotactic coordinate system. The tumor volume may then be sliced orthogonal to any specified surgical approach. Thus a complex three-dimensional structure is viewed as a series of two-dimensional slices.

Unfortunately, the data base derived from CT scanning may not necessarily represent the histologic limits of the tumor (1,5). Histologic examination of serial stereotactic biopsy specimens gives information on the histologic tumor boundaries only along the trajectory of the biopsy. Other imaging modalities, e.g., nuclear magnetic resonance (NMR), may present a more accurate picture on the actual limits of intracranial neoplasms in the future.

References

1. Daumas-Duport C, Monsaingeon V, Szenthe L, et al: Serial stereotactic biopsies a double histologic code of gliomas according to malignancy and 3-D configuration as an aid to therapeutic decision and assessment of results. J Appl Neurophysiol 45:431–437, 1982
2. Goerss S, Kelly PJ, Kall B, et al: A computed tomographic stereotactic adaptation system. Neurosurgery 10:375–379, 1982

3. Kelly PJ, Alker GJ: A method for stereotactic laser microsurgery in the treatment of deep-seated CNS neoplasms. Appl Neurophysiol 43:210–215, 1980
4. Kelly PJ, Alker GJ, Goerss S: Computer-assisted stereotactic laser microsurgery for the treatment of intracranial neoplasms. Neurosurgery 10:324–331, 1982
5. Kelly PJ, Alker GJ, Kall B, et al: Precision resection of intra-axial CNS lesions by CT-based stereotactic craniotomy and computer monitored CO_2 laser. Acta Neurochir (Wien) (in press)
6. Kelly PJ, Alker GJ, Zoll JG: A microstereotactic approach to deep-seated arteriovenous malformations. Surg Neurol 17:260–262, 1982
7. Kelly PJ, Olsen MH, Wright AE: Stereotactic implantation of iridium 192 into CNS neoplasms. Surg Neurol 10:349–354, 1978
8. Kelly PJ, Olsen MH, Wright AE, et al: CT localization and stereotactic implantation of iridium 192 into CNS neoplasms. In: INSERM Symposium No. 12, edited by G Szikla. Elsevier/North Holland Biomedical Press, Amsterdam, 1979, pp 123–128
9. Mundinger F, Birg W, Klar M: Computer-assisted stereotactic brain operations by means including computerized axial tomography. Appl Neurophysiol 41:169–182 1978
10. Mundinger F, Birg W, Ostertag CB: Treatment of small cerebral gliomas with CT-aided stereotaxic curietherapy. Neuroradiology 16:564–567, 1978
11. Mundinger F, Hoefer T: Protracted long-term irradiation of inoperable midbrain tumours by stereotactic curietherapy using iridium-192. Acta Neurochir (Wien) [Suppl] 21:93–100, 1974
12. Mundinger F, Metzel E: Interstitial radioisotope therapy of intractable diencephalic tumors by the stereotactic permanent implantation of iridium 192 including bioptic control. Confin Neurol 32:195–202, 1970
13. Schlienger M, Bouhnik H, Missir O, et al: Association of temporary interstitial ^{192}Ir implantation and external radiotherapy in the management of supratentorial tumors. In: INSERM Symposium No. 12, edited by G Szikla. Elsevier/North Holland Biomedical Press, Amsterdam, 1979, pp 117–121
14. Szikla G, Betti O, Blond S: Data on late reactions following stereotactic irradiation of gliomas. In: INSERM Symposium No. 12, edited by G Szikla. Elsevier/North Holland Biomedical Press, Amsterdam, 1979, pp 167–174
15. Szikla G, Schlienger M, Betti O, et al: Combined interstitial and external irradiation of gliomas: a progress report. In: INSERM Symposium No. 12, edited by G Szikla. Elsevier/North Holland Biomedical Press, Amsterdam, 1979, pp 329–338

12 CT-Adapted Leksell Stereotaxy

Jörgen Boëthius

The new imaging techniques, e.g., computerized tomographic (CT) scanning, positron emission tomography (PET) scanning, and nuclear magnetic resonance (NMR) have meant a dramatic improvement in the practice of stereotactic neurosurgery. Beyond this, a change in conceptual perspective emerges from the fact that the information in these techniques is contained in a tridimensional matrix similar to the one used to organize the information in stereotaxy. The new diagnostic modalities thus constitute natural matches to the older therapeutic systems. The next logical step in the development of stereotactic neurosurgery seems to be the achievement of a full tridimensional integration of the various diagnostic and therapeutic modalities presently in use. In the next stage of this development it seems feasible and desirable to have a further integration between the two most rapidly developing sections in neurosurgery, i.e., stereotactic neurosurgery and microneurosurgery.

In a fully integrated stereotactic system it is fundamental to create and retain an exact spatial orientation which remains unchanged throughout a number of therapeutic and diagnostic procedures. There are obviously many possible technical solutions to this problem, but at present some kind of mechanical device seems to be the most practical. In the Fixter system the spatial orientation is retained by a base plate (Figure 12–1) attached to the head of the patient with aluminum bars. The bars are sufficiently long to allow the base plate to be mounted below the head with screws in the skull or with a plastic helmet (6,9). To the base plate one may adapt various diagnostic and therapeutic stereotactic devices. These are mounted in holes constructed in such a way that all devices have an identical stereotactic coordinate system.

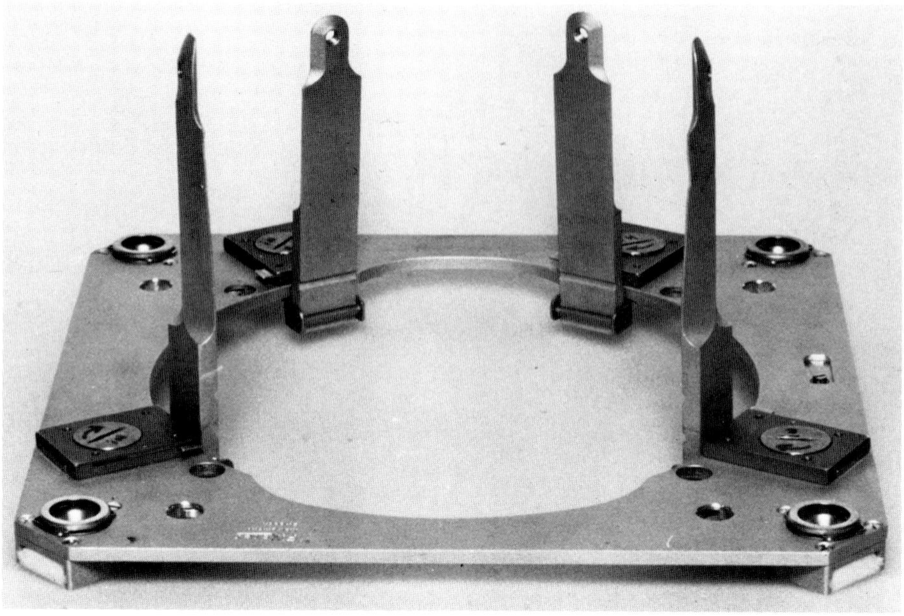

Figure 12–1 Base plate with attached aluminum bars for skull fixation. The plate carries three sets of holes which are used to fasten it to the holder and to mount localizing frames and stereotactic instruments.

Practical Applications

Mounting the Base Plate With Skull Screws

The patient is placed with his head in a special simulator of a scanner opening (6) or, alternatively, on the operating table with the head rest removed. Aluminum bars (Figure 12–2) of proper length are selected so that the screws are placed somewhat above the occipital protuberance occipitally and on the upper part of the temporal bone frontally. The base plate is placed in its proper position in relation to the head, in the simulator on performed plugs, and on the operating table with the aid of a special movable support functionally analogous to that which carries, for example, a Mayfield head clamp. The aluminum bars are angled inward with the aid of special locking devices on the base plate. When the tops of the bars are lying against the head (Figure 12–3), local

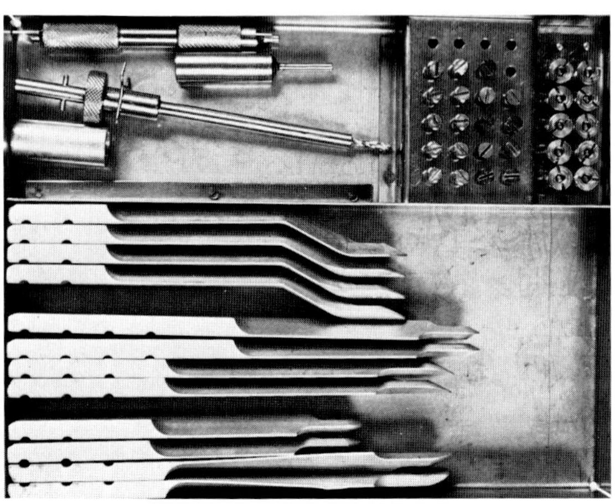

Figure 12–2 Set of aluminum bars, skull screws, and a drill with stopper which is used to make shallow holes in the skull bone for fixation.

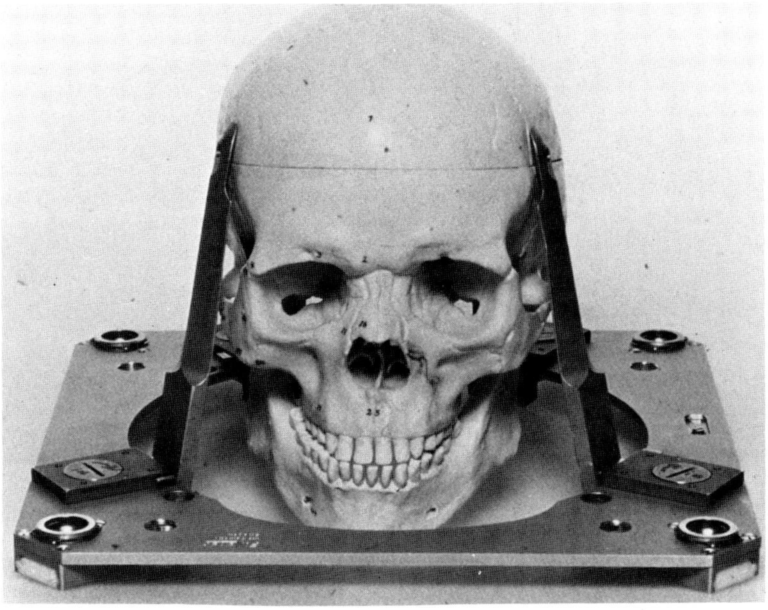

Figure 12–3 Base plate is attached to the skull with the aluminum bars angled inward to lie against the skull.

anesthetic is injected into the skin through the screw holes in the bars. To fix the head a special screw is used which consists of an outer aluminum part and a detachable inner stainless steel core. This core has a sharp point which penetrates into the outer tabula of the skull. The stainless steel cores are then removed in order to avoid artifacts on the CT scan. Shallow holes are then drilled into the skull bone and the stainless steel cores replaced with aluminum cores. The whole procedure typically takes about 20 min to perform.

Mounting the Base Plate With a Plastic Helmet

The helmet is made by winding a few turns of Light cast plastic tightly around the skull, after which it is cured with ultraviolet (UV) irradiation. For further stability a dental fixation is made by having the patient bite into a piece of Ortoplast which attaches to the Light cast helmet. The patient is now placed in the simulator, and the helmet is mounted on the base plate with aluminum braces. These braces are fixed to the helmet with an additional layer of Light cast plastic (Figure 12–4). The top of the head remains uncovered; when it is desirable to use the helmet repeatedly, it is cut open and easily removed and repositioned by widening the cut. When the helmet is repositioned, the cut is closed and fixed with a plaster.

Diagnostic Procedures

Localization With CT scanning

The patient, carrying the base plate, is positioned on the scanning table, and the ordinary head rest is exchanged for a special attachment which plugs into a special set of holes in the base plate. If a body scanner

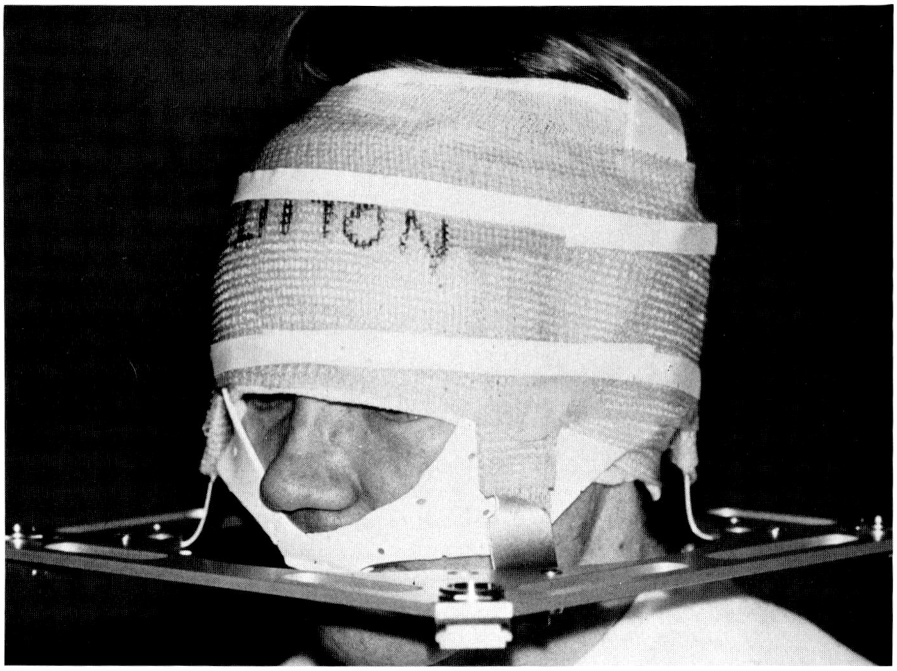

Figure 12–4
Patient mounted in a plastic helmet.

is used there are usually no problems, but with head scanners the base plate cannot be introduced in the scanner opening and care must be taken to ensure that the bars are sufficiently long to allow proper scanning of the head. In order to define the coordinate system, it is necessary to have some well defined structures visible in the picture. This is done by fixing a Perspex frame in the specially designed holes in the base plate (2). This frame and a picture resulting from its use are shown in Figure 12–5. The center of the stereotactic system in the anterior-posterior and the right-left direction is obtained by determining the middle of a rectangle with its corners at the marks caused by vertical aluminum strips mortised in the frame. The height coordinate is determined by measuring the scanned distance between a vertical aluminum strip and an aluminum strip running from the top of one vertical strip to the bottom of the other at a 45° angle. The coordinates can be measured on the CT picture directly or on the CRO screen of the scanner (6).

If the patient is not properly centered in the hole of the base plate, his head or one of the aluminum bars may interfere with the localizing frame so that its feet cannot be fitted in the holes in the base plate. It is therefore advisable to check the placement of the frame at the time the base plate is fixed to the head of the patient. The dimensions of the localizing frame are determined by the properties of the CT scanner.

Localization With PET Scanning

Localization with a PET scanner is performed in a fashion similar to that with a CT scanner (2). Figure 12–6 shows the localization frame for PET scanning. The frame is similar to the one used for CT scanning with the exception that a thin tube filled with a radioactive material is used to generate the visual marks on the picture in place of the aluminum strips. The tube is mounted in the same pattern as the aluminum strips, with sections running vertically in order to define the corners of the

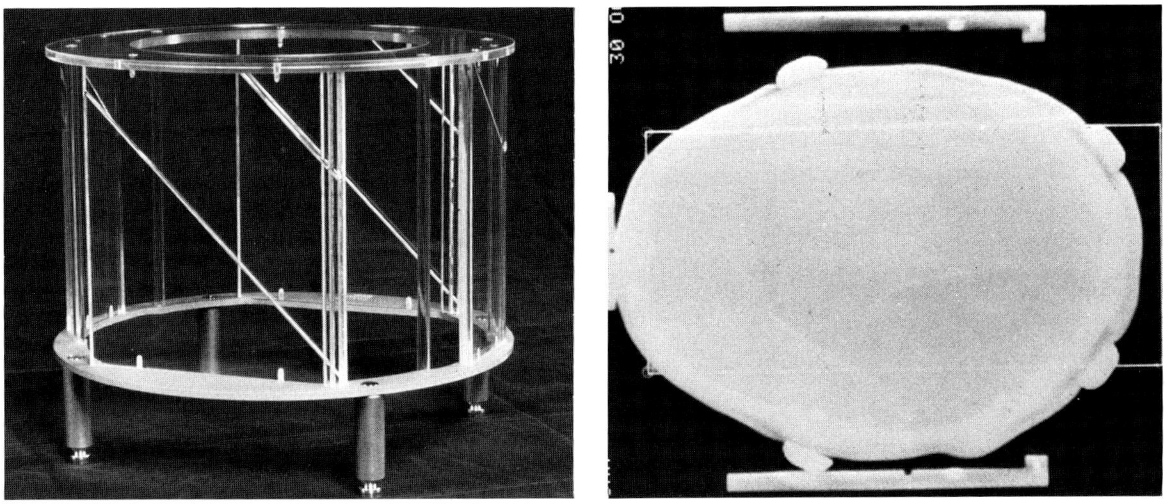

A B

Figure 12–5 A: Localization frame for CT scanning. The reference marks in the picture are caused by thin aluminum strips—four vertical ones and two running at 45° angles in the side pieces of the frame. **B:** CT scan taken with the frame on shows the marks caused by the strips which are used to define the stereotactic coordinates.

rectangle which determines the midpoint of the stereotactic coordinate system and two tube sections, one on each side, running at 45° angles to indicate the height coordinate. The PET scan frame is mounted in the same holes in the base plates as the CT frame.

Localization With Conventional X-ray Techniques

Conventional x-ray techniques include plain radiography, angiography, and encephalography. Localization with these modes is performed with yet another frame (Figure 12–7) which is rectangular and has milli-

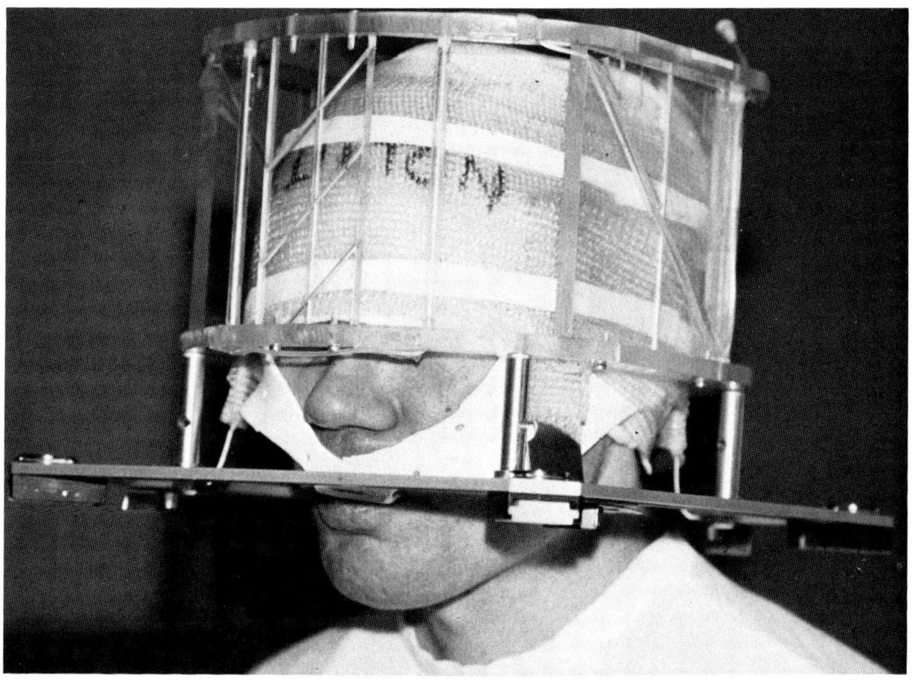

Figure 12–6 Localizing frame for PET scanning. The reference marks in the picture are caused by thin tubes filled with a radioactive liquid—four vertical ones and two running at 45° angles.

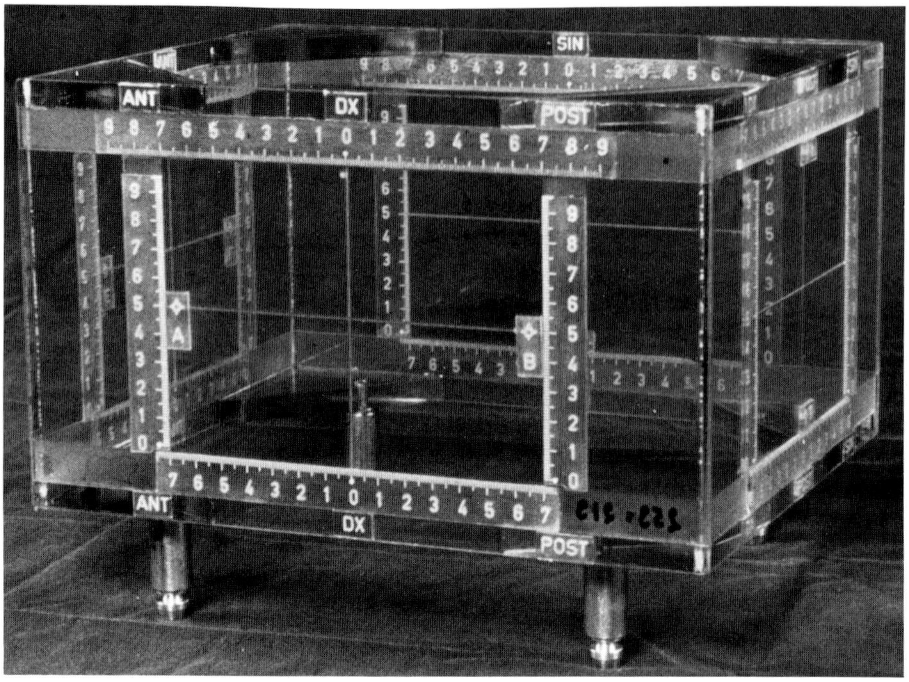

Figure 12–7 Localizing frame for conventional x-rays. The millimeter scales seen on x-rays are engraved on the four sides of the frame.

meter scales engraved on its four sides (3). The stereotactic coordinates of a target are obtained by doing one side and one frontal projection. In the pictures the scale closest to the x-ray source show up as the larger and the scale distal to the source as the smaller. For each axis a line is drawn at right angles to the scales through the target point. The millimeter values of the proximal and distant scales are read at the point where this line crosses the scales. The easiest way to obtain the true coordinates is to connect the values obtained this way in a diagram.

Localization With NMR

At present, NMR has not been used in conjunction with the system. However, there should be no problem of constructing a localizing frame similar to the ones used for CT and PET scanning with rods in a material appropriate to give good images with NMR.

Therapeutic Techniques

When the target coordinates have been determined, the localization frame is removed and a stereotactic instrument mounted in the same holes in the base plate. The coordinates are set on the instrument, and the stereotactic procedure is carried out.

Leksell Instrument

The Leksell frame was originally constructed to be fastened directly to the head. In the present system the Leksell frame is adapted with special feet which fit into the same base plate holes as the localizing frames. The feet are constructed to make the Leksell coordinate system identical to that of the localizing frames. With the Leksell frame in position (Figure 12–8), the stereotactic procedure can be carried out as usual; that is, the target coordinates are set, and the desired position of the craniotomy is selected. The arch of the Leksell system and the guidance system which is mounted on it is adjusted so that the stereotactic probe passes through the craniotomy and on down to the target. No additional calculations are needed because the target point in the Leksell system is always located in the midpoint of the half-sphere defined by the possible movements of the semicircular arch.

Riechert-Mundinger Instrument

The Riechert-Mundinger instrument is adapted to the base plate in a manner similar to that in the Leksell instrument; that is, the pins which are usually used to mount the ring on the skull are removed and replaced with feet which fit into four holes in the base plate. As in the case of the Leksell instrument, these feet are constructed to make the coordinate system of the Riechert-Mundinger instrument identical to that of the localizing frame. When thus mounted the instrument is used in a conventional manner.

Fixter Instrument

Both the Leksell and the Riechert-Mundinger systems have arches to carry the stereotactic probe, which make them difficult to use in conjunction with open surgery. Both systems also have dead angles, which puts some restraints on the number of possible trajectories which can be used to reach a target. To minimize these drawbacks a new stereotactic instrument has been constructed (8). This instrument consists of a ring which can be mounted on the base plate (Figure 12–9). At every 15° a screw hole is made in the upper surface of the ring in order to fasten

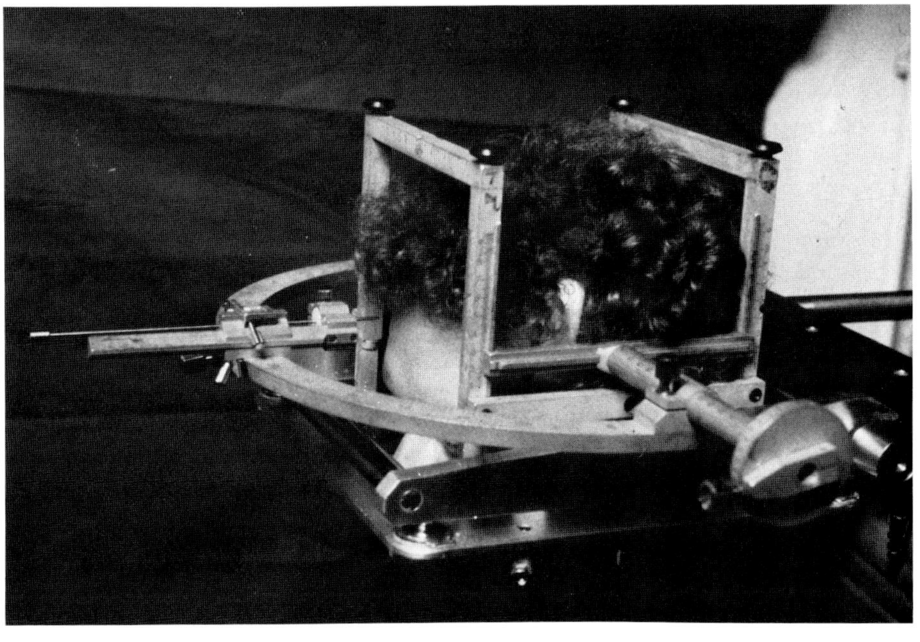

Figure 12–8 Leksell system mounted on the base plate ready for use.

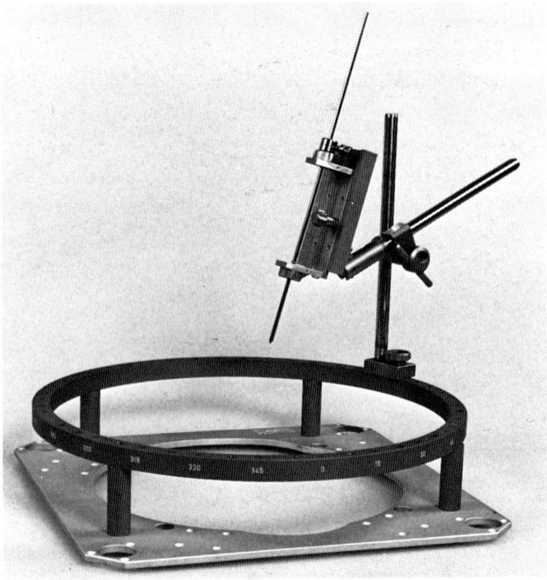

Figure 12–9 Fixter instrument on the base plate. The probe holder is mounted on the ring.

probe holders and other instruments. The coordinates are set with the aid of a phantom (Figure 12–10) which has a ring similar to the one used on the patient and a tridimensional scale system which is used to place a target indicator at the target position. If a predetermined probe trajectory is desired, a marker is mounted on the ring and brought down to the target point. The target indicator is then moved to some other point on the probe trajectory (Figure 12–11A). The stereotactic probe is then mounted on a probe carrier which is fixed in one of the holes in the phantom ring and adjusted so that its tip goes down to the target point indicated by a marker at the same time as it touches the second point of the trajectory indicated by the target indicator (Figure 12–11B). Because a trajectory is uniquely determined by two points along its course, the stereotactic probe is now mounted in its proper position. The probe holder is moved from the phantom ring and placed in a similar hole in the patient ring and the operation is performed. The craniotomy is made at the site indicated by the probe.

If it is desirable to reach a target from a preselected craniotomy,

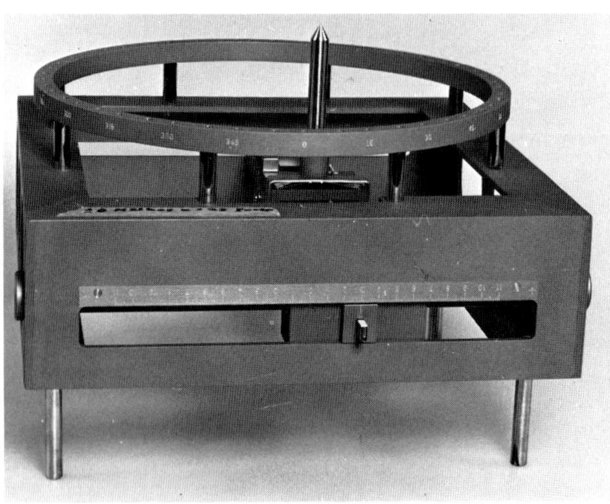

Figure 12–10 Fixter phantom used for target localization. The target indicator is set in a slide which can be moved along the two axes in the plane of the ring. The height coordinate is set by moving the target indicator up or down. The top of the phantom carries a ring identical to the one on the Fixter instrument.

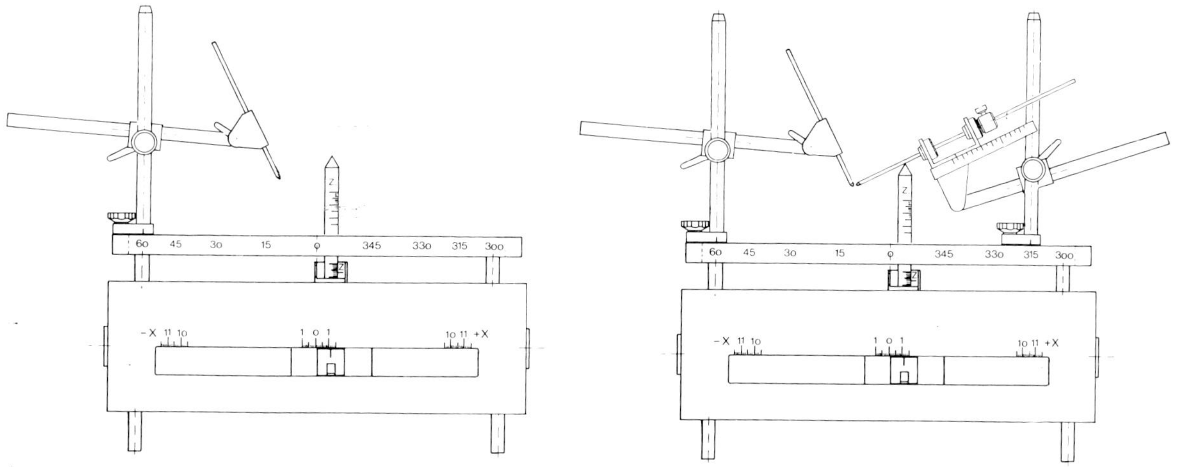

A B

Figure 12–11 **A:** Method to set a predetermined trajectory on the Fixter phantom. The target point previously set with the target indicator is now retained with a pointer mounted on the ring when the target indicator has been moved to some other point on the desired trajectory. **B:** Probe carrier mounted on the ring and adjusted to bring the tip of the probe to the target at the same time the probe shaft touches the second point on the trajectory indicated by the target indicator.

one proceeds as follows. The target is set on the phantom, and a marker is mounted on the patient ring so that it touches the craniotomy (Figure 12–12). This marker is then moved to the analogous hole in the phantom ring. A probe holder is mounted in an appropriate hole in the phantom ring, the desired coordinates are set, and the probe is adjusted so that its tip hits the target indicator while the shaft touches the marker indicating the position of the craniotomy. The probe is now ready to be used and is moved in its holder to the analogous hole in the patient ring. It will now pass through the craniotomy and reach the target point.

The instrument has the further advantage that it is possible to indicate a structure (e.g., on the brain of the patient), move this pointer to the analogous position on the phantom, and with the aid of the target indicator determine its coordinates by moving the indicator so that it touches the tip of the marker. It is possible to use these coordinates to see exactly what the point or area corresponds to on the CT scan, PET scan, or angiographic picture.

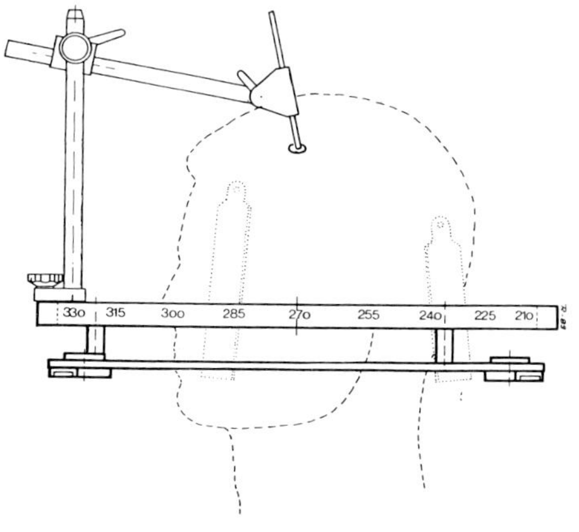

Figure 12–12 The point at which a target will be reached through a predetermined craniotomy is indicated with a marker mounted on the instrument. See text for further details.

Stereotactic Irradiation

The base plate system has been used to implement stereotactic irradiation with a linear accelerator. Such irradiation has been applied in cases of deep-seated surgically inaccessible tumors (4) and large arteriovenous malformations (AVMs) (11).

The patient is put in a plastic helmet. The appropriate (CT for tumors and angiography for AVMs) localizing frame is mounted on the base plate, and the stereotactic coordinates are determined. The plastic helmet can be removed from the head by cutting it open, and at later sessions it can be repositioned on the head of the patient with acceptable accuracy (10). The pictures are used by the physicist to plan the irradiation. That done, the helmet is repositioned and remounted on the base plate. The patient is fixed to the linear accelerator with an attachment for the base plate and irradiated. Stereotactically the procedure makes it possible to irradiate areas of different size with good protection of neighboring brain tissue against irradiation. Figure 12–13 shows the patient mounted in the linear accelerator for treatment.

Typical Procedures

Biopsy of Gliomas

Before the introduction of stereotactic CT scanning, evaluable biopsies were obtained in only about 70% of gliomas mainly because the nonevaluable biopsies contained only necrotic material. Experience with CT scanning has shown that it is important to obtain biopsy material from both high and low attenuating tumor areas. In order to achieve this we usually take several biopsies along one trajectory. This trajectory

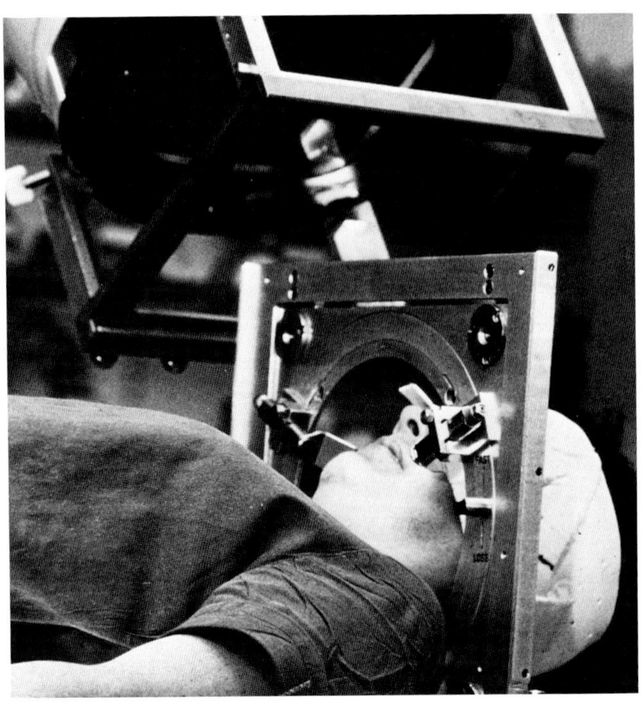

Figure 12–13 Patient in a linear accelerator mounted for stereotactic irradiation.

is designed to pass through various types of tumor tissue, both high and low attenuating. The simplest way to do this is to design the trajectory in the plane of a CT section. When this is not suitable it may be difficult to determine exactly where in the tumor the biopsies are taken. This difficulty can be minimized if the probe trajectory is perpendicular to the CT plane and the various biopsies placed in each CT section. With a Fixter instrument it is possible to localize the exact coordinate of each biopsy irrespective of the angle of the probe trajectory with the use of the procedure described above and also to determine what the spacing of the biopsies should be in order to make each biopsy fall in the middle of a CT section. Most biopsies have been taken with the Leksell instrument, which has been adequate even though it is sometimes difficult to get biopsies along a trajectory which goes at right angles to the side of the head.

As a biopsy instrument we have used a spiral needle (1). The complications have been few and usually minor. The spiral needle yields biopsies about 1 cm long with a diameter of about 1 mm. These biopsies are sufficiently large to enable a pathologist experienced in their evaluation to obtain paraffin sections, smears, and some material for tissue culture. In large tumors it is possible to use a larger spiral needle, one with an outer diameter of 4 mm. Biopsies obtained with this needle are large enough to allow flow cytometric determinations of the DNA distribution of the tumor (5). Biopsies can be performed with the patient fixed to the base plate with screws in the calvarium or with the plastic helmet fixation.

Cryosurgery

Small deep-seated tumors can be treated with cryosurgery if they are not close to the ventricular system. The cryosurgical lesion extends 1–1.5 cm out from the wall of the probe. The probes come in different dimensions and must be chosen with this restriction in mind. It is advantageous to do cryosurgery in the scanner because the ice of the lesion is easily demonstrated with the CT scanner. One can thus directly see the size of the lesion and determine whether it is appropriate. Our only experience is with the Leksell system, and the procedure is as follows (7).

The patient is mounted in the base plate, and a craniotomy is performed. The patient is then brought down to the scanner and the CT localizing box is adapted and the stereotactic target determined. The Leksell instrument is fixed on the base plate, the coordinates are set, and the arch and probe carrier are adjusted so that the probe will pass through the craniotomy. That having been done, the instrument is removed from the base plate without changing its settings. The patient is removed from the scanner, and a new base plate with the unchanged Leksell instrument mounted on it is put in the scanner. Because the Leksell instrument produces artifacts on the CT scan, it must be removed from the scanner and replaced by another mechanical system which retains the probe orientation. Two Perspex rods are mounted on the attachment which holds the base plate on the scanning table. From the top of these Perspex rods two "swanhalses" are brought down to the probe holder of the Leksell instrument and fastened to it with screws. The swanhalses are tightened and form a rigid attachment to the probe holder.

The arch of the Leksell system is removed from the probe holder, and then the base plate with the Leksell system is removed. There now remains only the probe holder mounted on the two swanhalses which are carried by the two Perspex rods. If the craniotomy is near the top of the head, all stereotactic hardware is now out of the x-ray path. The probe is introduced to its position and scanned in order to check that it is correctly placed in the coordinate system. The patient, still carrying the base plate, is again repositioned and the probe can now be introduced through the craniotomy into the tumor. Cryosurgery can be performed with the patient in the scanner (and being scanned when the freezing takes place), thereby making it possible to determine precisely the size of the lesion.

Open Stereotactic Exploration

Sometimes it is desirable to localize a small tumor stereotactically in order to minimize the operation's trauma and maximize the chances of finding the lesion, which is then removed by open surgery. A similar procedure can be used to localize and clip the feeding arteries of a large AVM. This operation, which is best performed with the Fixter instrument, is done as follows: The patient is mounted in the base plate and the coordinates of the lesion are determined with CT scanning or angiography. The patient is then moved to the operating room, and the Fixter instrument is mounted on the base plate. The target of the lesion and the trajectory are set on the phantom as described above, and a probe is brought down to the target from the probe holder mounted on the phantom ring. The holder is moved to analogous position in the patient ring and the probe is advanced to indicate the center of a small craniotomy. Because the craniotomy can be made small, it is usually not necessary to turn a skin flap; a vertical incision is sufficient. A small bone flap is turned, and for tumors a biopsy should now be taken through the dura to minimize any chance of displacement of the lesion by a possible tissue shift, e.g., one caused by brain bulging. The dura is then opened, and the stereotactic probe is used to indicate the precise location of the lesion, which is removed by conventional means. The patient ring can also be used to mount retractors and other instruments.

Discussion

Advantages and Disadvantages of the Base Plate System

The main advantage of the base plate system is that it makes it possible to have a fully integrated stereotactic system where all or most diagnostic and therapeutic modalities can be combined in a controlled manner within a defined tridimensional spatial system. The use of aluminum bars for mounting the base plate causes only minimal CT artifacts. At present, work is under way to replace the aluminum with plastic, which should abolish the minimal remaining artifacts. One disadvantage is a certain awkwardness in mounting the base plate. Obviously the degree of awkwardness has to do with the surgeon's familiarity with the equipment. Sometimes there are difficulties in fitting patients with very large heads into the CT localizing frame. It is our experience, however, that such patients are met with only rarely.

Screws Versus Plastic Helmet Fixation

The principal difference between fixation with screws directly in the calvarium as opposed to plastic helmet fixation is that the fixation is more rigid and changes less during the procedure. For high-precision stereotactic applications, screws therefore seem to be the fixation of choice. The possibility of reapplying the plastic helmet repeatedly makes this fixation the superior one for repeated treatments, e.g., stereotactic irradiation in the linear accelerator. It is also feasible to use the plastic helmet for biopsying gliomas.

Integration of Stereotaxy and Microneurosurgery

Every stereotactic surgeon has at times been frustrated by the limitations of ordinary stereotactic instrumentation, which makes it impossible to intervene effectively against pathologic lesions which are not physically very small or cystic. Similarly, conventional neurosurgeons have felt the limitations of their instruments when it comes to localizing small targets in brain tissue. A prime example of this difficulty is the excessive explorations which are too frequently used to find small metastatic tumors. The Fixter instrument makes it possible to combine the strong points of the two principal neurosurgical approaches, especially when used together with the operating microscope. The possibility of localizing the lesion with high precision allows the use of small flaps, and thus some of the time used for the stereotactic localization can be regained. The use of small flaps also diminishes the drawback of having the head mounted in four braces. However, sometimes the braces interfere with the "open" part of the procedure, and work is now in progress to make the mountings of the aluminum bars movable and thus to make the system more flexible. Even with the present system it is possible to place the bone flap at almost any position by adjusting the height of the bars and/or by rotating the base plate somewhat in respect to the long axis of the patient. The instrument is best suited for supratentorial interventions; we have never used it for lesions in the posterior fossa. Because of the small dimensions in this area, it has been thought that the need for "open" stereotactic surgery in the posterior fossa was insufficient to warrant the development of the special equipment which would be needed. This equipment is necessary only for "open" stereotactic surgery; for traditional stereotaxy the system is adequate for use in the posterior fossa.

References

1. Backlund EO: A new instrument for stereotactic brain tumor biopsy. Acta Chir Scand 137:825–827, 1971
2. Bergström M, Boëthius J, Eriksson L, et al: Head fixation device for reproducible position alignment in transmission CT and positron emission tomography. J Comput Assist Tomogr 5:136–141, 1981
3. Bergström M, Greitz T, Ribble T: A method for stereotaxic localization adapted for conventional and digital radiography. 1983 (in press)
4. Blomgren H, Berggren BM, Bergström M, et al: Preliminary experience with stereotactically placed isocentric irradiation from a linear accelerator on high and low grade gliomas. Acta Neurochir (Wien) 1983 (in press)
5. Boëthius J, Bergstrand G, Collins VP, et al: DNA-distribution in various parts of malignant gliomas assayed on stereotactic biopsies. J Appl Neurophysiol 43:216–221, 1980

6. Boëthius J, Bergström M, Greitz T: Stereotactic computerized tomography with a GE 8800 scanner. J Neurosurg 52:794–800, 1980
7. Boëthius J, Greitz T, Kuylenstierna R, et al: Stereotactic cryosurgery in a CT scanner 1983 (in press)
8. Boëthius J, Ribble T: A new stereotactic instrument which can be used in conjunction with open surgery. Acta Neurochir (Wien) 1983 (in press)
9. Greitz T, Bergström M, Boëthius J, et al: Head fixation system for integration of radiodiagnostic and therapeutic procedures. Neuroradiology 19:1–6, 1980
10. Kingsley DPE, Bergström M, Berggren B-M: A critical evaluation of two methods of head fixation. Neuroradiology 19:7–12, 1980
11. Steiner L, Berggren BM, Bergström M, et al: To be published, 1983

13

Contemporary Trends in Brain Tumor Treatment

Peter Dyck

> He who cares for patients suffering from brain tumors must bring to his problem much thought and stout action. There is a need also for a formidable optimism, for the dice of the gods are loaded.
>
> Foster Kennedy

It is humbling irony that, in spite of vast advances in a number of frontiers in medicine, Foster Kennedy's laconic admonition, which echoed the corridors of neurologic wards more than half a century ago, should be as true today as it was then. In spite of advances in neuroanesthesia and surgical technic, the prognosis of patients harboring malignant intracranial neoplasms has not improved a great deal. Having excluded neuroectodermal neoplasms associated with phacomatoses that are apparently genetically linked, the etiology of intracranial tumors remains unknown. In other words, although existing animal experimental models may help to elucidate oncogenesis in general, no specific chemical, viral, or other etiologic agent has been uncontestedly proved to produce cerebral neoplasm.

Almost one century ago Cohnheim implored his colleagues to consider that most likely all cancer arose unicentrically from a single cell gone "amuck" (4), yet this ipse dixit was not accepted without reservation. Commensurate with such skepticism, Willis, in 1967, proposed the so-called "field-theory" of oncogenesis, which held that not one but a number of cells may behave in a neoplastic manner, should the circumstances be favorable for such events. Extrapolating from this, the tumor bulk and its cell population would be the product not only of replicating centrally placed cells but also of the formation of peripherally situated new oncogenic tissue (38).

In support of such contentions, Russell and Rubinstein estimated that 6% of glioblastomas might be classified as multicentric in origin (26). In a recent pathologic study of 20 cases of glioblastoma multiforme treated premorbidly with teletherapy and chemotherapy, the widespread histopathologic alterations observed appeared to them to support multicentricity of neoplasia (3). No consideration seemed to be given by the authors to what role radiation or chemotherapeutic drugs might play in these histopathologic alterations. Such imperiousness, in my opinion, is based on assumptions that fail in both deductive logic and inductive reasoning.

To complicate matters, it is evident that fibroblast or lymphocyte chalones act to inhibit cell replication by controlling mitosis (12). These chalones are tissue, but not species, specific. Unfortunately, the chalone concentration has been observed to be decreased in rats with leukemia (27). Could the same be true of other malignant states, particularly in man? Folkman has shown that neoplasms have the capacity to produce a tumor angiogenesis factor (TAF), in order to facilitate neovascularization of the mass (8). To complement these observations, Kelly et al. have reported a high concentration of TAF in astrocytomas, tumors notorious for endothelial proliferation and neovascularization (16).

Finally, it might be said that, although no specific viral agent is known to produce human brain tumors, data to permit extemporaneous speculation exist. It is common knowledge that oncogenic virus infections of the brain result in progressive multifocal leucoencephalopathy (PML), particularly in patients harboring leukemia or lymphoma (24). Walker has shown that, when a JC strain of the papovavirus extracted from PML brain tissue is injected into newborn hamsters, malignant gliomas were induced in 83% of the animals (37).

So it becomes irksomely apparent that, certainly from an etiologic standpoint, the "dice of the gods" remain loaded against us, now as then.

Tumor Resection

When an intracranial mass reaches sufficient size to induce neurologic signs as a result of mass effect, surgical reduction is uniformly indicated. Such endeavor improves the immediate prognosis, but does it really prolong life in a patient with glioblastoma multiforme? This is a moot point, yet the practice of radical excision of infiltrative gliomas has replaced the "biopsy only" era and is in full swing today. McKenzie was probably its earliest proponent, when he proposed in 1936 the so-called "internal decompression" (19). It consisted of radical excision of tumor and injured brain followed by a cosmetic closure that included replacement of calvarial bone. Bucy and others have been strong advocates of such practice in present times. However, recent data cast some doubt on this teaching, as Seiler has shown (30). Excluding those instances where a mass effect itself portends patient demise, debulking for the sake of reduction in the neoplastic cell population does not appear to prolong life. Useful survival is probably determined more by the extent of preoperative neurologic deficit than by the size of the intracranial lesion.

The development of computerized microstereotaxy, as described by Sheldon et al., is an exciting and promising event (32). Such cerebroscopy is precise and allows for excision of a lesion while it is still small. The impact of this procedure on patient long-term survival is not presently known. This surgical technic lends itself to laser applications, and it is here where laser, in my opinion, will retain its advantage over other surgical modalities long after the fad dies down.

Chemotherapy

Not being an oncologist, being placed in a position to formulate an independent opinion about chemotherapy without condemnation or endorsement is not an easy task. In my opinion, the literature contains more desultory extemporization based on flimsy facts than true scientific observation. To illustrate the point, all preceding clinical observations are cast aside by an experiment by Gerosa et al. that combines BCNU and 5-fluorouracil (5-FU) (10). In this experiment, out of 113 rats injected intracerebrally with a tumor, the controls lived 30 days, and the 5-FU group fared no better. The BCNU-treated rats lived 50 days. Of 17 animals treated with BCNU and 5-FU, 10% (<2 animals) lived longer than those given only BCNU. Such data are then extrapolated to recommendations for therapeucis in man. The bibliography is totally devoid of contradictory references (see Chapter 9).

Seilers' recent monograph is an elegant and informed rendition of the therapeutic state of the art in the treatment of malignant gliomas and is highly recommended reading (30). It and the EORTC study (6) are probably most informative to the clinician who is intimidated or not well enough informed to sort out the endless protocols of the oncologist.

Teletherapy

Teletherapy, a word not commonly heard in the doctor's dining room, is derived from the Greek words "tēle" (far off) and "therapeuein" (to attend or treat). In contemporary medical jargon it equates to external radiotherapy. Chapter 8 is a gargantuan endeavor to present its contemporary role in the treatment of cerebral neoplasia. Here I wish only to underscore recently surfaced concern about external radiotherapy.

Druckmann, in 1929, was probably the first to observe adverse consequences of external radiation. He described a period of lethargy and irresistable somnolence after teletherapy (5). With regard to present concerns, Fukamachi et al. (9) published a study of brainstem necrosis following radiation for pituitary adenoma, with devastating late results, and an excellent literature review. Progressive white matter destruction following teletherapy has also been observed (25). In this case, the patient received 5000 rads of teletherapy in September for a metastatic left occipital lesion (Figure 13–1A). Four months later the metastatic deposit was absent on CT scan, but profound ex vacuo hydrocephalus was apparent (Figure 13–1B). The cortical surface had not been deleteriously affected as it was in a similar case (Figure 13–2). This 46-year-old woman was interstitially radiated after teletherapy, and prolonged chemotherapeutic failure was heralded by a recurrent cerebral metastatic lesion.

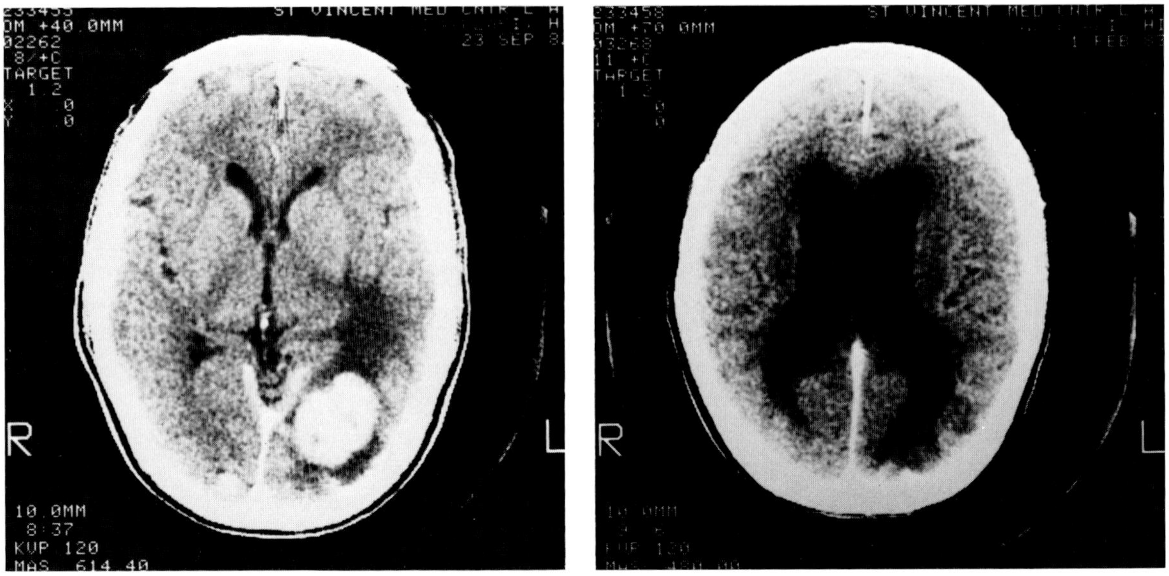

A B

Figure 13–1 **A:** A metastatic left occipital lesion. Teletherapy was begun at this time. **B:** Same case as in Figure 1A. Note the advanced ventriculomegaly resulting from white matter destruction following 50 Gy of teletherapy.

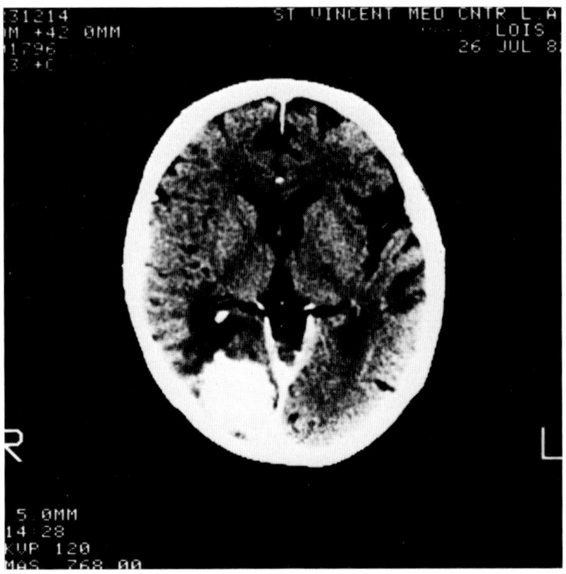

Figure 13–2 Metastatic mass in right occipital lobe that was nonresponsive to teletherapy. Note the advanced cortical atrophy.

Sundareson et al. from the Memorial Sloan-Kettering Cancer Center offered an epenetic review of this topic supported by an excellent bibliography (33). More disconcerting than that cerebral irradiation causes brain injury is the fact that chemotherapeutic adjuncts do not seem to potentiate a desirable effect on useful survival (17,29,31,36). In fact, in Seiler's recent monograph (30), 11.7% of patients treated by combined teletherapy and chemotherapy manifested some degree of brain injury. Yet nitrosoureas probably do have a role in the treatment of malignant cerebral neoplasms when all other therapeutic endeavors have failed. My intention here has not been to interpolate the benefits of external radiotherapy, but rather to make the reader aware of its potential harm as expressed in recent literature (2,7,18,39). Although one may reprobate the notion, it has been said that teletherapy is in some instances clinically beneficial to patients not by reducing tumor bulk but rather by reducing brain volume.

In spite of its disadvantages, ionizing irradiation provides us with the best therapeutic adjunct to surgical resection of a brain tumor that we have. In a scholarly review of the literature, Salcman (28) has shown that only 7.5% of patients live for 2 years after resection of a glioblastoma. The addition of teletherapy doubled the survival time, but it must be stressed that the 6-month survival rate was 70%. At 1 year only 10% of patients treated by surgical resection alone were alive, as contrasted with a 40% survival rate when teletherapy was added (28). The benefits of additional chemotherapy are marginal at best and possibly detrimental, as discussed in previous chapters. Hence it is incumbent upon us to develop the therapeutic potential of ionizing radiation to its maximal potential. Of necessity this includes a scholarly look at interstitial irradiation from an imaginative, innovative, but most of all open-minded perspective.

Interstitial Irradiation

Historically the word curietherapy is interchangeable with interstitial irradiation. Its etymologic derivation is self-evident to the reader of a text such as this. Fritz Mundinger probably deserves to be named the "Father of Curietherapy of Brain Tumors." To distinguish radiotherapy by permanent implantation of radioisotopes (curietherapy) from short-term irradiation, Mundinger (20) coined the word *brachycurietherapy*, meaning short-term intense irradiation of a lesion with a retrievable ionizing source. Its details have been previously discussed.

In the United States, Kelly et al. were probably the first to brachytherapeutically treat a patient with iridium-192 (15). The technique was a modification of that of Kelly's mentor, Professor Szikla of Paris (35). In 1981, Szikla et al. reported on 28 cases of focal low-grade gliomas treated by iridium-192 interstitial implantation, with encouraging results (34). Since that time Szikla's experience has been vastly expanded and his optimism prevails (14). Gutin et al. reported on their experience with interstitial radiation of 37 patients harboring various intracranial mass lesions (11). A number of isotopes were employed, culminating in a conclusion that high-energy iodine-125 was probably the most suitable radioisotope for interstitial irradiation.

Mundinger and his colleagues at the University of Freiburg im Breisgau, have been and remain the pioneers of interstitial irradiation of brain tumors to the present day (21; Mundinger, personal communication, 18 May 1983). Since January 1981 more than 500 CT-aided stereotactic procedures were performed at that institution for biopsy and/or interstitial radiotherapy of brain tumors (Mundinger, personal communication, 18 May 1983). By 1982, Mundinger and his colleagues had performed 1665 stereotactic biopsies of intracranial lesions and treated 1103 cases of brain tumor with curietherapy (22). There were 177 glioblastomas and 408 astrocytomas in the group. Sixteen meningiomas were treated by interstitial implant, as were 17 pinealomas. Only 20 metastatic cases were included in this group. The transient morbidity was reported as 3%, with a surgical mortality of 1.1%.

It must be remembered that many intracranial lesions lie deep within midline structures of the brain and are considered surgically inaccessible by conventional means. Of 285 cases stereotactically biopsied under CT guidance, 172 harbored lesions either in the basal ganglia, diencephalon, or midbrain or pons (20,23). In a group of patients treated by interstitial high-energy iodine-125 implantation from February 1979 to March 1981, 117 out of 146 patients were alive in 1982. Grouping all cerebral gliomas together, 80% of 119 cases were still alive when the chapter in Schaltenbrand and Walker's *Atlas* was written (20). However, the authors underscore the fact that not enough time has elapsed to make conclusive statements.

Brachycurietherapy employing iridium-192 has also been extensively used by the Freiburg group. Of 62 cases with glioblastoma, the mean survival was 8.3 ± 6.8 months (maximal survival 35.3 months) when radiosensitizers were used. By 24 months fewer than 10% of these patients were alive. Among the astrocytoma group, about one-half of the patients were still alive 2 years later, but by 4 years only 10% were alive (21).

The oligodendroglioma group fared better than the astrocytoma series. Metastases comprised only a small percentage of the brachytherapeutically treated series; mean survival was 9.1 ± 0.8 months, with the longest survival being in excess of 95 months. In Salcman's exponential model of survival with glioblastoma as a function of time (28), about 22% of patients were alive at 12 months when all modalities of treatment were combined. Only 9% were alive 1 year later when treated by surgical resection alone, compared with 32% when postoperative irradiation was added. That irradiation is beneficial was also supported by the prospective study done by the Brain Tumor Study Group (36).

Interstitial irradiation of brain tumors needs the close attention other modes of therapy have received. Victor Levin, in a review of the current trends in brain tumor therapy (17), reiterated the marginal benefits of chemotherapy in brain tumor treatment and emphasized a need to look elsewhere. Interstitial irradiation has promise, but no hard and fast guidelines have been determined on the exact role it plays in therapy.

Stereotactic biopsy is a low-risk procedure and, because tissue classification of neoplasms is essential, the benefits outweigh the hazard entailed. Also, with the introduction of the CT scanner, an intracranial lesion may be observed with greater accuracy without having to rely on clinical signs alone. Hence it is our present policy to interstitially irradiate low-grade astrocytomas and follow them with regular-interval CT scans.

Patients with glioblastomas receive 50 Gy to the periphery of the lesion. This is supplemented by 30 Gy in the form of external irradiation several weeks later. Metastatic lesions also receive 50 Gy to the CT-determined periphery of the lesion, teletherapy being added when other lesions appear on CT scan. Those patients who have persistence or recurrence of metastatic cerebral disease after having received prior external irradiation receive only brachytherapy.

Our data-time base with brachytherapy is not sufficient to make sweeping conclusions. Since the inception of this undertaking, our clinical experience now encompasses 35 cases, although only the first 20 cases were reviewed in the earlier chapters. Our optimism has not been daunted to date; the project will continue at our institution. Finally, I would like to emphasize that the best treatment of a brain tumor is excision, and irradiation should be reserved for those tumors that cannot be removed for whatever reason. It is here that interstitial irradiation probably plays a meaningful role.

CT Adaption of Stereotactic Equipment

It is appropriate to offer several comments about the adaptation of conventional stereotactic equipment to CT-guided stereotaxy. Just as CT scanners have improved since 1973 (1,13), so has adaptation of stereotactic apparati to CT scanning. Yet all equipment presently available is a customized adaptation of either the Leksell, the Trent-Wells, or the Riechert-Mundinger stereotactic systems to CT scanner guidance (see Chapters 4, 11, and 12.) The only exception is the in-scanner technic (described in Chapter 10) developed by William Glenn and his associates. Hence, presently available stereotactic systems are in reality custom-made for a particular institution. There is enough commercial pressure present to date, however, to facilitate improvements in design.

Because my contemporary experience with stereotactic apparati is with the Riechert-Mundinger equipment, I limit my comments to that equipment. Soon upon becoming familiar with the apparatus, its good and bad points became apparent. On the plus side, the equipment is well designed and almost foolproof. In the horizontal plane, it allows access to the calvarium through 140°. Along the Y axis or vertical plane, the inferior 40° offer limited access to the occipital brain because of a table-mount design for the base ring that is a holdover from the roentgen era of stereotaxy.

The value of the phantom apparatus is inestimable, but the Y axis adjustments encounter a mechanical impasse when paramedian lesions are represented on it. Hence, in order to facilitate free movement along the Y axis, the phantom ring has been redesigned by recessing the X-Y coordinate plane 5 cm below the 0 point of the original Z plane (Figure 13–3). The commercially available metallic calvarial fixation pins are sturdy and well designed, but are incompatible with CT scanning. Cus-

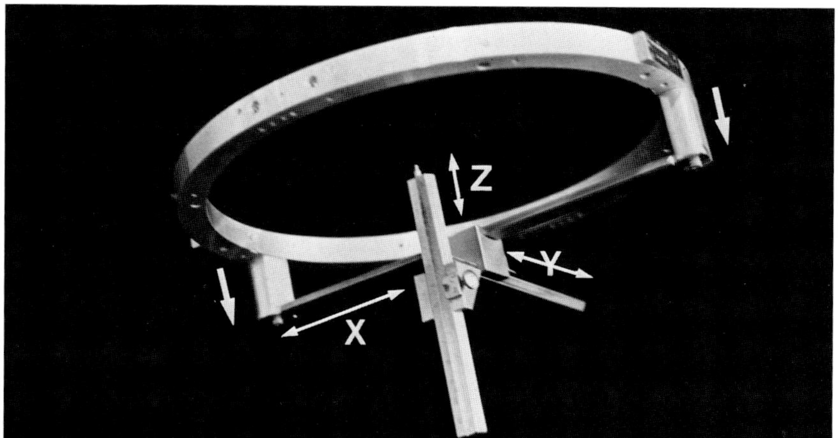

Figure 13–3 The phantom base ring is shown with modifications incorporated as shown by arrows on each side of the ring. This inferior displacement of the X-Y plane allowed unimpeded movement along the Y axis.

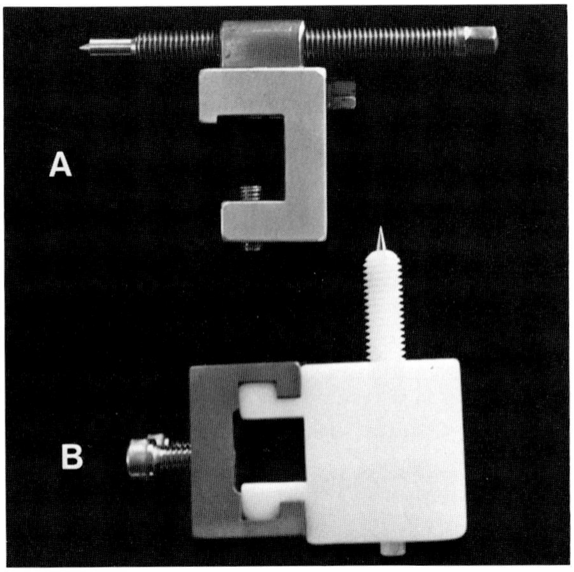

Figure 13–4 **A:** metallic commercially available calvarial pins and mount block. **B:** the author's modification to improve CT compatibility.

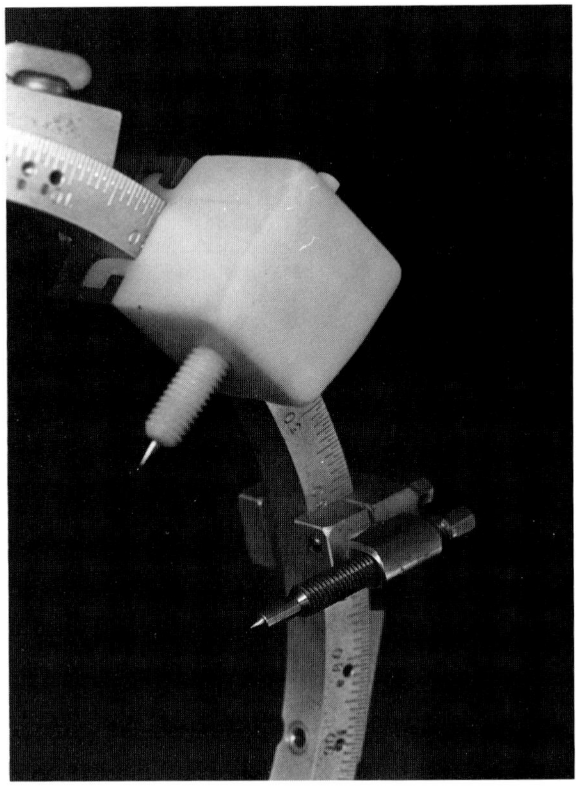

Figure 13–5 Illustration shows how the CT-compatible skeletal fixation pin mounts onto the base ring.

tom-made pins and mount blades were designed to circumvent this obstacle. The metallic and our own design of skeletal fixation are shown in Figure 13–4. These pins are mounted on the base ring as illustrated in Figure 13–5.

It is extremely uncomfortable for the patient to lie face down on an operating table while a direct approach is made to target a lesion in the posterior fossa (Figure 13–6). To improve this situation, it was decided that a sitting position would be most advisable. The universally available Mayfield pin head fixation mount was retooled to hold the patient's base ring (Figure 13–7). Thus by attaching the base ring mount, the patient need not stay in the face-down position, but may be placed in a conventional sitting position that allows ample access to the posterior fossa, even with the base ring attached high on the skull as shown in Figure 13–6. An endeavor is also underway to replace the commercially available CT scanner mount with one made of CT-compatible materials, so that the posterior fossa structures below the base ring may be scanned without imposing radiographic artifacts.

In order to allow stereotaxy with the Riechert-Mundinger apparatus on a Phillips scanner, all that was needed was rigid fixation of the base ring during CT scanning. This was accomplished by means of a base mount attached securely to the Phillips scanner table that allows precise stereotaxy, as attested by our preliminary trials (Figure 13–8). Further modifications in the phantom device are also in progress to allow easier representation of posterior fossa lesions or brainstem lesions when necessity dictates that the base ring be reverse-mounted high on the head. With the new custom-made calvarial fixation pins, this latter endeavor of reverse base ring mounting may be completely obviated in the future.

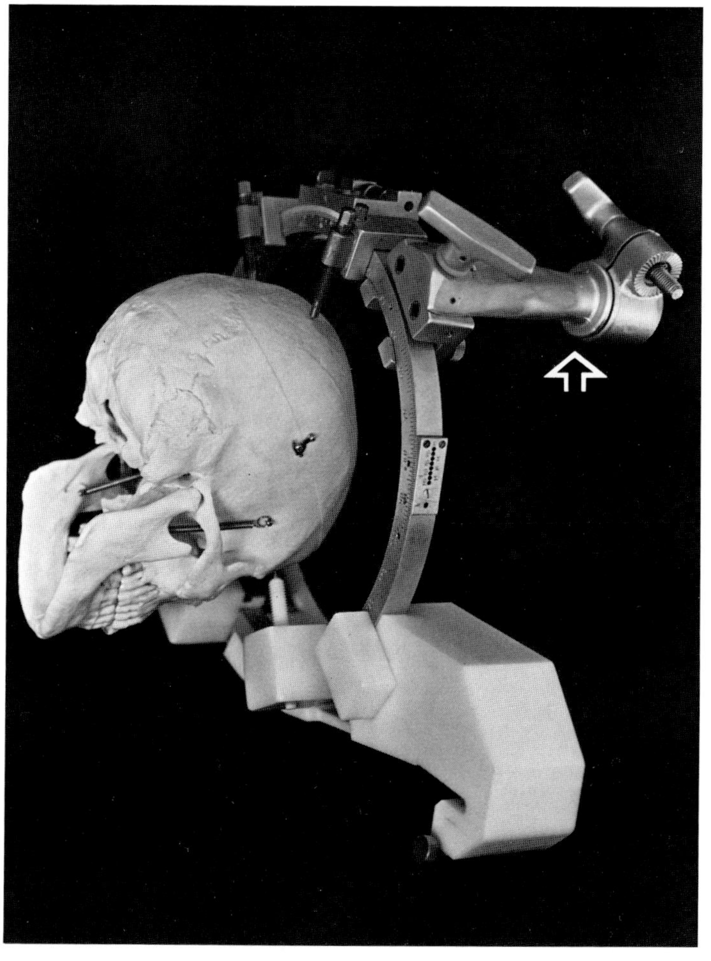

Figure 13–6 There are two options by which the posterior fossa may be stereotactically approached. The patient may remain face down as shown, or may be lifted into a sitting position. The base ring is then attached to the Mayfield headrest (*arrow*).

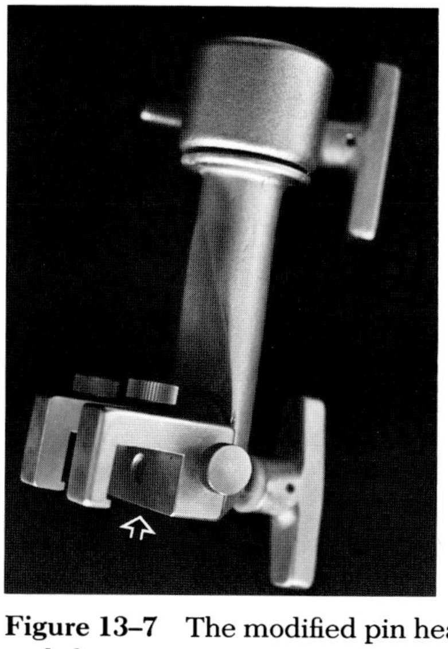

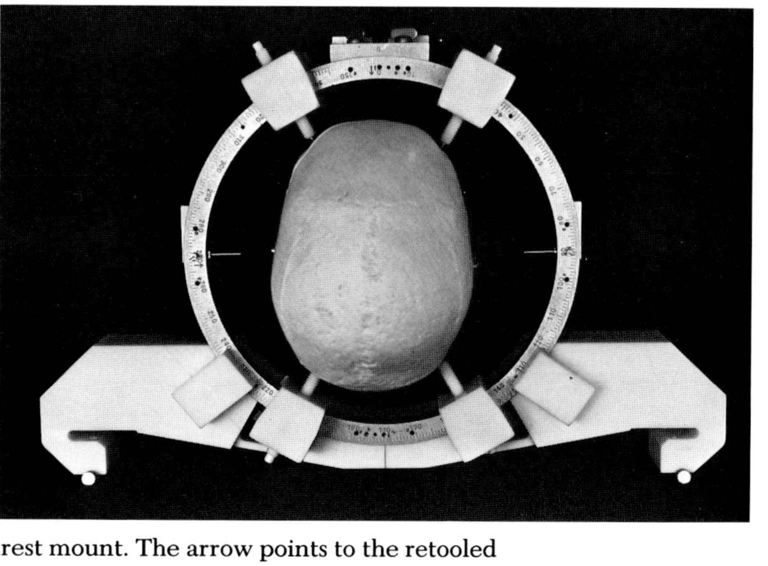

Figure 13–7 The modified pin headrest mount. The arrow points to the retooled end that attaches to the base ring.

Figure 13–8 View from the CT gantry showing how the base ring fits the Phillips CT scanner mount. Note the customized skeletal fixation device.

Summary

It is quite apparent that, although this book comes to an end, the work in this therapeutic field has only begun. It is hoped that this undertaking will stimulate greater interest in contemporary stereotaxy of brain tumors, because, if it does, more patients may be offered the priceless gift of additional life. There is no better reward than that for a paracelsian with compassion.

References

1. Ambrose J: Computerized transverse axial scanning (tomography) Part 2: Clinical application. Br J Radiol 46:1023–1047, 1973.
2. Boldrey E, Sheline G: Delayed transitory clinical manifestations after radiation treatment of intracranial tumors. Acta Radiol (Ther) 5:5–10, 1965.
3. Burger PC, Dubois PJ, Schold Jr SC, et al: Computerized tomographic studies of untreated, quiescent and recurrent glioblastoma multiforme. J Neurosurg 58:159–169, 1983.
4. Cohnheim J: Lectures on General Pathology. Translated from 2nd German edition by McKee. New Sydenham Society, London, 1889, p 746.
5. Druckmann A: Schlafsucht als Folge der Roentgenbestrahlung. Strahlenther 33:382, 1929.
6. EORTC Data Center, Institut Jules Bordet, Brussels: Evaluation of CCNU, VM-26 plus CCNU, and procarbazine in supratentorial brain gliomas. Final evaluation of a randomized study. J Neurosurg 55:27–31, 1981.
7. Eyster EF, Nielsen SL, Sheline GE, et al: Cerebral radiation necrosis simulating a tumor. J Neurosurg 40:267–271, 1974.
8. Folkman J: The vascularization of tumors. Sci Am 234:58, 1976.
9. Fukamachi A, Wakao T, Akai J: Brain stem necrosis after irradiation of pituitary adenoma. Surg Neurol 18:343–350, 1982.
10. Gerosa MA, Dougherty DV, Wilson CB, et al: Improved treatment of a brain-tumor model. Part 2: sequential therapy with BCNU and 5-fluorouracil. J Neurosurg 58:368–373, 1983.
11. Gutin PH, Phillips TL, Hosobushi Y, et al: Permanent and removable implants for the brachytherapy of brain tumors. Int J Radiat Oncol Biol Phys 7:1371–1381, 1981.
12. Houk JC, Kamagalingam K, Hunt C, et al: Lymphocyte and fibroblast chalcones; some chemical properties. Science 196:896, 1961.
13. Hounsfield GN: Computerized transverse axial scanning (tomography). Part 1: Description of system. Br J Radiol 46:1016–1022, 1973.
14. Kelly PJ: Seminar: Selected Topics in Contemporary Stereotactic Techniques. Buffalo, NY, June 2–5, 1982.
15. Kelly PJ, Olson MH, Wright AE: Stereotactic implantation of Iridium-192 into CNS neoplasms. Surg Neurol 10:349–354, 1978.
16. Kelly PJ, Suddith RL, Hutchinson HT, et al: Endothelial growth factor present in tissue culture of CNS tumors. J Neurosurg 44:342–346, 1976.
17. Levin V: Current status of brain tumor therapy. Paper presented to the California chapter of the American Endocurietherapy Society, Interstitial Brain Implant Symposium, June 11, 1983.
18. Martins AN, Johnston JS, Henry JM, et al: Delayed radiation necrosis of brain. J Neurosurg 47:336–345, 1977.
19. McKenzie KG: Glioblastoma: A point of view concerning treatment. Arch Neurol Psychiatr 36:542, 1936.
20. Mundinger F: Die stereotaktische interstitielle Therapie nicht resezierbarer intrakranieller Tumoren mit Iridium-192 und Jod-125. In: Kombinierte chirurgische und radiologische Therapie maligner Tumoren, edited by HW

Schreiber, F Gauwerky, HA Ladner. Urban & Schwarzenberg, Munich, Vienna, Baltimore, 1981, pp 90–112.
21. Mundinger F: Implantation of radioisotopes (curietherapy). In: Stereotaxy of the Human Brain, edited by G Schaltenbrandt, AE Walker. Georg Thieme Verlag, Stuttgart–New York, 1982, pp 410–434.
22. Mundinger F: CT-stereotactic biopsy of brain tumors. In: Tumors of the Central Nervous System in Infancy and Childhood, edited by D Voth, P Gutjahr, C Langmaid. Springer-Verlag, Berlin, Heidelberg, New York, 1982, pp 234–246.
23. Ostertag CB, Mundinger F, Weigel K: Biopsie stereotactique et radiothérapie interstitielle des tumeurs cérébrales. Med Hyg 39:1994–2008, 1981.
24. Richardson EP: Progressive multifocal leucoencephalopathy. In: Handbook of Clinical Neurology, edited by PJ Vinken, TW Bruyn. North-Holland, Amsterdam, 1970, Vol 9, p 485.
25. Rottenberg DA, Horten B, Kim JH, et al: Progressive white matter destruction following irradiation of an extracranial neoplasm. Ann Neurol 8:76–78, 1980.
26. Russell DS, Rubinstein LJ: Pathology of Tumours of the Nervous System (4th ed). Edward Arnold, London, 1977.
27. Rytömaa T, Kiviniemai K: Control of DNA duplication in rat chloroleukemia by means of granulocytic chalone. Eur J Cancer 4:595–597, 1968.
28. Salcman M: Survival of glioblastoma: Historical perspective. Neurosurgery 7:435–439, 1980.
29. Seiler RW: Late results of multimodality therapy of high-grade supratentorial astrocytomas. Surg Neurol 15:88–91, 1981.
30. Seiler RW: Die undifferenzierten Astrozytome des Grosshirns. Eine Übersicht der aktuellen Therapie-möglichkeiten. Springer-Verlag, Berlin, Heidelberg, New York, 1982.
31. Seiler RW, Greiner RH, Zimmerman A, et al: Radiotherapy combined with procarbazine, bleomycin and CCNU in the treatment of high grade supratentorial astrocytoma. J Neurosurg 48:861–865, 1978.
32. Sheldon CH, McCann G, Jacqués S, et al: Development of a computerized microstereotaxic method for localization and removal of minute CNS lesions under direct 3-D vision. J Neurosurg 52:21–27, 1980.
33. Sundaresan N, Galicich JH, Deck MDF, et al: Radiation necrosis after treatment of solitary intracranial metastases. Neurosurgery 8:329–333, 1981.
34. Szikla G, Betti O, Szenthe L, et al: L'expérience actuelle des irradiationes stéréotaxiques dans le traitment des gliomes hémisphériques. Neurochirurgia 27:295–298, 1981.
35. Szikla G, Peragut JC: Irradiation interstitielle des gliomes. In: Radiotherapie des Tumeurs du Systeme Nerveux Central, edited by JP Constans, M Schlienger. Neurochirurgia 21:187–255, 1975.
36. Walker MD, Alexander Jr E, Hunt WE, et al: Evaluation of BCNU and/or radiotherapy in the treatment of anaplastic gliomas: A cooperative clinical trial. J Neurosurg 49:333–343, 1978.
37. Walker DL, Padgett BL, Zurhein GM, et al: Human papovavirus (JC): Induction of brain tumors in hamsters. J Cell Sci 181:674, 1973.
38. Willis RA: Pathology of Tumours (4th ed.). Butterworth, London, 1967.
39. Wilson GH, Byfield J, Hanafee WN: Atrophy following radiation therapy for CNS neoplasms. Acta Radiol [Ther] (Stockh) 11:361–368, 1972.

Index

T